THE
PRIMAL
BLUEPRINT

MARK SISSON

The Primal Blueprint

Library of Congress Control Number: 2011919329
Library of Congress Cataloging-in-Publication Data
Sisson, Mark, 1953–

The Primal Blueprint: Reprogram your genes for effortless weight loss, vibrant health, and maximum longevity / Mark Sisson
ISBN 978-0-9822077-8-9
1. Health 2. Weight Loss 3. Diet 4. Physical Fitness

Writing/Consulting: Brad Kearns
Design/Layout: Caroline De Vita
Project Manager: Aaron Fox, Primal Nutrition
Text Editing: Laura Gabler, Greg Brown, Catherine Fisse, Amy Lucas
Consultants: Rudy Dressendorfer, PhD, R.P.T, Walter Kearns, M.D.

For more information about the Primal Blueprint, please visit primalblueprint.com
For information on quantity discounts, please call 888-774-6259

Publisher: Primal Nutrition, Inc.
23805 Stuart Ranch Rd. Suite 145
Malibu, CA
90265

TABLE OF CONTENTS

Disclaimer

The ideas, concepts and opinions expressed in this book are intended to be used for educational purposes only. This book is sold with the understanding that author and publisher are not rendering medical advice of any kind, nor is this book intended to replace medical advice, nor to diagnose, prescribe or treat any disease, condition, illness or injury. It is imperative that before beginning any diet or exercise program, including any aspect of the Primal Blueprint program, you receive full medical clearance from a licensed physician. Author and publisher claim no responsibility to any person or entity for any liability, loss, or damage caused or alleged to be caused directly or indirectly as a result of the use, application or interpretation of the material in this book. If you object to this disclaimer, you may return the book to the publisher for a full refund.

Welcome from Mark

The doctor of the future will give no medicine, but instead will interest his patients in the care of human frame, in diet, and in the cause and prevention of disease.
—**Thomas Edison**

When I began the journey to produce this book nearly five years ago, it felt like David versus Goliath redux. Yes, I had readers of my MarksDailyApple.com blog egging me on to produce a Primal manifesto attacking Conventional Wisdom (a recurring term throughout the book, akin to a yellow highway hazard sign), and had a few fitness books under my belt from years past, but this endeavor was doing battle against the mighty opponent of the status quo, Conventional Wisdom ... not to mention the staid publishing industry. More than a few doors were shut in my face and phones politely hung up as I breathlessly wrapped up my pitch. "Mark, you're not a doctor. You have no credibility." "Clever idea, but you need a celebrity attached or it won't go anywhere." "Ditching grains? Eating more fat? Making workouts slower or shorter? This stuff will never fly with today's reader."

After literally pounding the pavement for two days making the publisher/agent rounds in New York City, I collapsed in a heap in my hotel room. My feet ached from wearing real shoes for hours (ah, the side effects of a mostly Vibram FiveFingers lifestyle...), but I had a big smile on my face. I was ready for battle. If the mainstream channels wouldn't bow down to receive the exciting new *Primal Blueprint*, I would be distinctly honored to become my own author, agent, and publisher!

Now, I wouldn't call myself the gloating type, but I think the Primal community as a whole can gloat like crazy these days. The movement has grown from a wacky, extreme grass-roots scene to a movement with mainstream acceptance. The hardcover version of this book, published by an unknown outfit out of Malibu, CA (can ya get any further away from the publishing epicenter of Park Ave?), sold through seven printings (nearly 200,000 copies), climbed the charts to hit #2 overall best-seller on amazon.com in March of 2010, and occupied the number one spot on Amazon's Exercise & Fitness and Diet & Weight Loss lists, on and off, for nearly a year. Many of my friends in the primal/paleo/ancestral health community have also published popular books in the last couple of years. The influence of Conventional Wisdom on our collective psyche has never been more tenuous, as people are sick of being sick, fat, tired, and stressed. The time has come to ditch once and for all the methodology dispensed by the decades-long succession of gimmicky best-selling diet books, and return to our genetic roots as hunter-gatherers.

This work represents the culmination of my primal philosophy, which has taken shape over the past 20 years through extensive research and life experience. I'm not a scientist or doctor; I'm an athlete, a coach, and a student on a lifelong quest for exceptional health, happiness, and peak performance. I have an insatiable curiosity about what we need to do to achieve such goals and a growing mistrust of the answers that have been heaped upon us by the traditional pillars of health "wisdom" (Big Pharma, Big Agra, the AMA, the FDA, and other government agencies), the health and fitness profiteers glorified by Madison Avenue, and even the know-it-all multilevel marketer next door.

The *Primal Blueprint* is my effort to distill the information I've studied from the world's leading evolutionary biologists, paleontologists, geneticists, anthropologists, physicians, nutritionists, food scientists, exercise physiologists, coaches, trainers, and scientific researchers into a concise list of behavior laws that have promoted optimal gene expression and indeed survival over the course of human evolution. While the book you are holding is a product of the new millennium, the behavior laws are as old as the dawn of mankind; they merely reinform us about the fundamentals of health that seem to have been forgotten, or misinterpreted, in the modern world.

The content in this book comes to you unfiltered by pretense or decorum. I am not beholden to any employer, government agency, professional licensing board, or sponsor, or to any other higher power that might result in the filtering of my message. I don't have any agenda—except, I suppose, to sell you a book and change your life! I simply don't trust many of the major elements of Conventional Wisdom that we have blindly accepted as gospel for decades.

In my case, the mistrust has been well earned over the past 35 years of trying to "do the right thing" (another recurring theme) by diligently following Conventional Wisdom. For several years of my youth, I ran in excess of 100 miles a week with a single-minded focus toward competing in the 1980 U.S. Olympic Marathon Trials. At my peak, I was considered by many to be a picture of health: six percent body fat, a resting heart rate of 38 beats per minute, and a marathon time of two hours, eighteen minutes that had placed me fifth in the U.S. National Marathon Championships.

While I reached some notable heights during my endurance career, I also experienced some devastating lows. Soon after my best marathon performance, the monumental physical stress of my training regimen and the state-of-the-art "high-energy" diet that fueled it resulted in a succession of serious overuse injuries, illnesses, and burnout. While I looked like a picture of health, I was really an example of overstress and inflammation. I was the fittest guy my friends knew, yet I suffered from recurring bouts of fatigue, osteoarthritis in both of my feet, severe tendonitis in my hip joints, stress-related gastrointestinal maladies, and six or more upper respiratory tract infections each year.

Most people have traveled a less extreme path than I, yet nearly all of us have experienced similar results following the Conventional Wisdom of our time: weight-loss efforts doomed to a 96 percent long-term failure rate, workout programs leading to fatigue and increased appetites for sugar, and medications that exacerbate the underlying cause of pain while barely alleviating symptoms (not to mention the unpleasant side effects).

> **“** *The **Primal Blueprint** is the centerpiece of a vibrant community of people connected by the Internet and committed to living their lives to the fullest potential, challenging the status quo, and not being afraid to try something **old.*** **”**

I applaud your effort and desire to do the right thing, and I deeply empathize with your frustration at trying to succeed amidst a whirlwind of conflicting and confusing advice. My goal with the Primal Blueprint is to expose much of the lucrative health and fitness industry as ethically and scientifically bankrupt; to peel back the many layers of marketing blather, folk wisdom, and manipulative dogma, and to replace it with 10 simple Primal Blueprint behavior laws modeled after the evolutionary success of our ancestors.

Pause and reflect on the following simple statement for a moment, for it is the most powerful and compelling rationale for living according to the Primal Blueprint: Human beings prevailed despite incalculable odds by adapting to the selective pressures in their environment over thousands of generations. Our primal ancestors were lean, strong, smart, and productive, which enabled them to survive, reproduce, rule over more physically imposing members of the animal kingdom, and exploit virtually every corner of the earth. This is no mean feat, yet Conventional Wisdom has essentially dismissed the legacy of our ancestors in favor of quick fixes.

Today at the age of 61, I feel healthier, fitter, happier, and more productive than ever. I am no longer a marathon or triathlon champion (nor do I want to be), but I maintain a weight of 165 pounds (75 kg) with eight percent body fat. I eat as much delicious food as I want, am not beholden to regular meal times, exercise just 3 to 6 hours per week (instead of the 20 to 30 I put in back in the day), and almost never get sick. My personal clients (ranging from world-champion triathletes to ordinary citizens just trying to lose a few—or a lot of—pounds), as well as tens of thousands of readers at MarksDailyApple. com, report similar life-altering benefits from following the Primal Blueprint. Now it's your turn.

Your Way or the Highway

My intention in this book is to show you the immense personal power you have to control your health and fitness destiny and to give you the tools to reprogram your genes, reshape your physique, and enjoy a long, healthy, energetic, and productive life. The Primal Blueprint principles are wonderfully simple, practical, and inexpensive, and they require minimal, if any, sacrifice or deprivation. Unlike many of the gimmicky diet and exercise books that have graced the best-seller shelves in recent decades, the Primal Blueprint is intuitive and easy to follow—not just for the first 21 days or the first four months, but for the rest of your life.

I have a deep understanding and empathy for real-world concerns like lack of time, budget issues, motivational challenges, dysfunctional social circumstances, eating disorders, ingrained bad habits, and other powerful influences that can sabotage the picture-perfect diet plan served up by the celebrity of the moment. On numerous occasions, I've felt the disappointment of taking a plunge with my heart and soul into a new diet or athletic training regimen, only to fall well short of the ambitious goals I had set. Adding insult to injury, I often discovered later that I'd been given bad advice—by my government (thanks to the tainted influence of special interests), Madison Avenue, or a less-than-knowledgeable coach, peer, or professional expert. Few things in life are more frustrating!

With the Primal Blueprint, there's no need for trepidation. This is not a regimented program—I'm not going to shove my agenda down your throat and cajole you to go against your own common sense or pleasure-seeking human nature. My experience with the MarksDailyApple.com community has taught me the value of the collaborative approach to health and well-being. Whenever I raise an interesting discussion that's contrary to Conventional Wisdom, I immediately have thousands of readers contributing their unfiltered opinions. Many of these readers are forward-thinking doctors, scientists, researchers, or coaches whose valuable input and suggestions I could not have otherwise easily solicited.

This interplay often forces me to substantiate—or at times even restructure—my position. It always requires me to adapt my message to resonate with real people and their real-life experiences. The philosophical positions and practical guidelines that shape the message of this book have been heavily battle-tested, scrutinized, refined, and finally approved by thousands of "Primal" enthusiasts (as well as skeptics) at MarksDailyApple.com.

You see, the Primal Blueprint is more than just a book. It's the centerpiece of a vibrant community of people connected by the Internet and committed to living their lives to the fullest potential, challenging the status quo, and trying something *old*. I encourage you to participate at MarksDailyApple.com. Share your experiences with the program and connect with an audience that can relate to you in a way that goes beyond what a book or even a paid trainer can offer. Every day, I augment the foundation of the Primal Blueprint with easy-to-read, hard-hitting but lighthearted commentary on all manner of healthy lifestyle topics, including delicious recipes, workout tips and videos, evaluation of the latest research, and an extensive library of bite-sized inspiration and reminders to keep you eating, exercising, and living to your potential.

In this book, I detail a basic framework of diet, exercise, and lifestyle guidelines that you must observe to be successful. However, making the pieces fit comfortably into your own life is best left up to you. I strongly support you making allowances for, adjustments to, and occasional deviations from the Primal Blueprint based on your particular real-life concerns and constraints. After all, our ancestors had to adjust constantly to their unpredictable environment and gave us the tools to do the same. That's the primal part. The word blueprint in the title connects us to the familiar analogy of construction plans that provide the foundation for action but are often altered during the actual construction project. A program that allows you to go with the flow frees you to listen more deeply to your own intuitive knowledge, which is far more expert than any outside resource.

The fact that you are in control will give you the most powerful source of motivation you can imagine—instant and ongoing direct feedback that the Primal Blueprint is working. No more exercising until exhaustion or obsessing about the arduous restrictions common to popular weight-loss programs. The Primal Blueprint is a way of life that is attainable for everyone, not just the socialites in Palm Beach or the gym rats in Venice Beach. It's time to pursue your own unique peak performance goals and enjoy your life to the absolute maximum, carrying on a tradition that humans have pursued for tens of thousands of years. Thank you for agreeing to take this journey with me. Let's have some fun and get primal!

Mark Sisson
Malibu, CA
September 2014

Striving for Perfection with the 80% Rule

A central philosophical component of the Primal Blueprint is my "80 Percent Rule," which basically means that you can chill out and enjoy your life, rather than invite the additional stress and anxiety that comes from a perfectionist approach or an overly strict regimen. I believe that if you are aligned with the Primal Blueprint 80 percent of the time, you will experience great success and likely build momentum toward being even more compliant, with less effort, as time proceeds. Since this admonition is potentially controversial ("Sisson offers a cop out!"), I'd like to further explain the spirit of the rule. The 80 Percent Rule is not a license to make less than a full commitment to the Primal Blueprint—that is, to strive for a "B" grade as your ultimate goal. This is particularly true when it comes to moderating your insulin production and getting off the sugar high/insulin crash cycle that we will cover in great detail shortly. Even a couple of steps out onto a slippery insulin slope aren't so easy to recover from!

What I suggest is that you strive for 100 percent success—total compliance with the Primal Blueprint guidelines and zero tolerance for the unhealthy foods, exercise, and lifestyle habits that are prevalent today. With that in mind, please realize a couple of things:

- A perfectionist approach to healthy living compromises many of the intended benefits of a strict and disciplined "healthy" lifestyle.
- The forces of hectic daily life (cultural traditions, convenience, fast pace, limited/expensive healthier options) will divert you from your ideal often, and this is perfectly okay (just make smart adjustments!).

> *Perfection is impossible. However, **striving** for perfection is not. Do the best you can under the conditions that exist. That is what counts.*
> —*John Wooden*

I'm a big believer in enjoying life, and indeed this has been my overpowering inspiration for developing the Primal Blueprint. The 80 Percent Rule exists because I understand how difficult lifestyle change can be. I want you to make an honest and devoted effort, but I never want you to feel discouraged that you aren't measuring up to arbitrary standards created in your mind or by society. The late John Wooden, legendary UCLA basketball coach, captured the spirit of the 80 Percent Rule well when he said: "Perfection is impossible. However, *striving* for perfection is not. Do the best you can under the conditions that exist. That is what counts."

Primal Blueprint
Paperback—Additions

This streamlined edition of the hardcover *Primal Blueprint* (published in June, 2009) contains numerous updates and enhancements to the text reflecting the evolving Primal movement in 2012. Many of the revisions have been inspired by reader feedback and Internet forum commentary. Areas that were confusing to more than a few have been reworded or explained differently. Areas where I might have made points a few more times than necessary have been edited to keep the story flowing!

After extensive consultation with experts and my own research, I've clarified and/or elaborated upon some of my dietary positions. For example, the importance of balancing your dietary ratio of omega-6:omega-3 fatty acids warrants more selectivity on nuts and seeds than I communicated in the 2009 hardcover. Hence, in this book you'll see macadamia nuts earning special distinction above other nuts and seeds due to their favorable fatty acid profile. The year-round availability of highly cultivated, overly-sweetened fruit warrants more selectivity and moderation to be truly Primal-aligned, particularly if you want to reduce excess body fat. I've tried to assert these and other important points stronger than ever in this edition. Finally, at the end of the book you will find extensive bonus material as follows:

Common Stumbling Blocks: Derived from thousands of MarksDailyApple.com forum posts, we provide quick tips to help overcome the most common challenges to transitioning to a Primal lifestyle.

"Hacks" for each of the 10 Primal Blueprint lifestyle laws to promote quick results in body composition, fitness, athletic performance, daily energy levels, and to reduce disease risk factors and reliance on medication. These can be your marching orders at the end of the book!

Workout Suggestions: Detailed descriptions of the Primal Essential Movements: simple, scalable, bodyweight resistance exercises that integrate the Primal Blueprint strength-training principles. Sprint workouts for all ability levels that are safe, fun, and highly effective.

A Few Words About Diet and Dieting: I attempt to eliminate confusion about contrasting dietary advice by examining how the basic assumptions, and entire paradigm, of Primal eating differs from that of the Standard

American Diet, causing differing conclusions to be reached. I clarify some misconceptions about vegetarianism, low-fat eating, and programs that promote an amazing rate of weight loss.

Internet Appendix: MarksDailyApple.com has extensive supporting material, including text references, suggested reading (blogs, magazine articles, and books), resources for shopping and information, and wide-ranging Q&A about all aspects of the Primal Blueprint.

INTRODUCTION

What Is Going On Here?

Conventional Wisdom
vs. The Primal Blueprint

In the Primal Blueprint (PB), we reframe these major elements of Conventional Wisdom (CW). Consider these alternatives with an open mind; we will discuss each in detail throughout the text.

Grains—wheat, rice, corn, cereal, bread, pasta, etc.

CW: "Staff of Life." Foundation of a healthy diet. 6-11 daily servings recommended by US Government and numerous other experts.

 Main energy source for brain and working muscles. Whole grains provide extra nutrition and fiber.

PB: "Worst mistake in the history of the human race" (UCLA evolutionary biologist Jared Diamond). Drives excess insulin production, fat storage, and heart disease. Allergenic, immune-suppressing, nutritional value inferior to plants and animals. Whole grains possibly worse due to "anti-nutrients" that compromise immune and digestive function and promote systemic inflammation.

Saturated Animal Fat

CW: "Eating fat makes you fat." Heart disease risk factor. Replace saturated fats (meat, dairy) with polyunsaturated vegetable oils.

PB: Major dietary calorie source (from animal foods). No direct correlation with heart disease risk. Drove human evolution/advancement of brain function for two million years. Promotes efficient fat metabolism, weight control, and stable energy levels.

Cholesterol

CW: Strictly limit intake. Elevated levels = elevated heart disease risk. Take statin drugs and eliminate animal foods (especially eggs) if total is 200 or over or if you have a family history of heart disease.

PB: Essential metabolic nutrient, no direct correlation with heart disease risk. Only dangerous when oxidation and inflammation occur (from poor diet and exercise habits). Statins have considerable side effects and minimal, if any, direct benefit.

Eggs

CW: Minimize consumption due to high cholesterol content of yolk.

PB: No correlation between egg intake and blood cholesterol levels. Yolk among the planet's most nutritious foods.

Fiber

CW: Important dietary goal, derived mostly from grains. Improves gastrointestinal function, lowers cholesterol, speeds elimination, and helps control weight by minimizing caloric intake.

PB: Incidental fiber from vegetables and fruit is optimum. Grain-based diet causes excess fiber, inhibiting nutrient absorption and hampering gastrointestinal function and elimination.

Meal Habits

CW: Three squares (or six small meals) daily to "keep flame burning." Skipped meals = slowed metabolism, lower energy levels, muscle breakdown, sugar cravings, and future binging risk.

PB: No need for regular meals when insulin production is moderated and you reprogram your genes to become a fat-burning beast. Intermittent Fasting becomes effective weight management tool.

Strength Training

CW: Focus on form and deliberate work/return rhythm. Lift to "failure" in sequence through numerous stations (takes about an hour for a complete workout). Isolate body parts to get desired size, toning, and "cuts."

PB: Emphasize explosive movements over deliberate pace. Conduct full body, functional exercises to develop broad athletic competency and an excellent strength-to-weight ratio. Finish workouts in 30 minutes or less.

Cardio Workouts

CW: "60 minutes of moderate-to-vigorous intensity on most days of the week" (US Government recommendation). A consistent schedule of vigorous workouts helps control weight by burning tons of calories.

PB: US Government recommendation results in "Chronic Cardio," leading to overstress, fatigue, burnout, injury, accelerated aging, and increased disease risk. Calories burned during chronic workouts simply increase appetite (particularly for sugar)—ineffective for weight loss. Slow down for better health and peak performance!

Weight Loss

CW: High-complex carb/low-fat diet, regimented meals, portion control, and Chronic Cardio exercise. It's all about "calories in/calories out ..." and lucky genes!

PB: High-fat/ moderate protein/ low-carb diet; intuitive, sporadic meals; and a strategic blend of Primal workouts. Don't worry about portion control, regimented meals, fanatical workouts, or even family genetic predispositions. Eat Primal foods, ditch SAD foods, and reprogram your genes to enjoy effortless lifelong weight control.

Play

CW: Ah, brings back fond memories of childhood. But who has time these days?

PB: Integral component of overall health and balanced lifestyle. Outdoor, active, unstructured fun is appropriate for all ages. Scientifically proven to increase work productivity and help manage stress of hectic daily life.

Sun Exposure

CW: Avoid the sun to prevent skin cancer! Lather up with SPF 20, 30, 40, 50—all you got!

PB: Get plenty of sun to avoid skin cancer! Vitamin D synthesis promotes healthy cel- lular function and prevents all forms of cancer, including melanoma. Expose large skin surface areas enough to maintain slight tan, but of course avoid burning with clothing, shade, and sunscreen.

Footwear

CW: Sturdy, cushioned shoes minimize injury, improve comfort. Custom orthotics can provide additional support and protection.

PB: Get primal—go barefoot (or minimalist)! Perpetual use of "big" shoes increases impact trauma, weakens foot muscles, and increases pain and injury rates throughout lower extremities.

Prescription Drugs

CW: Relieve pain, speed healing, prevent/cure disease, and address genetic frailties. Everyday use can enhance quality of life (Viagra, etc.).

PB: Mask/exacerbate underlying causes, compromise homeostasis and thus health, and produce disastrous side effects. Simple lifestyle changes can replace vast majority of pills. Wonderful in case of emergency!

Goals

CW: Set specific, measurable goals to stay motivated and focused. "Consistency is key." Missed workouts = guilt, weight gain, and lost fitness.

PB: De-emphasize specific, results-oriented goals (potential to discourage—such as weight loss failure or "post-marathon blues"). Stay motivated by focusing on fun, and release attachment to outcome. Consistency = overstress. Vary routine to minimize stress and improve adaptive response by genes. Missed workouts drive recovery, improvement, and freshness.

Americans will always do the right thing—after they've exhausted all the alternatives.
—Winston Churchill

I'm going to ask you to forget most everything you thought you knew about diet, exercise, and health. There is a distressing amount of flawed Conventional Wisdom that confuses, misleads, manipulates, and complicates even the most devoted efforts to do the right thing: eat healthfully, exercise effectively, control weight, and avoid common health conditions like obesity, arthritis, indigestion, insomnia, diabetes, heart disease, and cancer.

In the *Primal Blueprint*, you will learn why eating a low-fat diet rich in whole grains such as bread, rice, pasta, and cereal can easily make you fat and malnourished. You'll learn why millions of joggers and gym-goers put in the time and effort to lose weight yet routinely compromise their health and accelerate the aging process as a direct result of their devotion to fitness. You'll learn why your cholesterol level and saturated fat intake are not the major risk factors for heart disease that we have been led to believe and why a relatively high-fat diet promotes health and longevity. I'll show how weight loss does not have to involve the suffering, sacrifice, and deprivation we've been conditioned to accept but instead is a matter of eating the right foods (plants and animals), avoiding the wrong foods (processed fats and carbs—including grains), and exercising strategically, for far fewer hours than you might assume, to reach your desired fitness goals.

All the answers are found in a set of 10 simple, logical Primal Blueprint diet, exercise, and lifestyle behaviors. Modeling your 21st-century life after our primal hunter-gatherer ancestors will help you greatly reduce or eliminate almost all of the disease risk factors that you may falsely blame on genes you inherited from your parents. Unfortunately, too many of us narrowly define genes as largely unalterable inherited traits—height, body type, eye color, physical or intellectual abilities, and "family history" health conditions and diseases. While some genes are indeed responsible for traits that are largely unaffected by lifestyle, many more play a bigger role in your health than you might realize. As coming chapters explain in detail, your genes—guided by what you eat, how you move, and even how you think—are the traffic cops that direct the functioning of every single cell in your body, every moment of every day.

Whatever you throw at them, your genes are going to respond in an effort to promote survival and, beyond that, homeostasis (the balanced and synchronistic functioning of all systems in the body). After all, this is the essence

> *Instead of falling victim to your genetic vulnerabilities, you can control how your genes express themselves in constantly rebuilding, repairing, and renewing your cells.*

of human evolution. However, be forewarned that when you are sitting on the couch late at night chowing down Cheetos® and Dr. Pepper®, your body will still valiantly pursue homeostasis (releasing insulin and stress hormones into the bloodstream), regardless of whether or not it benefits your long-term health. I am merely presenting the steps you can take to reprogram your genes and achieve (as the cover suggests) effortless weight loss, vibrant health, and boundless energy—if these happen to be of interest to you!

The idea that you can reprogram your genes through lifestyle behavior is the central premise of this book. It represents a clear departure from today's fatalistic Conventional Wisdom, which suggests that our genes, for better or worse, determine our destiny and that we have little say in the matter … unless prescription drugs or Human Genome Project discoveries can come to the rescue. True, you might have a genetic tendency toward accumulating excess body fat or a family history of type 2 diabetes, but you'll be more likely to see these traits expressed when you make poor lifestyle choices and send the wrong signals to your genes. Instead of falling victim to your genetic vulnerabilities, you can control how your genes express themselves in constantly rebuilding, repairing, and renewing your cells. Briefly, here are the most critical, life-altering elements of the Primal Blueprint:

Become a *Fat-Burning Beast* by eliminating processed carbohydrates from your diet to minimize your body's insulin production. This means eliminating not only sugars and sweets, but also grain products, including wheat, rice, pasta, cereal, and corn (yep, corn is a grain, not a vegetable), and even legumes (beans, soy, peas, peanuts). A diet that emphasizes meat, fish, fowl, eggs, nuts, seeds, and colorful natural carbs, such as vegetables and fruits, is the primary way to improve your general health, control your weight, and minimize the risk of heart disease, cancer, diabetes, arthritis, and other diet-influenced medical conditions.

If you are carrying excess body fat, it will disappear virtually effortlessly when you focus on eating the delicious, filling, nutritious foods that have nourished humans throughout the course of evolution. Seriously, it's as simple as choosing the right foods to moderate insulin production. You will not have to struggle or suffer to shed excess body fat.

Optimize Your Exercise Program by engaging in a blend of frequent, low-intensity energizing movement (walking, hiking, easy cardio); regular brief, intense strength-training sessions (I'll detail the Primal Essential Movements in the Bonus Material at the end of the book); and occasional all-out sprints that help improve body composition and delay the aging process.

This strategy is far superior to the Conventional Wisdom approach of following a consistent schedule of frequent medium-to-difficult-intensity sustained workouts, such as jogging, running, or cycling; cardio machines; or group classes. This Conventional Wisdom workout strategy, which I refer to as "Chronic Cardio," places excessive and prolonged physical stress on your body, leading to fatigue, injuries, compromised immune function, and burnout. Sometimes, less really is more.

Manage Stress Levels with plenty of sleep, play, sunlight, fresh air, and creative outlets, and avoid trauma that often arises from stupid mistakes. Rebel against the tremendous cultural momentum toward sedentary lifestyles, excessive digital stimulation, and insufficient rest. Honor your primal genes by slowing down and simplifying your life. Your ancestors worked hard to survive, but their regular respites from stress gave them the peace of mind and body that are so highly coveted today.

Is Dying of Old Age Getting Old, or What?

As you will soon discover, our genes were not only designed through evolution to keep us healthy, but they desperately want and expect us to be healthy. Today, with the hectic pace of the high-tech modern world, we struggle with how to do the right thing by our genes. The ensuing failure creates a level of frustration and confusion that causes many of us, whether overtly or deep down inside, simply to give up. Experience teaches us how difficult, if not impossible, it is to be lean, fit, energetic, and healthy following Conventional Wisdom. Instead, we succumb to the forces of consumerism designed to placate our pain with silly shortcuts, comforts, conveniences, and indulgences. Consequently, the popular "Hey man, life is short!" rationalization becomes a self-fulfilling prophecy.

> " *70 percent of today's health care expenditures are for lifestyle-related chronic diseases, such as obesity, diabetes, and heart disease.* "

The consequences of eating processed foods, exercising excessively (or, conversely, being inactive), and making poor lifestyle decisions work in concert against your genetic mandate for health. At the very least, you can experience excess body fat storage, subpar fitness results, aching joints, gastrointestinal problems, frequent minor illnesses, sugar cravings, energy level swings, and recurring fatigue. Sounds bad enough as it is, but continuing to misdirect your genes with bad choices over years and decades will likely result in obesity, diabetes, heart disease, cancer, and/or the vast majority of degenerative conditions requiring a doctor's care or medication. A huge percentage of all doctor visits today are a direct consequence of lifestyle choices that are misaligned with the environmental and survival conditions that shaped our primal genetic makeup.

These consequences are painfully obvious to most everyone, and our collective interest in doing the right thing has driven a booming fitness industry, incredible advancements in medicine, much greater awareness of healthy foods and lifestyle choices, sharp declines in smoking, and sharp increases in restaurants offering salad bars and smoothies. Ironically though, the collective health of America—and other Western countries that have adopted our fast-paced culture—is worse than ever. A study released in 2008 by Johns Hopkins University suggests that by the year 2030, 86 percent of all adults in the United States will be overweight or obese (up from the current estimate of 65 percent). What's more, a National Institutes of Health conference report stated that "our trends predict that *all* Americans will be obese by 2230!"

We reluctantly accept as fact that the normal human life span consists of growing up to reach a physical peak in our early 20s, followed by an inevitable steady decline caused by the aging process. Under this faulty assumption, we allow ourselves to gain an average of one and a half pounds of fat (two-thirds of a kilo) per year starting at age 25 and continuing through age 55[1] (we also lose half a pound of muscle per year, resulting in adding a pound of fat a year in the wrong places as we age). Our last decade or two (until we reach the average life span of about 78 years)[2] is commonly characterized by inactivity, insufficient muscle mass and excess body fat, assorted medical conditions, and a host of prescription drugs to alleviate the pain and symptoms of chronic disease. Twenty-seven percent of us will die from cardiovascular disease, and another 23 percent will die from cancer.[3]

I know that 100 percent of us will die from something, but personally, I'd prefer to actualize a motto I crafted in honor of our hunter-gatherer ancestors: *Live Long, Drop Dead!* Yes, many primal humans succumbed to primitive hazards (death by predator or infection from a deep cut) before they hit today's voting age, but many of those who avoided misfortune could live six or seven decades in exceptional health and fitness. In almost all cases, primal humans were healthy and strong for their entire lives, until they met their sudden demise. There was simply no such thing as today's abysmal decline into old age. After all, the clan couldn't support any excess baggage in its daily battle for survival. While 21st century longevity stats are vastly superior to those of any other time in human history, these increases are mostly due to science, not healthier lifestyle behaviors. Furthermore, modern longevity is often undesirably inflated by advancements that keep us alive but do not improve quality of life: hospital machinery, pharmaceuticals, and the ability to reel in the years doing little more than putting spoon to mouth and thumb to remote control.

Of the two and a half trillion dollars America spends annually on health care, the Centers for Disease Control and Prevention (CDC) estimates that 70 percent is spent on lifestyle-related chronic diseases, such as obesity, diabetes, and heart disease. A surprising number of people accept all this as a normal part of life, believing that some of us are just fortunate to have "good genes" and the rest must cross their fingers against bad luck.

Sure, millions of modern citizens contributing to these woeful statistics are completely disconnected from what's required to be healthy. It might be hard for you even to relate to this segment of humanity that hasn't a clue or a care about this stuff. However, even the most health conscious among us often struggle. Despite a sincere commitment to do the right thing by Conventional Wisdom, we have collectively failed to lose that last 5, 10, or 50 pounds. Injuries, fatigue, and burnout plague exercisers ranging from weekend warriors to professionals. We have been programmed by the health care establishment to reflexively turn to prescription drugs to treat symptoms of distress, even though most conditions are minor and easily corrected by simple dietary and lifestyle changes. In the process, we interfere with normal gene-driven metabolic processes and thwart our innate ability to heal naturally—paving our way to joining the masses on the wrong side of the stats.

The story is sad, but the good news is that your destiny for the most part is in your hands. By the time you complete this book, you will understand the big picture and all the necessary details of how to eat, exercise, and live in order to reprogram many of your genes for lifelong health. In the process, you will take control of your own body and your own life. This is really the only sensible way to counter the tremendous momentum pushing us away from health, balance, and well-being in our hectic modern world.

Chapter Endnotes

[1] Physiology of Sport and Exercise, by Dr. David Costill and Jack Wilmore.

[2] The Central Intelligence Agency's World Factbook reports that the 2008 U.S. overall life expectancy at birth is 78 (75 for males; 81 for females).

[3] The 2008 American Heart Association "Heart Disease and Stroke Statistics," available for download at americanheart.org, reported that in 2004, 869,000 deaths were attributed to heart disease and 550,000 to cancer. 2005 CDC stats indicate the percentage referenced, but recent headlines suggest cancer has surpassed heart disease as the number one killer. cdc.gov/nchs/data/nvsr/nvsr56/nvsr56_10.pdf

CHAPTER 1

The Ten
Primal Blueprint Laws

("Commandments" Was
Already Taken)

In This Chapter

I introduce the "re:evolutionary" premise that we should model our diet, exercise, and lifestyle behaviors after our primal ancestors from 10,000 years ago, adapting those behaviors strategically to the realities of high-tech modern life. The inexorable technological progress of civilization has diverted us from the healthy dietary habits and active, stress-balanced lifestyles that allowed primal humans to prevail under the harsh competitive circumstances of evolution. However, we are genetically identical (in virtually all respects relevant to human health) to our hunter-gatherer ancestors, owing to the fact that evolution ground to a halt when the major selection pressures of starvation and predator danger (eat or get eaten!) were eliminated.

Genes are more than just the largely inalterable inherited traits. They are the "traffic cops" that direct the function of all the cells in your body, at all times. Hence, you can reprogram them with healthy lifestyle behaviors and make irrelevant even strong genetic predispositions to disease, excess body fat, and other adverse health conditions.

The 10 Primal Blueprint laws are:
1. Eat Plants and Animals
2. Avoid Poisonous Things
3. Move Frequently at a Slow Pace
4. Lift Heavy Things
5. Sprint Once in a While
6. Get Adequate Sleep
7. Play
8. Get Adequate Sunlight
9. Avoid Stupid Mistakes
10. Use Your Brain

Nothing in biology makes sense except in the light of evolution.
— **Theodosius Dobzhansky**

The quote by Dobzhansky was also the title of a famous 1973 essay in which the noted evolutionary biologist and devout Russian Orthodox Christian acknowledged that, whether or not you believed in the existence of a higher power, you could not begin to understand even the simplest concepts in biology unless you understood how evolution had worked to shape and differentiate the genes of every single one of the several million species on the planet.

Within the past hundred years, tens of thousands of anthropologists, evolutionary biologists, paleontologists, epigeneticists, and other scientists have worked diligently to piece together a fairly detailed interpretation of the environmental and behavioral factors that directly influenced our development as a species. As a result, we now have a very good picture of the conditions under which we emerged as Homo sapiens.

Some seven million years ago, hominids (our prehuman ancestors) split from apes and branched out into various new species and subspecies. Then, about two million years ago, the humanlike species Homo erectus, with its large brain, upright stature, skilled use of tools and fire, and organized hunter-gatherer societies, began to take charge of the food chain. Over time, Homo erectus branched into various species and subspecies (Homo neanderthaensis, Homo habilis, Homo sapiens, and others). Most researchers believe that the modern Homo sapiens evolved in Africa between 200,000 and 100,000 years ago, prevailing over all in the Homo erectus family tree. Then, about 60,000 years ago, a small number of modern humans left Africa and began their great migration across the planet. Recent archaeological findings strongly support this "out of Africa"[1] theory: that the entire human population of the planet, amazingly, can trace their origins to a small pool of intrepid Homo sapiens in Africa. There were only an estimated 2,000 to 5,000 African humans at that time, and some scientists believe that only about 150 people crossed the Red Sea to begin the migration. Talk about six degrees of separation!

Civilization Cuts Both Ways

I hope you are sitting down to absorb one of the most critical—and quite possibly mind-blowing—tenets of the Primal Blueprint:

Our primal ancestors were likely stronger
and healthier than we are today.

"How can this be?" you ask. It's all about survival of the fittest. The human body is the miraculous result of millions of years of painstaking design by evolution. Through natural selection involving countless small genetic mutations and adaptations in response to a hostile environment, our ancestors were able to prevail over unimaginably difficult conditions and opponents and populate all corners of the earth.

"The development of agriculture and civilization caused humans to become smaller and sicker, leading to a dramatic decline in life expectancy."

Many anthropologists suggest that the human species reached its evolutionary pinnacle (in terms of average muscularity, bone density, and brain size) about 10,000 years ago. After that, we started to take it easy and get soft. Our physical decline was a natural consequence of a couple of things. First, we had already spent thousands of generations leveraging our increasingly proficient brain function to manipulate and tame the natural environment (with tools, weapons, fire, and shelter) to our advantage. The second factor is perhaps the most significant lifestyle change in the history of humanity: the gradual advent of agriculture. When humans began to domesticate and harvest wheat, rice, corn, and other crops, as well as livestock, the ability to store food, divide and specialize labor, and live in close civilized quarters eliminated the main selection pressures that had driven human evolution for two million years—the threats of starvation and predator danger. (The transition to agriculture happened independently around the globe, becoming prominent about 7,000 years ago in modern-day Egypt; North America was one of the last areas to implement agriculture, about 4,500 years ago).[2]

When humans no longer faced these constant selection pressures, evolution essentially ground to a halt in conjunction with the flourishing of civilization. Consequently, many researchers assert that today we are genetically identical to our primal ancestors, at least relating to behaviors that promote human health. Some challenge this assertion by pointing to examples of recent genetic variations, such as higher lactose tolerance rates among those of herding ancestry. This is indeed a very interesting example of genetic drift and environmental adaptation (see more details in the book's Q&A supplement at MarksDailyApple.com). For now, let's stay focused on the big picture: discovering the most important evolution-tested lifestyle behaviors that promote optimal gene expression—behaviors that have not changed in 10,000 years.

This idea that human DNA—the genetic "recipe" for building a healthy, lean, thriving human that resides in each of our 60 trillion cells—is almost exactly the same today as it was 10,000 years ago has been most notably promoted by the work of Dr. Boyd Eaton, chief anthropologist at Emory University in Atlanta and author of *The Paleolithic Prescription*, and the late James V. Neel, founder of the University of Michigan's Department of Genetics. It's a popular theory, supported by hundreds of other leading anthropologists, evolutionary biologists, and genetic researchers.

While our primal ancestors made the most of their genes (remember, they had no choice; the alternative was to starve or become some other creature's dinner!), we have fallen far short. The development of agriculture and civilization caused humans to become smaller (including our brain size) and sicker (originally due to contagious diseases, but lately more because of vastly inferior diet, exercise, and lifestyle behaviors).

Human life expectancy 10,000 years ago was about 33 years. While not too impressive by 21st-century standards, primal man actually lived longer than his civilized successors all the way into the early 20th century! Average life expectancy reached a low of 18 during the Bronze Age (~3300-1200 B.C., Ancient Egypt, etc.), rose only slightly to a range of 20-30 through Classical Greek (~500-300 B.C.) times, the Roman Empire (~0-500 A.D.), and the Middle Ages (~700-1500), and was still only between 30 and 40 as late as the early 20th century. Around that time, medical advancements (antibiotics, hospital and community sanitation, decreased infant mortality rates, etc.) helped life expectancy stats skyrocket.

Fossil records show that primal humans who could steer clear of fatal misfortune could routinely live six or seven decades in excellent health, and had a "maximum observed life span" of an astonishing 94 years![3] Among present-day hunter-gatherers (e.g., Ache, Hadza, Hiwi, and !Kung—groups that have almost no modern conveniences or medical care) it is not uncommon to see strong, healthy folks living well into their 80s. More than a quarter of the Ache (Ah-CHAY) people of Paraguay make it to 70. Moreover, 73 percent of Ache adults die from accidents and only 17 percent from illness. Think about the extraordinary implications of hunter-gatherer longevity: with no medications or medical care of any kind, a massive lifelong struggle for food, clothing, and shelter completely devoid of modern comforts, primal humans (and modern humans living primally) can still live to what even we softies consider old age.

> *The Ultimate Human award goes to **Grok**, my nickname for the prototypical preagricultural human being.*

Of course, the civilization-driven decline in life expectancy didn't matter in a pure evolutionary context. As long as civilized humans made it to reproductive age and had children, they could pass their genes along to the next generation without penalty. While progressing beyond survival of the fittest conditions is definitely a good thing, the sober reality is that today's technological age is enjoyed by the fattest, laziest humans in the history of humanity. Hence, the Ultimate Human award goes to Grok[4], my nickname for the prototypical preagricultural human being. Grok is the central character of both this book and my blog. He's a lean, smart, healthy character whom you will grow to love.

Unlike Grok, who ruled the planet with little more than a spear and a thatched hut in his portfolio, even the most impoverished humans of the last several thousand years, extending up to the present day's Third World inhabitants, have not really "competed" genetically. The presence of the most rudimentary modern influences, such as grain consumption, food storage, permanent shelters, and basic weapons to thwart potential predators, all suppress the true Darwinian survival of the fittest playing field that allowed Grok to thrive.

Sure, being a math whiz or a natural athlete may significantly influence your path through life and give you a competitive edge in pursuits to which you are inclined, but these genetic attributes no longer provide a survival advantage in the evolutionary sense. NBA superstar LeBron James has a genetically superior athletic skillset, but he could have easily cruised through life as a candy-chomping, video-gaming fat kid and still have reproduced successfully due to lack of selection pressure for human endurance in the modern world.

In fact, considering all the comforts and medical advancements of modern life, we could easily argue that we currently exist in a state of devolution. For the most part, this is great (many of us have suffered illnesses or traumas over the course of our lives that would have killed us a century ago, let alone 1,000 or 10,000 years ago). However, we must be vigilant not to let the advantages of modern life compromise our health (e.g., hitting the pharmacy instead of the gym to combat back pain).

The challenge is in applying the Primal Blueprint laws to modern life. How do we leverage the lessons and benefits of natural selection against the pressures of a complex modern society bent on promoting consumerism and quick fixes over the pursuit of health? How do we reprogram our ancient genes to recapture excellent health? We simply have to ask ourselves, "what would Grok do?"

You Have to Fit Your Genes to Fit into Your Jeans

In order to begin to understand the concept of "reprogramming" your genes, it will help to understand what they actually are and how they work. Each of your 50 or 60 trillion cells contains a nucleus with a complete set of DNA instructions divided into handy subsets called genes. There are approximately 20,000 different genes located on the long strands of DNA in each cell. These DNA strands are further organized into 23 pairs of chromosomes with which we are familiar. In any given cell, only a small fraction of the total number of genes is actively involved in carrying out the main "business" of that particular type of cell. Depending on environmental signals, genes trigger the manufacture of specific proteins and enzymes to perform the various tasks required of them. For example, the beta cells in your pancreas manufacture insulin but they don't grow bigger when you lift weights. Liver cells can synthesize nutrients, but they don't grow new bone tissue. And yet each cell has the entire "recipe" for a human residing on the DNA.

> *Genes don't know—or care—whether these environmental signals promote or compromise your health; they simply react to each stimulus in an effort to promote your immediate survival.*

The most important thing to understand here is that most genes are not self-determining. They do not turn on or off by themselves; they respond to signals they receive from their immediate environment. You have the power to turn on or turn off certain genes that have a profound influence on your health. You may not be able to reprogram your eyes from blue to brown, but you can certainly avoid getting a pot belly, even if your dad, grandpa, and brothers all exhibit a strong disposition in their familial genes for such an attribute.

Genes actively control cell function all the time, so the overall health and survival of your body is primarily dependent on which genes get turned on or off in response to their immediate environment. Genes don't know—or care—whether these environmental signals promote or compromise your long-term health; they simply react to each stimulus in an effort to sustain your short-term survival, just as they have been designed to do by evolution and by the precise behaviors of our ancestors.

Sprint or lift weights, and the biochemical "by-products" from that specific activity turn on certain genes that repair and strengthen the exercised muscle. Do too much exercise, and other genes promote excessive production of catabolic hormones, leading to prolonged inflammation and hindered recovery. An allergic reaction represents your body's (misdirected) genetic response to a perceived airborne or ingested threat. An autoimmune disease is often a genetic overreaction of that same system caused by unfamiliar foods (see Chapter 5). Type 2 diabetes typically develops after prolonged periods when your genes are trying to protect you from the dangers of eating too many carbohydrates.

Here's a great example of our genes' ability to switch on and off: researchers studying the link between smoking and lung cancer discovered that tobacco smoking causes hypermethylation (a complete or partial deactivation) of a single gene known as MTHFR. Turning off MTHFR triggers an opposite effect—hypomethylation (systemic dysfunction)—in many other genes, setting the stage for further cancer development.

The idea that the environment influences whether genes are turned on or off is not a new one. In 1942 geneticist and evolutionary biologist C. H. Waddington first coined the term epigenetics to describe how genes might interact with their surroundings to create a unique individual. Today the study of epigenetics is one of the fastest growing subdisciplines of genetics. Moreover, the burgeoning field of nutrigenomics has identified hundreds of ways that nutrients (foods or supplements) impact gene expression. You may be familiar with the direct influence folic acid has on reducing neural tube birth defects, which is why all pregnant women are advised to take supplemental folic acid. This is but one small example of the powerful influence diet can have on reprogramming genes.

An Australian study suggested that human genes are adversely affected by sugar ingestion for two weeks (genetic controls designed to protect the body against diabetes and heart disease are switched off as an acute reaction to eating sugar) and that prolonged poor eating can cause genetic damage that can potentially be passed through bloodlines! On an even grander scale, research shows that certain cells within the body called mesenchymal stem cells can become bone cells, fat cells, muscle cells, or even cancer cells in adults, depending upon the environmental signals they receive.

Clearly, your lifestyle behaviors can either destroy or support many aspects of your health and can often be far more relevant than inherited predispositions to allergies, diabetes, or even more serious conditions. Not to make light of the serious genetically influenced health challenges that many face over their lifetimes, I would argue that we are all predisposed to heart disease, cancer, arthritis, and today's other leading lifestyle-related health problems if we program our genes with the wrong diet, wrong lifestyle behaviors—even the wrong thoughts.

Obviously, you cannot grow your kids seven feet tall simply by feeding them healthy food and making sure they get plenty of sleep; we all have profound limitations in how our genes can express our unique individual potential. For confirmation, just take a look at the physical marvels in the Olympic 100-meter dash or on an NFL or NBA roster, collections of the most physically gifted athletes on the planet. These athletes might be one in a million genetically, but they are still an example of optimal gene expression. The choices they have made—the foods they've eaten, how they've trained, even how they've thought—have all helped them make the most of their natural-born talents to rise to the top of very competitive arenas. This is all you ought to be concerned with—making the most of your own genetic recipe to enjoy a long life of excellent health and peak performance through the 10 Primal Blueprint laws.

The chapters that follow will explore the rationale, benefits, and practical suggestions for living according to the 10 simple Primal Blueprint laws. These laws represent the specific behaviors that led directly (shaped by two million years of evolution) to the genetic recipe for a healthy, lean, fit, happy human being. Almost nothing has changed in this recipe since preagricultural times—except the endless new ways we modern humans mismanage our genes and compromise our health.

By understanding how these behavioral "laws" shaped our genome, we can reprogram our genes to express themselves in the direction of health. And when I say "simple laws," I really mean it. If you read just this chapter and never open the book again, you'd have all the information you need to live a long, healthy, disease-free life. Here then is a brief description of the laws of living 10,000 years ago, and a quick primer on how to adapt them to a healthy 21st-century lifestyle.

Primal Blueprint Law #1: Eat Plants and Animals

Plants and animals encompass everything our ancestors ate (from a huge list of individual foods) to get the protein, fats, carbohydrates, vitamins, minerals, antioxidants, phenols, fiber, water, and other nutrients necessary to sustain life, increase brain size, improve physical fitness, and support immune function. Ironically, the human diet throughout our evolution differs greatly from what Conventional Wisdom recommends. Because the various diet camps passionately argue conflicting positions to a confused public, it's essential to reflect on how profoundly important and logically sound it is to model our diets after the diets of our ancestors, whose bodies evolved to survive, reproduce, and thrive on these foods. Talk about a lengthy and severely scrutinized (as in, "life or death") study protocol!

For one, primal humans across the globe ate widely varied diets due to environmental circumstances, such as climate, geography, seasons, and activity level. There is no single regimented diet of narrowly defined foods that trumps all. Once you subscribe to the broad guidelines of the Primal Blueprint (eat plants and animals, avoid modern foods foreign to your genes), personal preference will be the driving force behind your food choices each day.

Also notable about our ancestors' diets was that they ate sporadically—mostly due to the lack of consistent availability of food (not a big issue in the developed world these days, eh?). Consequently, we became well adapted to store caloric energy (in the form of body fat, along with a little bit of muscle and liver glycogen) and burn it when dietary calories were scarce. You may be disturbed about possessing the genetic trait to store extra food calories efficiently as fat. However, by simply eating the right kinds of foods, you can leverage this bank account "savings and withdrawal" mechanism to your advantage—maintaining ideal body fat levels and stabilizing daily appetite and energy levels. Hint: it's mostly about moderating the wildly excessive insulin production resulting from the Standard American Diet (SAD).

Today similar principles apply for healthy eating. Focus on quality sources of animal protein (local, pasture-raised or organic sources of meat, fowl, fish, and eggs), an assortment of colorful vegetables and fresh fruits, and healthy sources of fat (animal fats, avocados, butter, coconut products, nuts and seeds, olives and olive oil). Realize that a significant amount of Conventional Wisdom about healthy eating is marketing fodder that grossly distorts the fundamental truth that humans thrive on natural plant and animal foods or that relies on gimmicks to support the dogma of flawed, manipulated "research." For example, eating at particular times (three squares or six small meals a day), combining or rotating specific food types at meals, structuring your meals according to pre-programmed phases or stages, eating foods supposedly aligned with your blood type, striving for specific macronutrient ratios, or keeping score of your portions and weekly treat allowances are all gimmicks that have no credibility in the context of evolutionary biology.

Furthermore, regimented programs are virtually impossible to enjoy and stick to over the long term, because they run counter to human nature. We humans thrive on eating a variety of natural foods that satisfy and nourish us, in times, amounts, and variations that fluctuate according to personal preference, environmental circumstances, activity levels, stress levels, and many other factors. I suggest you enjoy eating as one of the pleasures of life and reject most everything you've ever heard about when and how much you should eat. Instead, eat when you are hungry and finish eating when you feel satisfied. Realize that Primal foods are intrinsically the most delicious, because they satisfy your cravings and distinct tastes, stabilize mood and energy levels, and promote health and well-being.

Primal Blueprint Law #2: Avoid Poisonous Things

The ability of humans to exploit almost every corner of the earth was partly predicated on consuming vastly different types of plant and animal life. Primal humans developed a keen sense of smell and taste, along with liver, kidney, and stomach function, to adapt to new food sources and avoid succumbing to poisonous plants that they encountered routinely when foraging and settling new areas. For example, the reason we have a sweet tooth today is probably an evolved response to an almost universal truth in the plant world that anything sweet is safe to eat.

While we have little risk of ingesting poisonous plants on walkabouts today, the number of toxic agents in our food supply is worse than ever. By toxic I mean human-made products that are foreign to your genes and disturb the normal, healthy function of your body when ingested. The big offenders, including sugars and sodas, chemically-altered fats, and heavily processed, packaged, fried, and preserved foods, are obvious. It's not a stretch to directly compare the poisonous berries of Grok's day with much of the stuff shelved at eye level in your local supermarket.

What's more insidious as dietary "poisons" are cultivated grain foods (wheat, rice, corn, pasta, cereal, and derivative products such as bread, chips, crackers, muffins, pancakes, tortillas, waffles, etc.); cooking grains such as barley, millet, rye, and amaranth; and—to a slightly lesser extent—legumes (beans, lentils, peanuts, peas, and soy products). These global dietary staples are generally inappropriate for human consumption because our digestive systems (and our genes) have not had ample time to adapt to both the unfamiliar protein structure of grains and the excessive carbohydrate load of all forms of cultivated grains and legumes. The advent of grains and civilization has eliminated the main factor that's made humans healthy: selection pressure to reach reproductive age—and to care for ourselves, and others, beyond!

Ingesting grains (yep, even whole grains, as we'll discuss in detail in Chapter 5), legumes, and other processed carbohydrates causes blood glucose levels to spike (both simple and complex carbs get converted into glucose—at differing rates—once they enter the body; we'll use the accurate term blood glucose to convey what many call blood sugar). This spike is a shock to your primal genes, which are accustomed to natural, slower-burning foods. Your pancreas compensates for this excess of glucose in the bloodstream (a condition that is toxic and can quickly become life-threatening, as experienced by diabetics) by secreting excessive levels of insulin. While insulin is an important hormone that delivers nutrients to muscle, liver, and fat cells for storage, excessive insulin released in the bloodstream causes glucose to be removed so rapidly and effectively that it can result in a "sugar crash": mental and physical lethargy and (because the brain relies heavily on glucose to fuel it) a strong craving for quick replacement energy in the form of more high-carbohydrate food. This leads to a vicious cycle of another ill-advised meal, another excessive insulin response, and another corresponding blood glucose decline.

Because insulin's job is to transport nutrients out of the bloodstream and into the muscle, liver, and fat cell storage depots, its excessive presence in the bloodstream inhibits the release of stored body fat for use as energy. Insulin's counterregulatory hormone, glucagon, accesses carbs, protein, and fat from your body's storage depots (muscle, liver, fat cells) and delivers them into the bloodstream for use as energy. When insulin is high, glucagon is usually low. You don't have energy in your bloodstream, so your brain says, "Eat now! And make it something sweet so we can burn it immediately!" The mobilization of stored body fat has been humans' preferred energy source (and weight-control device) for a couple of million years, and now you've just bypassed that whole process. It's as simple as this: you cannot reduce body fat on a diet that stimulates high levels of insulin production—period.

> *The mobilization of stored body fat has been humans' preferred energy source (and weight-control device) for a couple of million years. It's as simple as this: you cannot reduce body fat on a diet that stimulates high levels of insulin production—period.*

Beyond the weight-loss frustrations, overstressing your insulin response system over years and decades can lead directly to devastating general system failure in the form of type 2 diabetes, obesity, cardiovascular disease (thanks to vascular inflammation, peripheral oxidative damage, and other insulin-related troubles we will learn more about later), and diet-related cancers. Chapter 5 will explain in detail that even whole grains (brown rice, whole wheat bread, etc.) are not particularly healthy, because they still trigger excessive insulin production, contain anti-nutrients that promote inflammation and hamper digestion and immune function, and (even though they have more nutritional value than refined "white" grain products) displace the far more nutritious plants and animals as the caloric emphasis of your diet.

Primal Blueprint Law #3: Move Frequently at a Slow Pace

Grok spent several hours each day moving about at what today's exercise physiologists might describe as a very low-level aerobic pace. He hunted, gathered, foraged, wandered, scouted, migrated, climbed, and crawled. This low-level activity prompted his genes to build a stronger capillary (blood vessel) network to provide oxygen and fuel to each muscle cell and readily convert stored fat into energy (fat is the main fuel used for low-level aerobic activity). His daily movement also helped develop strong bones, joints, and connective tissue.

What Grok did not do was deplete his energy and muscle glycogen supply with regularly scheduled sustained efforts of moderate-to-difficult intensity. This counterintuitive behavior could have left him vulnerable to a predator, starvation, or some other misfortune. You may have heard the recently popularized sentiment that humans were "born to run"? More accurately, we were born to walk extensively and run (long distances or sprint) once in a while—after or away from something when life depended on it.

Today most of us either are too sedentary or conduct workouts that are too stressful and misaligned with our primal genetic requirements for optimum health. The exercise gospel for decades has been to pursue a consistent routine of aerobic exercise (jogging, cycling, cardio machines, group classes, or any other sustained effort), supposedly leading to more energy, better health, and weight control. However, too many lengthy workouts at elevated heart rates (above 75 percent of maximum) can put you at risk of exhaustion, burnout, injury, and illness. The high-carbohydrate diet required to perform these workouts day-in and day-out only adds to the problem. At the extreme—such as with the overtrained marathon runner or ironman triathlete—a commitment to fitness can actually accelerate the aging process and elevate the risk of heart disease.

Overexercising is a common scenario when you consider how our active population has such strong focus, dedication, and willpower to push through signs of fatigue. Our bodies are simply not adapted to benefit from chronic aerobic exercise at intense or even mildly uncomfortable heart rates. Neither are our bodies designed to slog through exhausting circuits of resistance machines several days a week. The mild to severe difficulty of these Chronic Cardio or strength workouts overtaxes the stress response (commonly referred to as the fight-or-flight response) in your body. Here, your pituitary gland tells your adrenal glands to release cortisol into your bloodstream. Cortisol is a powerful stress hormone that is critical to a variety of physical functions and energy production. The spike of cortisol in the bloodstream from a stressful event increases respiration, heart rate, blood circulation, and mental focus and even converts muscle tissue into glucose for quick energy.

This is a great example of how we abuse a system that was genetically designed to respond to emergencies, such as Grok facing a predator. Even today the fight-or-flight response is highly desirable and effective in the face of true danger or peak performance stimuli, such as an Olympic sprinter crouching in the starting blocks or an emergency worker summoning super-human strength for a rescue effort. Unfortunately, when the stress response is triggered repeatedly (by the constant hectic pace of modern life, overly-stressful workouts), your adrenal glands can so overproduce cortisol that they eventually become fatigued and release less-than-normal levels of cortisol and other hormones critical to many aspects of health. Thyroid hormones and testosterone also decrease from prolonged stress, resulting in a decline in energy levels, loss of lean muscle tissue, a suppressed immune system, and the general condition best described as burnout.

What our genes truly crave is frequent movement at a slow, comfortable pace: walking, hiking, easy cycling, or other light aerobic activities with a heart rate range of 55 percent to no more than 75 percent of maximum. These efforts are far less taxing than the typical huffing and puffing, struggling and suffering exertion level that we've been conditioned to think leads to fitness. Find ways every day to move more often—walking (even across parking lots, instead of cruising for a close space; take the stairs instead of the elevator—it all adds up over a lifetime!), hiking, swimming, easy cycling, or anything else that moderately elevates heart rate. Strive to accumulate two to five hours per week of low-level exercise. More is better as long as you have the time and can resist the temptation to "go hard." If possible, make an effort to go barefoot frequently to develop natural balance, flexibility, and lower extremity strength.

Primal Blueprint Law #4: Lift Heavy Things

 Grok's life demanded frequent bursts of intense physical effort— returning gathered items (firewood, shelter supplies, tool material, and animal carcasses) to camp, climbing rocks and trees to scout and forage, and arranging boulders and logs to build shelter. The biochemical signals triggered by these brief but intense muscle contractions prompted improvements and adaptations in muscle tone, size, and power.

Today, following a strength-training program featuring natural, total-body movements (squats, pushups, pull-ups, etc.) helps you develop and maintain lean muscle mass, increase metabolism to maintain low levels of body fat, increase bone density, prevent injuries, and enjoy balanced hormone and blood glucose levels. An approach of short-duration, high-intensity workouts—conducted fairly regularly but without excessive regimentation (always aligned with your energy levels)—will produce superior results to a routine of going to the gym too often for workouts that last too long. The latter is a recipe for fatigue and undesirable gene expression. You can enjoy extraordinary benefits doing as little as two focused, intense 25-minute sessions per week, with minimal risk of overtraining or mental burnout.

Primal Blueprint Law #5: Sprint Once in a While

In a primal world where danger lurked around every corner, Grok's ability to run was a strong indicator of whether he would live long enough to pass those superior genes down to the next generation. Whether he was dashing off to avoid a charging herd of mastodons or running down small game for dinner, Grok's sprints triggered gene expression within fast twitch muscle that allowed him to go a little faster the next time.

Today, occasional maximum effort sprints help increase energy levels, improve athletic performance, and minimize the effects of aging by promoting the release of testosterone and human growth hormone (these are beneficial for women as well as men). Once every 7-10 days, when energy and motivation levels are high, choose a simple, brief sprint workout and go all out! Novices can choose low-impact options (stationary bike), and work up to actual running sprints.

Primal Blueprint Law #6: Get Adequate Sleep

Our ancestors' activity and sleep patterns were shaped by sunrise and sunset. Days started early (they actually caught the worm … and ate it!), and after the sun went down, it was safer to huddle together and rest. Furthermore, hunter-gatherers required plenty of downtime to repair and rejuvenate from their active lifestyles. Sleep researchers believe evolution wired us for bi-phasic sleep patterns: a major nighttime chunk (likely interrupted in primal times by security or family issues) along with a mid-day siesta, well-timed to correspond with a natural circadian rhythm dip that we all experience in the afternoon hours.

Today, with life exponentially more hectic and stressful than at any other time in human history, adequate sleep and restoration are widely neglected. Primarily to blame is excess artificial light and digital stimulation after dark, along with ingestible toxins (e.g., sugar, alcohol, and prescription and over-the-counter medications), and, of course, the ubiquitous alarm clock. It's critical to minimize your exposure to artificial light after dark, create calm, relaxing transitions into sleep time, and then obtain sufficient hours of sleep such that you wake up naturally (no alarm) refreshed and energized.

Adequate sleep helps the immune system function optimally, promotes release of the key hormones that enhance brain and endocrine function, and plays a major role in regulating appetite and metabolizing fat optimally. Go to sleep at the same time each night after a calm, deliberate wind down—no television, heavy exercise, big meals, or other high stimulation before bed. Your sleep requirements will vary according to lifestyle circumstances (early airplane flights, etc.) but establishing a solid foundation of excellent habits is essential.

Don't be afraid to take naps when your afternoon energy levels lull. The world will not miss you while you grab a few quick winks, and you will refresh the optimum balance of brain chemicals to increase productivity when you get back at it. Even a 20-minute siesta can provide awesome benefits when you are deficient in sleep.

Primal Blueprint Law #7: Play

Our ancestors spent hours every day involved in various forms of social interaction not related to their core "careers" of securing food and shelter and caring for their young. Studies of modern hunter-gatherers, such as the !Kung Bushmen of the Kalahari Desert in Africa, reveal that they generally work far fewer hours and have more leisure time than the average 40-hour-plus modern worker. Anthropologist Marshall Sahlins's popular theory of the "original affluent society" argues that hunter-gatherers are able to achieve affluence (indeed a more literal definition than the consumerism-tainted one that we are familiar with) by *desiring little and meeting those desires in normal daily life.*

Once the day's catch was complete or the roots, shoots, nuts, and berries had been gathered, it was time for Grok to play. Youngsters might have chased each other around and wrestled, vying for a place higher up in the tribe's social strata. Primal humans might also have practiced spear- or rock-throwing for accuracy, chased small animals just for sport, or spent time hanging out and grooming each other. The net effect of their play was to support family and intergenerational bonding, unwind from frequent life-threatening stress, and keep their bodies primed for the physical challenges of daily life.

Today *play* is a four-letter word. We still pick blackberries in our spare time, but now they're on a Web site and come with various calling plan options and messaging features. The unrelenting stimulation of modern life, combined with the consumerism mentality of the free market economy, makes play more important than ever—yet more difficult to schedule. Take some time every day to unplug from the office or daily chores and have some unstructured fun. Particularly if you have children, you can model that play is a lifetime endeavor—and learn a few things from them while you're at it! Besides being fun and socially redeeming, play offers biochemical benefits in the form of endorphins released into the bloodstream, and provides a healthy cognitive balance to the excessive stimulation thrust upon us in the digital age.

Primal Blueprint Law #8: Get Adequate Sunlight

Cavemen (and women) didn't spend their days inside caves; they were outdoors pursuing their various survival and leisure endeavors. Regular sun exposure allowed Grok to manufacture plenty of vitamin D (technically a precursor hormone, not a vitamin), which is critical to healthy cell function. Adequate vitamin D is nearly impossible to obtain from diet alone; we must manufacture this agent internally through the exposure of large skin surface areas to sufficient amounts of sunlight over the long term (vitamin D can be stored up in summer and dispensed during the winter months).

Today getting plenty of sunlight—and hence vitamin D—is nowhere near a given, what with our penchant for spending much of our time in confined spaces, such as cars, offices, and homes—and screening obsessively when we do venture out into the big, bad sun. Experts believe a variety of serious health problems result from this relatively abrupt change in human lifestyle (sound familiar from our advent of agriculture discussion?). Besides the critical vitamin D requirement, sunlight also has a powerful mood-elevating effect, which can enhance productivity at work and interpersonal relations.

Getting regular sunlight implies that you are spending time outdoors, appreciating open space and breathing fresh air. Taking time to enjoy these positive environmental surroundings (perhaps during your daily moderate exercise sessions!) balances any confinement in spaces with artificial light and stale air. Your cells become truly energized on a biochemical level when you obtain regular doses of sunlight, fresh air, and open space. While burning is certainly not healthy, maintaining a slight tan over much of the year indicates that you have adequate vitamin D exposure.

Primal Blueprint Law #9: Avoid Stupid Mistakes

Our ancestors required a keen sense of observation and self-preservation to avoid danger. They were always scanning, smelling, and listening to their surroundings, ever aware of potential trouble from saber-toothed tigers, falling rocks, poisonous snakes, or even a twisted ankle from a careless step. Hypervigilance and risk management were premium skills honed to perfection every day. Even minor mistakes could prove disastrous, such as scraping a knee on a rock and dying from an ensuing infection gone unchecked.

Today vicious tigers are not a life-threatening safety concern but we humans carelessly (can you say, multitasking?) find ways to invite pain and suffering of a different nature into our lives. Buckle your seat belt; don't drink, text, or talk and drive; and be prepared and hypervigilant when you go backpacking in the wilderness, descend a steep hill on your 15-pound racing bike, or use a blowtorch, chain saw, or tile cutter. Devote a little more attention and energy to risk management in your daily choices so you can enjoy a long, happy life and pass your own superior genes to the next generation.

Primal Blueprint Law #10: Use Your Brain

One of the most important things that separates humans from all other animals is intellectual ability. The rapid increase in the size of our brains over just a few thousand generations was the combined result of optimum dietary choices (including high levels of healthy fat and protein—see Law #1) and a continued reliance on complex thought—working the brain out just like a muscle. The best proof of this is the fact that hunter-gatherers all around the world developed language, tools, and superior hunting methods independently.

While you might argue that we use our minds plenty to navigate and make a buck in today's world, the reality is that many of us are stuck in unfulfilling or rote jobs or are otherwise disconnected from continued intellectual challenge and stimulation. Numerous studies of general intelligence qualities identify *curiosity* as one of the most profound intelligence markers. Opportunities for intellectual stimulation are everywhere in daily life. Commit to some personal challenges, such as learning a new language, playing a musical instrument, or taking an evening college class. Research indicates that risk of devastating mental conditions including depression, dementia, and Alzheimer's can be reduced by keeping your brain active as well as your body.

> *[My] greatest error has been not allowing sufficient weight to the direct action of the environments [upon evolution], i.e., food, climate, etc., independently of natural selection.*
> *—Charles Darwin*

Learn Them, Know Them, Live Them!

Law #1 - Eat Plants and Animals: Enjoy the natural, satisfying foods that fueled two million years of human evolution.

Law #2 - Avoid Poisonous Things: Avoid processed foods (trans and partially hydrogenated oils, sugars, grains—even whole grains—and legumes) that are foreign to our genes and make us fat and sick.

Law #3 - Move Frequently at a Slow Pace: Enhance fat metabolism and avoid burnout by keeping active but taking it easy.

Law #4 - Lift Heavy Things: Brief, intense sessions of functional, full-body movements support muscle development and delay aging.

Law #5 - Sprint Once in a While: Occasional all-out sprints trigger optimal gene expression and beneficial hormone flow.

Law #6 - Get Adequate Sleep: Avoid excessive artificial light and digital stimulation after dark to align your circadian rhythm with the sun and enjoy optimal immune, brain, and endocrine function.

Law #7 - Play: Balance the stress of modern life with some unstructured, physical fun! Both brief breaks and grand outings are essential to mental and physical well-being.

Law #8 - Get Adequate Sunlight: Don't fear the sun! Adequate sun exposure helps synthesize vitamin D to ensure healthy cell function.

Law #9 - Avoid Stupid Mistakes: Cultivate hypervigilance and risk management to avoid the stupid mistakes that bring "avoidable suffering" to modern humans.

Law #10 - Use Your Brain: Engage in creative and stimulating activities to nurture your mental health and overall well-being.

That's It

Aside from—ahem—the reproductive act, I challenge you to name any other significant behavior that shaped our genes and currently plays a critical role in our health and well-being. Could it really be this simple? Could the prevention of and cure for obesity, diabetes, heart disease, physical decline, most cancers, and the general overstressed existence of the modern human be contained in our genes? While you may be able to find detractors to extract bits and pieces of this blueprint and offer up a critical view, the premise is unassailable: our genes are suited for a hunter-gatherer existence, because that is how we Homo sapiens have spent the great majority of our time on earth.

The same genes that turn against you to develop heart disease, diabetes, atherosclerosis, high blood pressure, high cholesterol, arthritis, and most other degenerative dieases can also be reprogrammed to unlock a leaner, fitter, more energetic body, a substantial slowing of the aging process, and a reduced risk of illness, injury, and burnout. The secret is to *do the right thing*: follow lifestyle habits that promote desirable gene expression and avoid those that promote negative outcomes.

That statement alone—do the right thing—is no revelation. The revelation here is how easy, natural, and fun the lifestyle behaviors are that will help you build your ideal body. Now you can enjoy delicious, nutrient-dense foods that promote health and effortless weight management by moderating insulin production. Now you have permission to back off from uncomfortable workouts and regimented schedules and instead enjoy an active lifestyle with regular low-intensity aerobic movement punctuated by occasional brief and very intense efforts. You can even hang out in the sun and take a nap in the name of health!

You will notice the benefits of the Primal Blueprint lifestyle laws in a matter of days, not weeks or months. Your genes are active all the time, either helping you build, regenerate, and maintain homeostasis or unintentionally tearing you down. It's all based on the environmental signals you provide them through your food, exercise, and lifestyle choices.

Chapter Summary

1. Grok: Survival of the fittest drove two million years of evolution to create the ultimate human being…10,000 years ago! *Grok* is the nickname for our primal human lifestyle role model, who was bigger, stronger, and in many respects healthier than us. Soon after Grok's time, the advent of agriculture across the globe eliminated the main selection pressure on humans: starvation. Civilization effectively resulted in a slowing of our evolution, and we have gone soft as a consequence. However, because our DNA is virtually identical to Grok's, we can adapt his evolutionary-based lifestyle behaviors into our 21st-century lifestyle to pursue optimum health.

Your health depends upon how genes respond to signals in their immediate environment. The Primal Blueprint consists of 10 simple behavior laws that direct your genes to build a healthy, energetic, happy, lean, strong, bright, productive modern human.

2. Diet: Eat plants and animals! Avoid processed foods (sugar products, grains, legumes, and manufactured foods with chemically-altered fats). Grains, while a global food staple long believed to be healthy, stimulate an excessive release of insulin and are less nutritious than vegetables, fruit, nuts, seeds, and animal foods. A diet emphasizing grains (and legumes, to a lesser extent) inhibits fat metabolism and paves the way for serious disease.

3. Exercise: Move frequently at a slow pace (walking, jogging, hiking—avoiding excessive medium-to-high intensity cardio), lift heavy things (regular strength-training sessions that are brief and intense), and conduct occasional all-out, short-duration sprints to stimulate growth hormone release, build muscle, reduce fat, and delay the aging process.

4. Lifestyle: Get adequate sleep (restores muscles and rejuvenates the brain). Find time in your busy schedule for unstructured play (relieves stress and improves emotional and mental well-being on a chemical level). Get plenty of sunlight (stimulates production of important vitamin D and helps balance the negative effects of spending excessive time confined indoors). Avoid stupid mistakes by practicing hypervigilance and risk management for today's hazards. Use your brain for creative pursuits that balance the often repetitive or intellectually rote elements of your existence.

5. Blueprint for Success: The Primal Blueprint laws are simple and intuitive, unlike many elements of Conventional Wisdom that suggest you have to struggle and suffer to attain your fitness and weight-loss goals. You will notice the benefits of Primal Blueprint living immediately—more even energy, better immune function, more enjoyable eating and exercising—as your genes direct your cells to function optimally at every moment.

Chapter Endnotes

[1] **Origin of Man**

The "out of Africa" theory is also known as the Recent Single-Origin Hypothesis (RSOH), Replacement Hypothesis, or Recent African Origin (RAO) model. The theory, originally proposed by Charles Darwin in his *Descent of Man*, modernized by Christopher Stringer and Peter Andrews, and strongly supported by recent studies of mitochondrial DNA, says that anatomically modern humans evolved solely in Africa between 200,000 (first appearance of anatomically modern humans) and 100,000 years ago, with members leaving Africa 60,000 years ago and replacing all earlier human populations, including Homo neanderthalensis and Homo erectus.

[2] **Origin of Agriculture**

Dr. Jared Diamond, evolutionary biologist, physiologist, and Pulitzer Prize-winning professor of geography at UCLA, is the author of *Guns, Germs and Steel: The Fates of Human Societies*, which discusses the advent of agriculture and its effects on civilization and human health. Chapter 5 of *Guns, Germs and Steel* details agriculture's origin (including which crops were cultivated) in several locations around the globe.

The *Emergence of Agriculture* by Bruce Smith details the great transition of humanity from a hunter-gatherer lifestyle to agriculture and thus civilization. *Guns, Germs and Steel* and Richard Manning's *Against the Grain* detail the negative aspects of humankind's shift to agriculture, blaming it for large-scale disease, imperialism, colonialism, slavery, and an inexorable progression to global warfare. All this thanks to the abuse of "free time" resulting from the specialization of labor and the pursuit of power over resources, humans, and geography—goals that were previously irrelevant in the largely egalitarian hunter-gatherer societies.

[3] **Primal Human Life Span**

The estimate of "maximum lifespan potential" from Homo sapiens 15,000 years ago of 94 years is actually higher than the corresponding figure attached to modern humans of 91 years! This material comes from the work of Dr. Richard G. Cutler, molecular gerontologist and longevity expert, who has produced more than 100 papers on the subject. Dr. Cutler was a research chemist at the Gerontology Research Center at the National Institute on Aging, National Institutes of Health for 19 years. Dr. Cutler's estimate is derived from laboratory analysis of skeletal material, with particular emphasis on the ratio of body weight to brain size. Other factors involved in making accurate life span calculations are age of sexual maturation to life span ratio (a 5:1 ratio is common among humans) and rates of caloric intake and expenditure.

[4] **Grok**

In Chapter 2 we talk about Grok as the patriarch of a primal family. However, in the interest of political correctness and ease of reading, you can view Grok as a not necessarily gender-specific euphemism for primal ancestor(s) whom we aspire to emulate in lifestyle behaviors. For example, "Grok never ate sugar, and neither should you."

CHAPTER 2

Grok and Korg

From Indigenous to Digital: One Giant Step (Backward) for Mankind

In This Chapter

We will examine the contrasting daily lives of Grok and his primal family with their modern-day antithesis, the Korg family. No, not to see who can travel 20 miles quicker (the Korgs' SUV beats Grok's bare feet with a few hours to spare…although the story might be different if it were a footrace!), but to examine the benefits of adapting primal behaviors to the modern world and the damage caused by living in conflict with our genetic predisposition to be fit, healthy, and happy.

The extremely unhealthy saga of the Korgs might seem embellished, but it's actually a statistically accurate indicator of many lifestyle trends today: hectic schedules compromising quality family time; processed foods emphasized in place of natural foods; prescription drugs used in place of lifestyle change; digital entertainment replacing physical activity; and overly stressful exercise programs that cause even the most devoted to fail with weight loss and fitness goals.

While the story is distressing, the good news is that with some simple, enjoyable lifestyle modifications, the momentum can turn immediately in the direction of better health (including freedom from dependence on prescription medications), higher energy, successful long-term weight loss, and a more enjoyable life for you and your family.

A man's health can be judged by which he takes two at a time—pills or stairs.
                                                        —Joan Welsh

As we contrast Grok and Korg, we must refrain from the common knee-jerk rationalizations about the superiority of today's technological world. While infant mortality rates and death from tiger attacks are way down, it is sobering (pun intended) to consider that motor vehicle accidents (heavily influenced by alcohol use) are the leading cause of death for youth ages 15 to 24, followed by suicide and homicide. While no one is arguing that we should disavow our worldly possessions and go back in time to mud huts and spears, we must take a hard look at our lifestyles and absorb some powerful lessons offered by the legacy of our ancestors.

Livin' Large 10,000 Years Ago

Your impression of primal human life might be negatively colored by sensationalized portrayals of precivilization humans as filthy, grunting savages dwelling in caves or by the harrowing vision of a primal human potentially meeting his doom in the jaws of a beast or by the fangs of a snake. Unpleasant camping experiences (you know—too many mosquitoes, strange night noises, or no hot showers) might add to a dark vision of what it might have been like to live in hunter-gatherer times. Indeed, life was rough in many ways—much time and energy was devoted to getting food and other basic essentials that we take for granted. However, in many other ways—including the most simple and fundamental areas necessary for a healthy, happy life—Grok actually had it pretty good.

Ten thousand years ago, a time period coinciding with the ending of the last major ice age, the continent of North America was populated with small bands of hunter-gatherer tribes. Many theorize that this migration into North America originated from Russia and moved very slowly eastward over dozens of generations across the Bering Land Bridge (which became submerged about 10,000 years ago) and then south into Canada and the United States. This population expansion across the continent was probably driven by the tracking of big game herds. These tribes typically numbered 10 to 30 people comprising nuclear or extended families. While the average human life expectancy was about 33 in Grok's time,[1] if Grok had been able to avoid misfortune by accident, predator, or illness, his life expectancy would have increased dramatically.

Shortly after Grok's time, the advent of agriculture drastically changed the nature of human life on earth and caused numerous markers of human health to steadily decline as previously mentioned. Matt Ridley, author of *The Agile Gene*, reports that average brain size in 50,000 B.C. was 1,567 cc for males and 1,468 cc for females. Strange as it may seem, average brain sizes today are 1,248 cc for males and 1,210 cc for females, with the onset of the shrinkage closely related to the advent of agriculture.

Grok's Walk

Grok and his longtime mate have two children, a 12-year-old boy and a one-year-old girl. Two other children didn't make it past infancy, a traumatic yet unavoidable part of primal life. Grok and his small band of 20 relatives live in what is now known as the Central Valley of California. It's a cool, moist climate supporting vast pine forests, owing to the lower mean temperatures of the era (mean earth temperatures have continued to rise over the last 10,000 years).

The gathering of berries and other fruit, leaves, roots, nuts, and seeds provide the bulk of Grok's food supply. Grok also hunts a variety of animals and probably enjoys a fair amount of fish and mollusks, being well positioned in the watershed of the Sierra. He probably scores some big game (mammoth, mastodon, bison, bear, lion, saber-toothed tiger, wolf, deer, and moose), but because many of these animals were at the end of their era, more food likely came from small mammals, such as beaver, rabbit, squirrel, and mole.

Naturally, we'll start our day with Grok at sunrise. Grok and his family awaken easily to the sound of birds chirping. They have a simple but comfortable shelter: a thatched, dome-shaped hut made with branches and brush. Grok's family begins the morning routine amidst the ageless singsong babble of a one-year-old. First things first—time to put together the morning meal. Grok's mate provides the baby the most nutritious food ever known to humankind—breast milk. The baby will begin to eat solid food within a few months but will continue to rely heavily on breast-feeding for three years. This provides nutrition for physical growth and gives her immune system a head start in dealing with potential health issues her mother has already been exposed to and overcome.

Grok's son will also enjoy a power breakfast. Because it's now late summer, special treats abound in the form of fat grub worms and local berries in their narrow ripening window. The current bounty is a far cry from the severe reduction in their typical food supplies the previous winter, caused by unusually heavy rains. Fortunately, Grok and his family had tapped into their genetic ability to efficiently mobilize their stored body fat and make up for the caloric deficits in their diet. The family had also adapted to their winter circumstances by sleeping more and reducing their daily activity level.

The son gladly handles the chore of picking a basket of berries and quickly returns to camp. After breakfast, they turn their attention to preparing items for their daily endeavors: tidying up woven storage receptacles, sharpening rudimentary weapons like spears, and packing food rations (mostly nuts and seeds) for their planned journey. Today they are going for a long walk, heading east toward the Sierra foothills to gather more berries and perhaps score some small game. Everyone is eager—even though the temperature will be warm and the walk will be longer than their typical daily wanderings—because they will get to enjoy a cool dip in the river at the midpoint of their journey.

After a nutritious breakfast, the family heads out, mother carrying the baby and the preteen keeping busy harassing squirrels with rocks. Arriving at the river, they feast on more berries and a few freshwater clams, sip clean water, and blissfully bathe, splash, and jump off rocks into the crystal clear and brisk river. Grok's occasional brief exposure to cold water offers more than fun.[2] He doesn't know it, but this activity is considered a "positive natural stressor" that helps boost immune function and antioxidant defense, decreases inflammation and pain, and increases blood flow and lymphatic function, something particularly therapeutic for tired muscles.

After his splash, Grok lounges on a sunbaked rock. His eyes gradually begin to shut, and he nods off for a power nap. As soon as his eyes fully close, positive hormonal changes occur in Grok's body.[3] Humans have adapted to obtain great benefits from even brief naps. One reason is the need for continued vigilance during the night (predators and other dangers made a "good night's sleep" hard to come by until recently). Another is because the relaxed pace of primal life lent itself to afternoon shut-eye opportunities. Grok quickly drifts into the deepest, most restorative "delta" sleep cycle. Stress hormone levels are moderated and his brain chemicals are rebalanced, allowing him to wake up 20 minutes later refreshed and relaxed. The daughter takes the opportunity to doze off for far longer, even as she is hoisted up into her carrying sling as the family heads off.

Clad in skirts made of plant fiber and animal skin, the family moves effortlessly in bare feet over undulating terrain and makeshift animal trails. The ground is covered with rock and plant debris, including sharp burrs discarded by native plants, but they deftly cruise along for hours without so much as a cramp or stubbed toe. Even at 12, Grok's son has already developed excellent cardiovascular endurance, muscle strength, and balance. And because a physically challenging life is routine to him, he probably doesn't moan or complain about the length of the journey or the boredom factor ("Are we there yet?"). After all, no video games await indoors.… The parents pause on numerous occasions to teach him about native plant life, point out animal markings, and dispense other environmental lessons that will serve him well and keep him safe as he grows to assume ever-more challenging and valuable hunter-gatherer responsibilities.

Typical of humans 10,000 years ago, Grok and his family are of similar height and weight as a modern family, but with far more muscle and less body fat! Grok sports a single-digit body fat percentage and the well-balanced physique of today's Olympic decathlete. Pardon the expression, but Grok's mate, by today's standards, would probably qualify as a hottie. Her active lifestyle gives her striking attributes of a ballerina, a gymnast, and an ironman triathlete rolled into one enviable primal physique.

> *Typical of humans 10,000 years ago, Grok and his family are of similar height and weight, but with far more muscle and less body fat!*

While Grok initially had planned to return to their permanent settlement that same evening, he chats briefly with his mate to discuss a spontaneous change of plans—to rest for the day and camp out. Because expectations and complexities are so minimal in Grok's life, the family easily goes with the flow of significant decisions like these without a second thought—this despite being unprepared for an overnight stay. It simply means a couple hours' additional work to gather up materials and construct a temporary shelter, build a fire, and get some dinner. No worry—they are safe together and accepting of every circumstance nature brings them.

Grok and his son head out for a quick hunt. We'd be surprised how primitive their weapons are, but the duo are able to leverage their extraordinary intelligence and instinct about the natural world to quickly procure a couple of rabbits for dinner. Walking back to camp, their celebratory banter is rudely interrupted by the appearance of a brown bear, drawn by the smell and wishing to make an unfair trade of lives for rabbits. A surge of fight-or-flight hormones flood the bloodstreams of Grok and his son. Grok immediately delivers a stream of detailed instructions to his son (back up slowly, maintain eye contact, etc.). His son nods calmly, naturally stifling his instinct to scream or run in the interest of survival. Grok, seemingly fearless in the face of this menacing creature, calmly lays the rabbits down on the ground and carefully joins his son in deliberate retreat. The bear issues a couple of loud roars just to be sure everyone knows who's boss, gathers his "kill," and moseys along. For good measure, Grok and his son take off on a dead sprint for 60 seconds, until they are safely out of the predator's sight.

Twenty minutes later, the fight-or-flight chemicals have worn off, the father-and-son debriefing is complete, and Grok arrives back at camp with empty hands and, most likely, a smile and shrug of the shoulders. This gesture epitomizes the requisite disposition for the uncertainty of primal life. It's a coping mechanism we have hardwired into our genes: "Don't worry, be happy."

Grok's mate has discovered some leafy green vegetation that they will eat raw or cook briefly over the campfire with a few wild potatoes. A computer analysis of the nutrient content of the food they consume, even without the rabbits, over the course of a typical month (a sufficient time period to account for the feast-or-famine realities of primal life and our graceful genetic ability to deal with it effectively) would reveal optimum levels of carbohydrates, protein, fat, vitamins, minerals, fiber, antioxidants, and other elements needed to sustain a lifetime of exceptional fitness and vibrant health. Similarly, if we were to draw Grok's blood for laboratory analysis, this primitive human would likely come up a big winner by today's health standards: free of disease

> *Don't bother about being modern.*
> *Unfortunately it is the one thing that,*
> *whatever you do, you cannot avoid.*
> *—Salvador Dalí*

markers such as high C-reactive protein levels (indicative of undesirable systemic inflammation); possessing ideal levels of cholesterol, triglycerides, blood glucose, and insulin; and exempt from common modern-day nutrient deficiencies.

After dinner, the family lingers around the campfire for perhaps an hour or two, relaxing, telling stories, and winding down the day as the sun sets. This routine of quality family time in the evening is likely more than today's average working parents spend with their children in an entire week (families average 19 minutes together per day of quality time—free from television and other distractions).[4] As the sun sets, Grok and his family are ready for a good night's sleep.

The American Dream—Unplugged (Or Should We Say, "Plugged In?")

Our modern family, the Korgs (that's Grok spelled backwards; fitting when you consider their dramatic departure from Grok's simple, healthy lifestyle), live where Grok did in California's Central Valley, in what is now known as Stockton. Stockton is a medium-sized, middle-income community located on the Sacramento River delta, only an hour's drive from the metropolitan San Francisco Bay Area, which has a population of some seven million. The Korgs—and thousands of other families like them in bedroom communities outside the Bay Area proper—believe they have the best of both worlds: an "easy" commute to Bay Area salaries combined with affordable housing (Stockton's median home price is several hundred thousand dollars less than most comparable homes in the Bay Area), less congestion, and good recreational, educational, and cultural opportunities. Ken Korg's two hours a day in the car seem like a routine cost of living the American Dream.[5]

An Alarming Morning

Waking up naturally with the sun? Not the Korgs. Ken's wife, Kelly, is up and out of the house when it's still dark, heading to the gym for a 6 A.M. Spinning class. It's a struggle for her to get her butt onto the bike seat for that class three days a week, but Kelly knows that her only chance to get a workout—or, for that matter, to enjoy some personal time—is before the family stirs and the responsibilities pile up. Besides, Kelly has struggled all her life with her body weight and would dearly love to drop the 20 or more pounds suggested by her physician to get her body mass index (BMI) into the healthy range.

When the alarm clock emits its digital chirping bird signal (very similar to Grok's; you can also choose breaking waves or wind chimes!) in the darkness of 5:15 A.M., an immediate stress reaction initiates throughout Kelly's body. Even the benign digital birds jolt her abruptly out of a restful sleep cycle and stimulate a mini fight-or-flight response by spiking her cortisol levels. Rising in the dark further disrupts her circadian rhythm (since a variety of hormones and brain chemicals are sensitive to light and dark cycles), resulting in a stressful start to Kelly's day—ironic in that her early morning workout is part of her sincere commitment to become more healthy.

The rest of the Korg family avoids Mom's cortisol spike, but due to a host of other factors, they have their own issues waking up. Ken is already awake when his alarm sounds at seven o'clock, but his mind and body are in no hurry to get up and out of bed. Part of his situation is psychological—he is not terribly excited to face an hour on the freeway. Other factors influencing his body's sluggish start are the medications he's taking and the previous night's late dessert—a generous slice of cheesecake made with 60 grams of processed carbohydrates, partially hydrogenated vegetable oil, and assorted unpronounceable chemical preservatives.

Ken's cheesecake spiked his blood glucose just as he was attempting to fall asleep, interfering with the release of melatonin that naturally triggers sleepiness. Instead of spending the first hour in bed drifting into ever deeper cycles of sleep, Ken was fidgeting and twitchy because of the excess blood glucose in his system. Besides the glucose coursing through his veins, Ken's brain waves were jacked up from spending the final 90 minutes of his evening watching television. Even though he was exhausted and thus attempting to wind down after a long day, the fast-moving, flickering images on the screen (often violent or otherwise arousing) caused irregular stimulation to Ken's retina. This type of stimulus is transferred directly to the brain via the optic nerve and disturbs the normal function of the hypothalamus, the control center for many vital body functions, including the initiation of proper sleep patterns.[6]

Alas, Ken is one of more than 30 million Americans who holds a prescription for sleep medication,[7] which he reaches for on occasions like these. The quick-acting sleep medication combined with the eventual heavy insulin release to counter the cheesecake has Ken dead to the world within 20 minutes of taking the pill. Seven hours later, with optimal sleep cycles disturbed and with the sedative effects of Ambien still trying to clear his bloodstream, Ken feels sluggish and groggy instead of naturally refreshed and energized.

Nevertheless, it's time to get the Korg clan moving, so Ken drags himself out of bed and heads over to the bedrooms of his 14-year-old son and 6-year-old daughter. Rousing them is not an easy task. Kenny Korg is experiencing his greatest need for sleep since infancy, and, like most modern teenagers, isn't getting enough.[8] Kenny is also affected by a couple of other common adolescent conditions: drowsiness during the day and a delayed circadian phase, which has him naturally wanting to stay up later and wake up later. Kenny would feel fantastic with a regular afternoon power nap, but of course napping isn't cool, so he usually fights his body's need by ingesting a caffeine-laced energy drink or soda. He effortlessly stays up late playing computer games, cruising Facebook, and texting his friends. Because he often doesn't power down until 11 P.M. or midnight, the 7 A.M. alarm comes far too early for him to feel rested and energized.

Young Miss Cindy Korg has her own troubles waking up. The mind-numbing effects of the cherry-flavored antihistamine/decongestant/cough suppressant/analgesic over-the-counter medication her mom had given her the previous evening are still lingering after a fitful sleep. She wakes up groggy, with blocked sinuses, but must rally to get to school on time. Cindy's third upper respiratory tract infection this year was chalked up to "the bug that's going around." However, bugs are always going around; it was really her suppressed immune system—weakened by the excessive consumption of processed carbs and sugars in her diet—that prevented her from easily containing the virus after the first contact.

Kelly, always wanting to do the right thing as a mother, unknowingly prolonged little Cindy's ordeal by giving her a common cold "remedy" that was intended to ease her suffering but that interfered with her daughter's natural defenses. Pounding the cough syrup every four hours for a few days likely doubled the time required for complete recovery, quelling the low fever her body had naturally developed as a first assault (mild fever is a primary defense in helping to kill viruses), blocking the production of mucus intended to drain the virus into the stomach (where it can easily be killed by stomach acid), drying out the sinuses so she could breathe easier (but thereby causing them to swell to the point that she can't breathe out of her nose at all this morning), and suppressing a productive cough that might have kept her up some at night but would have allowed her lungs to expel the virus-laden mucus. All these "symptoms" were actually Cindy's potent gene-based natural defenses—thwarted by modern medicine.

Cindy's tendency to get sick more often than other kids her age is partly due to immune-suppressing dietary factors but also may be associated with Kelly's choice to breast feed for a shorter period than is optimal. By contacting the baby's skin and picking up any pathogens on the body, the mother's immune system manufactures the antibodies and immune cells required to resist infections. She then passes those antibodies and lymphocytes ("natural killer" white blood cells) to the baby through breast milk. With infant formulas so highly touted by television, magazines, and physicians today, we typically see infants switching over long before optimal nutritional and immune benefits have accrued from breastfeeding, which World Health Organization experts recommend for two years or more. At any rate, Cindy finally summons the strength to get dressed and head downstairs.

Kelly bursts through the door as the family is shuffling around trying to get ready for the day. She's chipper and energized from her 50-minute class, which elevated her heart rate to 85 percent of maximum or higher for most of that time period. The intensity of the effort has released a flood of stress hormones into her bloodstream, so she's on an "exercise high" due to the effects of natural painkilling endorphins as she greets her family. Kelly quickly sticks three waffles into the toaster. Trying to shop healthy, she always chooses the whole grain waffles for her family.

Kelly dutifully cracks open a can of Slim-Fast meal-replacement drink. Main ingredients: skim milk powder, sugar, fructose, and cacao (pronounced "Kuh-Kay-Oh"), along with plenty of chemicals, synthetic vitamins, and vegetable oils—not much nutrition but plenty of simple carbs (38 grams) to raise blood glucose temporarily and stimulate an energy-sapping insulin surge soon after. The "good" news: it contains only 240 calories. A minute later, the Korgs' power breakfast is ready: orange juice and whole grain waffles with a polyunsaturated (and thus pro-inflammatory and immune suppressing) butter-like spread and "low-sugar" maple syrup made with artificial sweeteners[9] and woefully far removed from the sweet nectar that flows out of a hole drilled in a Vermont maple tree.

Kelly's second shake at lunch will result in a total of only 480 calories consumed since seven o'clock the previous evening—a period of 17 hours. While our bodies are adept at supplying adequate energy through intermittent food consumption (such was the reality of daily life for Grok), Kelly's long-term reliance on dietary carbohydrates for energy, her high-intensity dawn workout, and the energy demands of her busy day make it the wrong time to skimp on healthy food. As a consequence, her metabolic rate will slow and the appetite center in her brain will send a strong message to consume quick-energy carbohydrates.

Unlike Grok, Kelly's calorie-restriction efforts will not result in the burning of stored body fat, because the frequent insulin spikes after her high-carb shakes, eating binges, and typical American meals can inhibit fat burning and, in fact (with high-insulin eating habits followed over time), produce metabolic changes that make it increasingly difficult to mobilize stored fat for energy. This condition is obviously affecting Kelly, an active, disciplined person miserably failing to reduce body fat. The net effect of Kelly's punishing (elite athletes spend a substantially lower percentage of total exercise time at elevated heart rates than Kelly)[10] early morning workouts and devoted calorie restriction is a reduction in muscle mass (which further lowers her metabolic rate and certainly doesn't improve her physique), an increase in body fat (due to the binge eating and slowed metabolic rate), and recurring fatigue, mood swings, and frustration.

The sting of failure is intensified every time Kelly sees her peppy neighbor Wendy, who has dropped eight pounds (3.6 kg) in two weeks since following her new multilevel marketing-driven cleansing diet. Upon further examination of these remarkable results, however, it's evident that the eight pounds consist almost entirely of reduced water retention from the depletion of muscle glycogen (every gram of stored glycogen binds with four grams of water in the body) and lean muscle tissue. The eight pounds will return in a matter of days when exhaustion causes a return to normal, or supernormal, calorie intake.

"*That* Problem"...Among Others

Ken hates these first few minutes after Kelly gets home from her morning workout, because her energy level is such a stark contrast to the slow-moving household. On the flip side, Kelly typically shuts down around 8:30 P.M., after the stress hormone buzz wears off and insulin floods her system following dinner. With Ken's contrasting late-evening pattern, time for couple intimacy is virtually nonexistent. Furthermore, Ken has recently been experiencing "*that* problem" but is hesitant tell anyone, let alone make an appointment with a physician to receive a prescription for Viagra. After all, Ken is still in his 40s and thinks Viagra is for old guys. Ken would be surprised to learn that about a third of all erectile prescriptions are dispensed to men under 50 and that use by men under age 45 tripled between 1998 and 2002.

Biochemically, Ken has several issues that contribute to his condition. The sustained high levels of cortisol in his bloodstream from his stressful lifestyle factors, such as inadequate sleep and job stress, suppress testosterone production, leading to diminished energy levels, weakened immune function, and, of course, reduced sex drive. His higher-than-optimum body fat levels and excessive insulin production from his high-carb diet and insufficient exercise also contribute to low testosterone, poor blood circulation, and other common-but-curable impotency factors.

Oh, I almost forgot Ken's Lipitor (the world's best-selling drug with nearly $12.4 billion in sales in 2008), a statin medication he takes for "high" cholesterol that can cause muscle and liver problems, deplete CoQ10 (coenzyme Q10; a natural antioxidant and cofactor that is critical to cellular energy metabolism), and, yes, inhibit sexual performance. Ken only recently (and reluctantly, to his credit) started on Lipitor, at the behest of his doctor, who was concerned about his total cholesterol count of 205. Not in the high-risk range by any means, but enough for the doc to want to bring it down some, which the statins manage to do quickly. Unfortunately, statins also produce serious side effects,[11] mainly by blocking the production and flow of CoQ10 into cell mitochondria. This disturbance of mitochondria hampers the body's ability to generate normal amounts of energy (hence the common patient complaint of weakness and fatigue), as well as fight free radicals and moderate inflammation. Furthermore, statins do not affect triglyceride (blood fat) levels or LDL (the so-called bad cholesterol) particle size, nor do they decrease risk of death in any women, in men over 65, or in men under 65 who have not had a heart attack.

Kelly, in turn, struggles with her body image, leading to reduced desire for intimacy. Furthermore, her stressful exercise regimen and poor nutritional habits interfere with healthy female hormone balance and contribute to the reduction of her drive.

Ken fills his commuter mug with coffee, hustles Cindy (with her cold medication hangover) into the car, and they depart. The first stop is four-tenths of a mile away at Cindy's elementary school.[12] It's four minutes until the tardy bell, and the front entrance is mobbed with a conga line of cars waiting to reach the drop-off zone. By the time Ken's car reaches its destination, Cindy is in a panic, as she will once again chase the tardy bell. Fear of a tardy slip may not be on par with a surprise visit from a bear, but the same fight-or-flight response occurs in Cindy as it did in Grok. The parting is anything but warm and comforting—a few choice words from the first grader and a quick admonishment in return from Ken: "Fine, maybe I'll just make you walk next time!" An excellent idea, considering the short trip from home to classroom by auto has taken six minutes, whereas even a leisurely walk (say, the pace that Grok and his family maintained for several hours, while trading off carrying a small child) from home to classroom would not have taken much longer.

Ken extracts his sedan from the campus swarm and soon begins his navigation of interstate freeways. As he drives up and over the small mountain range that marks the geographic boundary of the Bay Area, Ken spends his hour of "solitude" listening to talk radio—bouncing back and forth between sports and news talk—and taking several phone calls from friends or coworkers in the office. This constant and distracted stimulation to a brain still experiencing the effects of Ambien leads to mental fatigue before he even sets foot in the office. What's more, at the 40-minute mark of Ken's journey, he is suffering from heartburn and bloating (from his regular consumption of fried and fatty foods, dairy products, alcohol, sugars and desserts, sodas and other carbonated beverages, and substantial caloric intake in the evenings) as well as his typical recurring back pain (an affliction he shares with 60 to 80 percent of the general population).

Ken reaches into his briefcase and whips out his pill container, extracting a purple pill and a white capsule. The "healing purple pill" is Nexium (the third best-selling drug in the world with $5.7 billion in sales in 2005), which is used to treat the increasingly common condition known as gastroesophageal reflux disease (GERD) and its main symptom of heartburn. Nexium, classified as a *proton pump inhibitor*, blocks the production of hydrochloric acid in the stomach. This provides immediate relief for Ken's pain but seriously inhibits the digestive process, which relies on hydrochloric acid and other powerful acids to break down and assimilate nutrients from food.

Next is the white capsule Celebrex, a popular nonsteroidal anti-inflammatory (NSAID) prescription medication that reduces levels of hormone-like substances called prostaglandins that are part of a natural inflammation response occurring in Ken's body. Ken takes it to alleviate the back pain that accompanies the inflammation. He will pop another Celebrex this evening per the recommendation of his physician, who also suggested at his last visit that he schedule an appointment at a physical therapy clinic to obtain a customized back and core strengthening exercise routine. He's been meaning to schedule that but hasn't yet found the time.[13] Instead, Ken grabs some exercise here and there when the stars align and gaps open up in his schedule. Owing to his athletic youth, his competitive appetite is bigger than his physical condition. His forays into adult pickup basketball at the club usually produce more tweaks and pulls than inspiration to pursue a regular, balanced total-body fitness program.

If Ken proceeds with the typical behavior pattern, he will use these prescription NSAIDs for years and neglect sufficient regular exercise. Down the road, owing to Ken's long-term use of such a powerful systemic anti-inflammatory medication, the drug's impact will diminish (at which point his doctor will probably put him on something stronger) and his body's natural ability to control all types of inflammation will have been steadily decimated. This will set the tone for a variety of serious health conditions to potentially take root, including—owing to his poor diet and lifestyle habits—many types of cancer and heart disease. Yep, that's right—studies suggest a significant increased risk of heart attack when taking NSAIDs. Vioxx was a very popular NSAID taken by 80 million people worldwide from 1999 until 2004, when it was taken off the market due to concerns about side effects that increased heart attack risk. Celebrex sales skyrocketed as a result, until research suggested it posed similar risks. Celebrex sales then dropped sharply but steadily resumed to exceed $2 billion in 2006.

> *The idea on the medical horizon is that chronic inflammation is a root cause of degenerative disease. If physicians are trained to use "food as medicine" they may not need to rely on drugs and their distressing side-effects to treat the inflammatory process.*
> —*Dr. Andrew Weil*

Spreadsheets and Chow Mein

After an hour and eight minutes of driving from the elementary school, Ken arrives at his office. He works as an accountant for a software company. The hours are regular (unlike many of his coworkers, who are selling or developing software and routinely working 10- to 12-hour days), and he makes a third more than he could in the same position in Stockton. Aside from the set hours and compensation benefits, the working conditions are challenging. Executives and division sales managers constantly enroll the accounting team in their hyperdrive mentality. They have a penchant for requesting ridiculously fancy presentations on short notice or strolling into Ken's office and literally breathing down his neck to obsessively review sales figures in the days counting down to quarterly close.

The perk of being able to leave promptly at 6:00 P.M. each evening is muted by the mental exhaustion that overcomes Ken as soon as he opens his car door in the parking lot. In his previous position (closer to home and for significantly less pay), Ken would take a leisurely lunch hour to eat a sandwich in the park or even join a coworker for a light workout at the gym. He'd return to work refreshed and proceed at a sensible pace through the afternoon hours, pausing often to share a laugh with coworkers. Lately, he has stayed at his desk to eat lunch, typically procured via a 40-second drive to a busy nearby intersection with numerous quick refueling options.

Ken, inspired by Kelly's commitment, is also making a concerted effort to "do the right thing" and eat healthier. He eschews McDonald's® and Burger King® for Chinese buffet, which sounds healthier but is actually far from it. He returns to the office armed with chow mein noodles and sweet-and-sour chicken, trying not to spill the predominantly simple carbohydrate meal onto his spreadsheets. Laughter in the hallways has been replaced by the discernible buzz of anxiety, the unspoken fear that heads will begin to roll out the door if Ken's spreadsheets don't impress stockholders and executives.

In contrast to the few brief moments of Grok's life-or-death encounter with a bear, Ken's workplace is essentially a daily nine-hour grind of unrelenting moderate stress. Ken and the rest of us would still choose the spreadsheets over being scared sheetless by a bear, but the impact of prolonged chronic stress is far more destructive to human health (and misaligned with our genes) than a pattern of brief intermittent stresses coupled with adequate downtime.

The midafternoon, post high-carb lunch sugar crash hits Ken hard, so he scarfs down one of the PowerBars® (better than a Snicker's, right?) Kelly threw into his briefcase ((PowerBar Energize Tangy Tropical has 42 grams of carbs—25 of them sugar; Snickers has 34.5 g total carbs—29 g sugar… whoops!) and heads to the break room for his daily afternoon cup o' joe. Ken consumes two cups of coffee and one to two diet sodas each day, a total of about 250 milligrams of caffeine.[14] Not quite enough to classify him as an addict (actually, that's about the daily average for Americans), but it's definitely another substance, along with the several prescription and over-the-counter meds, that he depends on to make it through his day.

Love, Money, and Insulin

Even while making a comfortable income by any reasonable definition, the Korgs are experiencing financial stresses familiar to many.[15] After paycheck deductions for taxes, 401(k), and, of course, the incredible employee stock purchase program (which entices five percent of his gross income to be fed back to the monster), a third of his annual net goes to mortgage and related tax and insurance costs. Other healthy chunks go to car payments and insurance, groceries and dining out, medical expenses not covered by Ken's skimpy company policy, and the occasional whopper, such as five grand to straighten Kenny's teeth, two grand for a major surgery at the vet, two grand for Kenny's school field trip to Washington, D.C., 800 bucks for Kelly's last-minute bereavement trip to the East Coast for a family friend's funeral, a C-note for a weight-loss "starter kit" that gung ho neighbor Wendy basically forced upon them, and so on.

Kelly contributes to the family's bottom line, running her own stimulating but stressful business as a freelance graphic designer. The flexible hours are great, although the healthy boundary between work and personal life often gets blurred. One favorite ritual is picking up her daughter from school every day and taking her out for a treat—carrying on a fond family tradition she and her sisters enjoyed with their mother. As Eric Schlosser details in *Fast Food Nation*, Kelly is cooperating with the food industry's institutionalized exploitation of American families that allows parents to replace quality time (particularly the nearly extinct family home mealtime…and also the guilty conscience that goes with being too busy for family time) with instant gratification—and therefore love—for their children.

The treat time coincides with Kelly's daily affliction of the afternoon blues. The colorful, peppy, healthy lifestyle messaging inside the local Jamba Juice franchise helps Kelly rationalize her impending insulin flash flood. She confidently orders up a 24-ounce Strawberry Surf Rider for herself and a 16-ounce Mango-a-go-go for her daughter. Cindy excitedly suggests adding a couple baked goods from the child-eye-level display case to the tab. Ever vigilant, Kelly scans the choices to pick the healthiest one and settles on the reduced-fat blueberry-lemon loaf, "part of a complete breakfast—complement with a smoothie or fresh squeezed orange juice," says the Jamba Juice menu. Each loaf offers 290 calories, 73 percent of which come from processed carbohydrates (lead ingredients: sugar and flour) with virtually zero nutritional value and a guaranteed strong insulin response. Cindy finishes only half her loaf, but Kelly makes sure it doesn't go to waste.

The discipline of Kelly consuming fewer than 500 calories in the previous 19 hours is no match for a depleted brain and body. While the 24-ounce Strawberry Surf Rider will provide Kelly with some much deserved antioxidants and other healthy nutrients from the frozen fruit, 87 percent of its 490 calories come from sugar. Along with one and a half blueberry-lemon loaves, Kelly has ingested 925 calories (make that an even thousand, counting a few long pulls on her daughter's straw to try the Mango-a-go-go), including 187 grams of refined carbohydrates (that's more than the Primal Blueprint's recommended range of 100 to 150 grams for an entire day!). Her sugar/insulin roller coaster will again hamper her fat-burning efforts for hours after this onslaught and lead to fatigue and sugar cravings come dinnertime.

> *Studies suggest that overweight kids are highly likely to become overweight adults and consequently suffer from serious health problems and life-threatening diseases.*

Young Cindy Korg's drink and half loaf send more than 100 grams of sugar into her little body, stressing her insulin system—and her immune system—yet again. The previous day, at a classmate's birthday party, she had consumed typical party fare of two slices of thin-crust cheese pizza (460 calories), a small slice of chocolate cake (235) with a small scoop of vanilla ice cream (150), 130 calories from some box juices with high fructose corn syrup (she opened three over the course of the party and drank only half of the fluid—typical ratio, as any parent who's hosted a birthday party can confirm), and several assorted bite-sized candies from the take-home party favor bag (150 calories). Her total calories in the three-hour period came to 1,125, more than half in the form of simple sugar. That's enough to stimulate a significant insulin response in a 300-pound man, let alone a 55-pound child.

Naturally (owing to family genes, her parents rationalize), young Cindy is already significantly overweight. Fortunately (from a psychological perspective only), unlike in past generations, her plump physique is shared by many of her fellow first graders.[16] While this certainly protects her self-esteem, it makes it difficult to change the popular chartered course of this young ship, sailing toward peril and doom. Studies suggest that overweight kids are highly likely to become overweight adults and consequently suffer from serious health problems and life-threatening diseases.

Kenny's World

We haven't heard much about the Korgs' teenage son, Kenny, which is appropriate because he is already emotionally disconnected from his busy family and pulled by the powerful force of peer influence in directions that create conflict with stable family life. In his early years, Kenny was naturally active and spent hours outside running and playing. Unfortunately, each passing preteen year saw more sedentary technological distractions commandeering his time and innocent backyard play being exchanged for competitive organized sports.[17]

While Kenny has some innate athletic ability, he lacks the naturally healthy aggression and competitiveness that allow young athletes to move to the front of the pack. Lacking time to connect with his son, Ken makes the common mistake of overpressurizing his son's athletic experience with misplaced emotion and "encouragement" that feels to his son like results expectations and criticism. By the time Kenny becomes a teen, he is finished with organized sports and deep into a new cultural phenomenon called massive multiplayer online role-playing games,[18] such as World of Warcraft and Runescape, where a player creates a digital persona and interacts with many others in a virtual world, often immersed for eight or 10 hours at a time. At school, he maintains grades that are decent yet below his potential, but he is misbehaving frequently in class. During a telephone conversation with the school counselor, the topic of attention deficit hyperactivity disorder (ADHD) is broached as a potential reason for Kenny's misbehavior.

Kenny's feelings of alienation are exacerbated at the dinner table that evening, when Ken peppers him with the exact same questions heard at the breakfast table about his son's decision to skip freshman basketball tryouts. The teen is naturally offended, unaware that one of the most common side effects of Ambien is short-term memory loss and that Ken truly has little recollection of the conversation from 12 hours prior (and some 8 hours after popping the Ambien).

The exchange escalates into a blowout covering various pent-up resentments. Ken decides to make an appointment for his son to visit a psychiatrist. After two sessions, the shrink diagnoses Kenny with ADHD and promptly prescribes the amphetamine Adderall[19]—this despite growing controversy surrounding its overprescription to children who lack serious symptoms and a true clinical diagnosis, the potential link to serious cardiovascular side effects, and the high incidence of abuse among teenagers using the stimulant recreationally. (An estimated seven million American kids take stimulants prescribed for attention disorders, a 500 percent increase since 1991.)

It's more likely that emotional factors, lack of sufficient vigorous exercise, and poor dietary habits (sugar binges, regular caffeine intake, and lack of healthy fats) are to blame for Kenny's adverse classroom behavior. Unfortunately, Kenny now has another hurdle on the path to getting his mind and body back into balance for the challenging high school years ahead: the powerful effects of stimulant medication on his growing body.

When critiquing the particulars of kids and their exercise, sleep, dietary habits, and school high jinks, you might default to thinking, "What's the big deal?" Kenny and millions of his peers will continue their mildly objectionable ways, but they'll get through high school just fine (provided they heed Primal Blueprint Law #9, Avoid Stupid Mistakes). They'll go off to college and pull all-nighters fueled by pizza, Red Bull, and Top Ramen, then they'll unwind after exam pressure with lots of alcohol, more pizza, and maybe a few cupcakes at the Kappa Kappa Gamma bash. I don't think previous generations can claim they are unfamiliar with this routine.

It's true, young people are incredibly resilient, in case you've forgotten. With metabolism accelerated and the endocrine system flooding the bloodstream with peak levels of key growth and reproductive hormones, the raw (indeed, primal) energy of youth can often override any potential insulin-driven fatigue from a Red Bull buzz wearing off. We can all attest to the difference between being at our physical peak and being beyond it. At 61, I'm stoked to be able to (more or less) hang with my son Kyle, a collegiate Ultimate competitor.

However, if we consider the concept that our genes—even young genes are predisposed to all kinds of problems if we give them the wrong environment (and, hence, the wrong signals), we can conclude that it's just a matter of time. Remember in college those frat boys with six-pack abs drinking pony kegs every weekend? A decade later, you can find most of them with pony keg guts drinking six-packs every weekend. As a parent or an influential figure in a child's life (or perhaps an evolved young person reading the Primal Blueprint!), you can assert the importance of having a foundation of healthy lifestyle habits and a deep respect for and understanding of how to get the best out of your body. This will pave the way for a different future than today's extremely disturbing one in which many experts predict a shorter life expectancy for children than their parents—for the first time in recorded history.[20]

"We Have Met the Enemy, and He Is Us"

This classic quote uttered by Walt Kelly's popular comic strip character Pogo captures the Korgs' plight perfectly: their well-intentioned efforts to do the right thing seem continuously sabotaged by cultural norms and misguided Conventional Wisdom. We are conditioned by the powerful forces of consumerism to pursue flawed solutions to our problems and ailments. The prescription and over-the-counter drugs downed by Ken, Kenny, and Cindy, Kelly's overly stressful exercise routine and overly restrictive diet, the massive amount of unhealthy food ingested by the family on a daily basis, and the lack of simple, quality family time might be disturbing to read about, but they are absolutely the norm today.

If you felt the Korgs' tale was an appalling, melodramatic, and unrealistic example of a modern family, you have lifestyle reference points that are significantly more healthy and balanced than those of the average American family. Extensive references to the Korgs' daily routine, prescription drug use, weight-loss battles, eating and exercise habits, childhood obesity, teenage behavior challenges, and digital media use are offered at the end of this chapter.

As they say, your kids grow up—and you grow old—before you know it. A lack of awareness, a lack of knowledge, and sometimes, sadly, a defiant, ignorant stance of disrespecting the essentials of health and well-being (including our genetic programming) tragically degrades the precious time families have together. This loss plays out every day and touches virtually every family in the modern world. It's time to stand up and take control of your health and well-being, to honor your genes by living according to the Primal Blueprint, and, finally, to reject many tenets of Conventional Wisdom that are flawed and hazardous to your health. In this book, we will do just that, further building momentum and crushing obstacles in our path as we march toward the ultimate expression of our human potential.

How Grok Probably Spent His Day

Hunting or gathering food..5 hours
Sleep, nap, rest, relax..10 hours
Habitat-, shelter-, basic human
needs-related chores...3 hours
Leisure time consisting of play
and family or group socializing....................................6 hours

Estimates derived from studies of the modern hunter-gatherer culture of the !Kung Bushmen in Africa.

How Ken Korg Spends His Day

Workplace...9 hours
Commute..2 hours
Sleep...6.7 hours
Television, computer, digital entertainment................ 4 hours[21]
Grooming, household chores, free time.........................2.3 hours

(free time components: leisure/educational reading: 24 minutes; meaningful conversation with child: 3.5 minutes)

Estimates derived from TV Free America in Washington, D.C. and American Time Use Survey Summary (U.S. Department of Labor, Washington, D.C.).

Chapter Summary

1. Grok's Lifestyle: Grok faced unimaginable hardships in primal life but in many ways enjoyed superior health to that of modern humans. While rates of infant mortality and death by predator or accident were far higher than they are today, if Grok were able to avoid such tragedy, he could enjoy robust health and supreme physical fitness into his 60s or 70s.

Grok's hunter-gatherer existence involved a diet of plants and animals, hours of low-level aerobic exercise every day, and occasional short bursts of maximum strength or speed efforts. Primal existence was simpler and slower paced, with life-or-death stressful events coming infrequently and lasting only briefly. This type of existence is more aligned with our genetic makeup than is the unrelenting stress of modern life.

2. Korg Lifestyle: Our modern suburban family, the Korgs, have diverged dramatically from the lifestyle basics modeled by Grok that are essential for good health. Long commutes, packed schedules, and excessive digital entertainment compromise family camaraderie. Financial pressures, insufficient sleep and downtime, extensive use of prescription drugs, poor dietary habits, and exhausting exercise programs lead to an excessively stressful modern existence and consequent health problems.

The Korgs' diet features excessive processed foods and insufficient nutritious foods. In particular, they eat too many simple carbs and grains that lead to excess insulin production. These dietary mistakes lead to assorted health problems, particularly undesirable body composition, beginning in childhood and continuing for a lifetime. Kelly Korg's well-meaning devotion to exercise and careful dieting does not lead to fat loss, because the workouts are too stressful and she regularly has excessive insulin in her bloodstream (from consuming too many carbs), which inhibits fat burning. Ken's lack of exercise, poor eating habits, work-related pressures, and reliance on prescription drugs to counter lifestyle errors make him tired and stressed and put him on the path to the eventual onset of serious disease. The Korg children are victimized by the disastrous cultural trends of today's youth, such as insufficient activity, excessive digital media use, high-insulin diets, and overpressurized athletic and academic experiences that lead to alienation and rebellion.

3. Your Family: It's critical to depart from these harmful cultural trends and create a different reality for you and your family. Modifying dietary habits to Primal Blueprint recommendations and placing limits on technology and jam-packed schedules in favor of relaxing family interaction will help reverse the appalling family dynamics characterized by the Korgs' story.

Chapter Endnotes

Grok Family References

[1] **Life Expectancy:** Life expectancy during the Paleolithic era (2.5 million years ago to 10,000 B.C) was around 33 years, factoring in the high rates of infant mortality. If Grok reached puberty, life expectancy increased to age 39 and if he reached 39, he could expect to live until 54. And this was a ripped, energetic 54, not the 54 of a guy struggling to hang on. The fatal hazards that befell Grok during his lifetime were entirely primitive: infections, accidents, and predators—not heart disease, diabetes, or obesity.

The advent of agriculture and civilization caused life expectancy to drop significantly, reaching a low of 18 during the Bronze Age of 3,300 B.C. to 1,200 B.C. Life expectancy remained low (between 20 and 30) through 1500 A.D. and then climbed only gradually, reaching 30 in 1800 and 40-50 in 1900 in the USA and Europe. The past century has seen a dramatic increase in lifespan in civilized countries, thanks mainly to medical advances that limit infant mortality and protect against disease plagues.

A 2004 study published by Rachel Caspari at the University of Michigan and Sang-Hee Lee at the University of California at Riverside revealed that a dramatic increase in human longevity that took place during the early Upper Paleolithic Period, around 30,000 years ago. The scientists studied dental information derived from molar wear patterns of *Australopithecines, Homo erectus,* and *Neanderthals* and discovered a five-fold increase in the number of individuals surviving to an older age (defined by doubling reproductive age—so humans could become grandparents) around that time period.

The scientists speculated that "this trend contributed importantly to population expansions and cultural innovations that are associated with modernity." Elders could pass on critical life knowledge to younger generations, social networks and family bonds were strengthened, and Grok could generally become a better parent by living longer. "There has been a lot of speculation about what gave modern humans their evolutionary advantage," Caspari said. "This research provides a simple explanation for which there is now concrete evidence: modern humans were older and wiser."

[2] **Cold Water Benefits:** The healing properties of water have been recognized for thousands of years. Public baths were a common feature in ancient civilizations. The Romans, Greeks, Egyptians, Turkish, Japanese, and Chinese all believed water was helpful for muscle recovery, sleep, and immune protection. In the early 1800s Vincent Priessnitz, an Austrian farmer, pioneered the use of hydrotherapy as a medical tool. During the mid to late 1800s, a Bavarian monk named Father Sebastian Kneipp gained wide recognition for his water therapy work. He cured himself of pulmonary tuberculosis (a common and typically fatal condition referred to then as "consumption") by regularly plunging into the icy Danube River to stimulate his immune system. Kneipp wrote extensively on the subject of hydrotherapy and other natural healing topics, gaining notoriety that attracted people from across the world to visit his clinic.

Several studies support the historical anecdotes that cold water offers health benefits. One study conducted by the Thrombosis Research Institute at London's Brompton Hospital found that exposure to cold baths boosted sex hormone production, improved fertility, chronic fatigue conditions, immune function, and blood circulation—reducing cardiovascular disease risk. Numerous studies indicate that the invigorating effect of cold water stimulates the release of endorphins by the autonomic nervous system. Anyone who has taken a plunge and emerged energized can attest to the powerful effects of cold water on the body.

[3] **Napping:** Data from the National Sleep Foundation suggests that "a well-timed afternoon nap may be the best way to combat sleepiness." Gregory Belenky, MD, Research Professor and Director of the Sleep and Performance Research Center at Washington State University, says naps can help make up for insufficient sleep, and that "it's even possible that divided sleep is more recuperative than sleep taken in a single block," noting how popular the afternoon siesta is in countries across the world. Dr. Mark Rosekind's studies with NASA pilots indicated that napping pilots had a 34 percent increase in performance and 54 percent boost in alertness that lasted for two to three hours. Harvard University studies show that 60-90 minute naps help the brain integrate new knowledge in the same manner as nighttime sleep. A study published in the research journal *Sleep* suggests that naps ranging from 10 to 30 minutes are optimal for improved cognitive performance and alertness.

The Center for Applied Cognitive Studies says that "the length of sleep is not what causes us to be refreshed upon waking. The key factor is the number of complete sleep cycles we enjoy. Each sleep cycle contains five distinct phases, which exhibit different brain-wave patterns." Leading sleep researcher Dr. Claudio Stampi found that naps taken in the afternoon (a common low energy period in our circadian rhythms) were comparatively higher in the most restorative slow-wave sleep. During a 10-20 minute afternoon nap, your brain cells reset their sodium and potassium ratios, which are thrown out of balance after long periods of intense brain arousal, as in a typical busy day. "This is the main cause of what is known as 'mental fatigue'," the Center says about this nutrient imbalance. "A brief period in Theta (slow wave sleep) can restore the ratio to normal, resulting in mental refreshment."

[4] **Quality Time:** The Office of National Statistics "Time Use Survey" study indicates that today's average working parent spends 19 minutes of digital distraction-free quality time per week.

Korg Family References

[5] Commuting: The Public Policy Institute of California reports that 18 percent of Californians commute over 45 minutes each way. 3.4 million Americans commute 90 minutes or more each way. The US Census reports that the average commute time nationwide is 25.5 minutes each way, with Californians commuting 10 percent longer than the national average. Tracy, CA, near the Korg's home of Stockton, had one of the longest average commute times in the state in 2000: 42 minutes each way.

In a United Kingdom survey of over 400 people by the International Stress Management Association, 44 percent said that rush-hour traffic was the most stressful part of their lives. A Hewlett Packard study of UK commuters found that blood pressure and heart rate were "higher than those experienced by fighter pilots going into combat and police officers facing rioting mobs."

A study by researchers at the New York University Sleep Disorder Center found that "long commuters"—those who travel 1 hour and 15 minutes or longer—have more sleep disorders and other health problems than the general population. There is also a significant danger of multitasking while commuting. The Harvard Center for Risk Analysis found drivers using cell phones are responsible for 2,600 traffic deaths per year and 330,000 traffic injuries (motorists on the road make 40 percent of all cellular telephone calls).

[6] **Digital Media Disturbing Sleep:** Daniel Reid's *The Tao of Health, Sex and Longevity* details how television disturbs the ocular-endocrine system. A US study showed that rats exposed to invisible television rays (screen was blackened) for six hours per day became hyperactive and extremely aggressive for about a week, then suddenly become totally lethargic and stopped breeding entirely. A Columbia University Study conducted in New York suggests that "watching late night television may put people in a state of heightened alertness and physiological arousal, preventing them from falling asleep with ease. In addition, being exposed to many hours of the bright light of the television screen may throw people off their sleep-wake cycle, while too little physical activity may cause people to become restless and struggle with sleep."

A Rhode Island study published in the journal *American Academy of Pediatrics* suggests children's sleep is disturbed by watching TV before bedtime—causing them to become "over-stimulated, disturbed or frightened by the content of programs... particularly those containing violence."

[7] **Sleep Medication:** 30 million people in the US take sleep medications (*American Academy of Sleep Medicine*), an estimated 50 percent jump since 2000. With an ode to the "over x billion served" signs adorning McDonald's franchises, Sanofi-Aventis, maker of Ambien, boasts an aggregate total of 12 billion nights of patient use worldwide. Two billion was spent on the drug worldwide in 2004. According to LiveScience, global sales for sleeping pills are estimated at five billion annually. Daniel Kripke, UC San Diego psychiatry professor and author of *The Dark Side of Sleeping Pills*, conducted a revealing six-year sleep study with over one million adults. Kripke reported that the health risk of taking sleeping pills daily was not much different that the risk of smoking a pack of cigarettes a day! A study by researchers at Beth Israel Deaconess Medical Center and Harvard Medical School found that treating insomnia with habit and attitude modification was more effective—both immediately and over the long term —than using Ambien. The sleep success techniques Kripke recommends include: don't go to bed until you're sleepy, get up at the same time each morning, avoid excessive stimulation or worry before bed, avoid caffeine for six hours before bed, avoid alcohol before bed, and spend adequate time outdoors.

[8] **Teenage Sleep:** A 2007 Mayo Clinic article suggests that teenagers require about nine hours of sleep to maintain optimal daytime alertness, but few actually get that much sleep due to jobs, homework, friends, digital media, and other distractions. The National Sleep Foundation reports that 25 percent of teens report sleeping 6.5 hours per night or less. "Puberty changes a teen's internal clock, delaying the time he or she starts feeling sleepy until 11 P.M. or later ("before adolescence, circadian rhythms direct most children to naturally fall asleep around 8 or 9 P.M."). "Staying up late to study or socialize can disrupt a teen's internal clock even more."

The article also notes that sleeping in or forcing an early bedtime are not adequate solutions, since they are not aligned with the teen's unique circadian rhythm. The Mayo Clinic staff suggests that you darken rooms at desired bedtime and expose teens to bright light in the morning, discourage naps longer than 30 minutes, discourage caffeine use and establish a consistent, quiet relaxing routine before bed—free of digital media.

[9] **Artificial sweeteners:** An on-line review mentioned by Dr John Briffa indicates that "100 percent of industry funded studies proclaim aspartame to be benign; more than 90 percent of independent studies and reports in the scientific literature say otherwise." Numerous studies suggest that intense artificial sweeteners increase appetite for sweet foods, promote overeating, and may even lead to weight gain. One study with rats from Purdue University concluded that "consuming a food sweetened with no-calorie saccharin can lead to greater body-weight gain and adiposity than would consuming the same food sweetened with higher calorie sugar." However, there are some other studies that refute the concept entirely. Perhaps the most relevant evidence is how obesity rates continue to climb even with the advent and increased used of artificial sweeteners in the modern diet.

[10] **Cardiovascular exercise heart rates:** My position that Chronic Cardio is harmful and that low-level aerobic work is beneficial is based on personal experience over three decades as an elite athlete, personal trainer to clients of all ability levels, and coach to elite professional triathletes. The extensive work of legendary coach Arthur Lydiard is a major influence as well. Lydiard, who pioneered the concept of overdistance endurance training for track and field athletes, developed numerous Olympic gold medalists and world record holders in his home country of New Zealand and for various other national teams. Elite athlete/authors like former professional triathletes Mark Allen (*Total Triathlete*) and Brad Kearns (*Breakthrough Triathlon Training*), former Olympic marathon runner and popular author and speaker Jeff Galloway, and Joe Friel's popular series of "Training Bibles" for various endurance sports all echo these fundamental principles of endurance training:

- Building a base of comfortable aerobic activity is critical for success
- High intensity exercise should be strictly limited as a small percentage of total exercise volume and conducted only when a sufficient aerobic base is present

Conversely, the American College of Sports Medicine recommends exercise intensities of 55-90 percent of maximum heart rate, a ridiculously disparate range that stimulates vastly different metabolic responses in the body. Sadly, this information is widely circulated by health clubs, personal trainers, group exercise programs, books, and magazines to the detriment of the average fitness enthusiast. Exceeding 75 percent of maximum heart rate regularly (particularly for a non-elite athlete) will greatly inhibit the development of a strong aerobic base and invite increased risk of injury and burnout. Your cardio exercise range should be 55-75 percent of maximum heart rate, with occasional high intensity sessions where heart rate approaches maximum during short sprints.

[11] **Statin Side Effects:** A Columbia University study published in the *Archives of Neurology* suggests that even short-term statin use depletes CoQ10 levels, a possible explanation for common statin side effects like exercise intolerance, muscle pain, and other indicators of muscle dysfunction.

The Conventional Wisdom connection between cholesterol levels and disease risk (and thus the popularity of cholesterol-reducing statins) is increasingly being called into question. Seventeen studies on lowering dietary cholesterol were assessed in a 2005 *Annals of Internal Medicine* article. Overall, the studies led to an average 10 percent decrease in cholesterol levels, but there was no decrease in overall risk of death.

A long-term study published in the *New England Journal of Medicine* (in 1986, 1987, and 1991) showed that people who are taking multiple cardiac medications have a 40 percent higher risk of mortality after four years than those who take nothing. Several other large studies (10,000 men in Europe, published in the *European Heart Journal*, 1986; 61,000 men in Europe, conducted by the World Health Organization and published in *Lancet*; 12,000 men in America, published in the *Journal of the American Medical Association*; a study in Finland published in the *Journal of the American Medical Association*, 1991) reported the same conclusion—medication either increased mortality or didn't increase survival time.

[12] **Walking To School:** CDC indicates that the percent of children who live within a mile of school and who walk or bike to school as their primary means of transportation has declined almost 25 percent over the past 30 years (from 87 percent to 63 percent) and that children who walk or bike from any distance has declined 26 percent (from 42 percent to 16 percent).

[13] **Poor compliance** with doctor prescribed exercise programs is a major reason for the widespread condition of lower back pain, poor recovery from surgery, and prolonged elevated risk factors for heart disease and cancer.

A 1998 *Journal of the American Medical Association* article noted that even when it comes to taking medication, the average compliance rate is only 50 percent. An article from AlignMap - Beyond Patient Compliance, further suggests that "noncompliance is underreported, typically hidden, and rarely detected by clinicians," and "research studies consistently reveal high levels of inadequate adherence to treatment recommendations throughout the healthcare spectrum, including cases of life-threatening illnesses. The indisputable conclusions are that medical noncompliance is, by any measure and from any perspective, pervasive, and that healthcare's failure to successfully address such a problem comes at the cost of diminished outcomes, unnecessary expense, and avoidable patient morbidity and mortality."

One Canadian study of heart attack victims published in the *Canadian Medical Association Journal* indicated a 43 percent noncompliance rate with rehabilitation and treatment recommendations. A Texas study of bariatric surgery patients revealed a noncompliance rate of 41 percent (female) and 37 percent (male).

[14] **Caffeine:** The average American uses about 230 milligrams of caffeine per day according to the Mayo Clinic. Side effects of consuming too much caffeine vary by individual (based on body weight, levels of physical and psychological stress, and other drug use—according to MayoClinic.com), but can include "increased heart rate and urination, anxiety, headaches, nausea and insomnia," according to the online medical encyclopedia provided by the U.S. National Library of Medicine and the National Institutes of Health. The Mayo Clinic calls caffeine the "most popular behavior-altering drug," with 9 out of 10 Americans consuming some type of caffeine regularly.

[15] **Family Finances:** A 2003 book by Elizabeth Warren and Amelia Warren Tyagi called *The Two Income Trap: Why Middle Class Mothers and Fathers are Going Broke*, details the financial challenges faced even by working families who enjoy income levels far higher (even adjusting for today's dollars) than previous generations. While many point to the "*Affluenza*" mentality (the widespread cultural ill of excessive consumption habits detailed in John De Graaf's book of the same name) for the middle class's financial challenges, the authors make the convincing case that the larger, less optional expenses are the biggest culprit. Expenses for child care, car payments, college tuition, and suburban homes result in millions living in financial distress. Homes sold to families with children skyrocketed 79 percent in inflation adjusted dollars from 1983 to 1998. The two income couple (comprising some three-quarters of all married couples) is a key component of the skyrocketing inflation of suburban home prices over the past 25 years. Hence, a vicious circle emerges: home prices rise because many two-income couples can afford them… because they have two incomes! This sounds like "keeping up with the Joneses" times fifty million.

The New York Times, in 2003, revealed that a "typical household" (two income earners and one or two children—a demographic responsible for half the nation's personal consumption expenditures) making $60,000-$80,000 per year spends 70 to 75 percent of its take home pay on essentials such as home costs, groceries, vehicles and fuel, education, and health care. The authors of *The Two Income Trap* point out that the figure for these expenses was only 54 percent in the early 1970s. Furthermore, the remaining 25 percent of disposable income, typically categorized as "discretionary," is further eaten up by expenses that might be better defined as "essential" due to social pressures and norms: cell phones, cable or satellite TV, Internet service, high definition TV sets, and digital entertainment like iPods. Arguably the category could extend to fashion, cosmetics, and popular diversions such as movies and vacations.

[16] **Childhood Obesity:** The CDC reports that nine million kids ages 6-19 are overweight or obese, and the American Academy of Pediatrics reports that 33 percent eat fast food every day. The prevalence of children (ages 6 to 11) who are overweight has increased from about 4 percent in the 1960s to almost 19 percent in 2004 (Dr Richard Troiano and Dr Cynthia Ogden).

[17] **Children Recreation:** Dr. Sandra Hofferth and colleagues report that the way children spend their discretionary time has changed—less time is spent in unstructured activities (e.g., free play) and more time is spent in structured activities (e.g., sports and youth programs). Other changes of interest include a doubling of computer use.

[18] **Massive Multiplayer Online Role-Playing Games:** The popularity has skyrocketed from zero in 1998 (due to poor graphics quality, slow Internet connections, and a consequent lack of interest) to an estimated 30-60 million active users in 2007, according to a Giga Omni Media article. Some consider this a vast underestimate, due to millions of Chinese playing in Internet cafés for four cents per hour but not registering as paid monthly subscribers. World of Warcraft (8.5 million users), Hobbo Hotel (7.5 million), and Runescape (5 million) are the leading games. Pre-teen games Club Penguin (4 million) and Webkinz (3.8 million) are also extremely popular. A survey published on Adpoll.com indicated that 45 percent of kids play for 10 or more hours per week.

[19] **ADHD Prescriptions:** Diagnosis rates of Attention Deficit Hyperactivity Disorder (ADHD) have skyrocketed 500 percent since 1991, according to the Drug Enforcement Administration. An estimated seven million schoolchildren are being treated with stimulants for ADHD, including 10 percent of all 10-year-old American boys, according to an article published in the *Journal of the American Medical Association*.

A 1998 study by researchers Adrian Angold and E. Jane Costello found that the majority of children and adolescents who receive stimulants for ADHD do not fully meet the criteria for ADHD. The efforts of neurologist Dr. Fred Baughman, ADHD diagnosis critic, led to admissions from the FDA, DEA, Novartis (manufacturers of Ritalin), and top ADHD researchers around the country that "*no objective validation of the diagnosis of ADHD exists.*" A Maryland Department of Education study found that white, suburban elementary school children are using medication for ADHD at more than twice the rate of African American students.

[20] **Life Expectancy of Today's Child:** A 2005 report published in the *New England Journal of Medicine* suggests that the prevalence of obesity is shortening average lifespan by a greater rate than accidents, homicides, and suicides combined. Children today will lose some two to five years of life expectancy due to the prevalence, and earlier onset of, obesity-related diseases like type 2 diabetes, heart disease, kidney failure, and cancer. Dr. David S. Ludwig, director of the obesity program at Children's Hospital

in Boston, said in the report, "obesity is such that this generation of children could be the first basically in the history of the United States to live less healthful and shorter lives than their parents. There is an unprecedented increase in prevalence of obesity at younger and younger ages without much obvious public health impact. But when they start developing heart attack, stroke, kidney failures, amputations, blindness, and ultimately death at younger ages, then that could be a huge effect on life expectancy."

[21] **American Television:** A.C. Neilsen reports that the average American watches 28 hours of TV per week and that 66 percent of households have three or more televisions at home (A.C. Nielsen Co.). Dr Donald Roberts and colleagues and Victoria Rideout and colleagues with the Kaiser Family Foundation report that children between the ages of 8 and 18 years spend an average of nearly 6.5 hours a day with electronic media.

CHAPTER 3

The Primal Blueprint
Eating Philosophy

*"Do These Genes Make Me
Look Fat?"*

In This Chapter

I present the philosophy, rationale, and benefits of Primal Blueprint eating, emphasizing the importance of moderating insulin production by limiting the intake of processed carbohydrates—not only sugars, but all cultivated grains (yep, even whole grains). This simple dietary modification—perhaps the single most critical takeaway action item from the Primal Blueprint—will allow you to avoid the unpleasant physical effects of high-carbohydrate eating, succeed with long-term weight-loss goals, and prevent most common lifestyle-related health problems and diseases.

You will learn why the Conventional Wisdom story about cholesterol as a direct heart disease risk factor is deeply flawed. The true culprits that trigger the development of atherosclerosis are oxidation and inflammation, created largely by the Standard American Diet of excess carbohydrates and chemically-altered fats. I detail the dietary steps you can take, including regulating your omega-6:omega-3 (O6:O3) balance to prevent systemic inflammation and virtually eliminate your risk of heart disease.

I discuss how each macronutrient (protein, carbohydrate, fat, and the "fourth fuel" of ketones) affects your eating strategy, energy levels, and overall health. The Primal Blueprint Carbohydrate Curve reveals how carb intake impacts your health and weight management success. The concept of "eating well" means more than just making healthy food choices; it means eating sensibly and intuitively, in a relaxed environment conducive to maximum appreciation of food, and avoiding regimented, restrictive diets that lead to negativity, guilt, and rebellion. Finally, I offer tips on how to succeed in converting to Primal Blueprint eating without causing the stress or disappointment that is so common with unrealistic diet programs.

*I bought a talking refrigerator that said "Oink" every time I opened the door.
It made me hungry for pork chops.*

—Marie Mott

Primal Blueprint eating offers many health benefits, which served Grok and his ancestors well for over two million years. The most important goal of eating like Grok is to minimize the wildly excessive insulin production caused by the Standard American Diet. Making this simple change will allow you to lose unwanted fat, maintain an ideal body composition for the rest of your life, and virtually eliminate the major disease risk factors that will kill more than half of all Americans. Here are some other major benefits of the Primal Blueprint eating style:

Fat-Burning Beast: When you reduce your consumption of grains, sugars, and other simple carbohydrates in favor of plants and animals, your levels of insulin and glucagon will be in an ideal balance, enabling you to utilize fatty acids (from both food intake and stored fat) as your preferred fuel source. This helps regulate daily energy levels, even if you skip meals. In contrast, excess insulin production from a sugar-burner diet requires that you eat every few hours to bump up blood glucose levels that have crashed.

Effortless Weight Management: Plants and animals are much more nutritionally dense than processed carbohydrate foods, which comprise a large percentage of calories in the Standard American Diet. Eat like Grok and you'll meet your nutritional needs with fewer calories and dramatically boost your antioxidant intake. Second, the protein and fat you will be eating have been shown by food scientists to provide deeper and longer lasting satisfaction levels—what they call satiety—than you get from a high-carb diet. Finally, when you consume fewer carbohydrates and, as a result, produce less insulin, your hunger and cravings (caused by insulin removing glucose from the bloodstream after high-carb meals or snacks) will subside, and you'll intuitively moderate your caloric intake.

Enhanced Cellular Function: The high quality fats found in Primal foods provide optimal structural components for cell membranes and encourage your body to convert stored fat efficiently into energy. This includes the well known omega-3s, monounsaturated fats such as avocados, coconut products, macadamia nuts, and olive oil, and even the saturated animal fat that Conventional Wisdom has warned us to avoid.

Lean Muscle Development and Maintenance: The high-quality protein found in Primal foods will help you build lean muscle mass, achieve ideal bone density, and control your body's day-to-day repair and renewal requirements. When you moderate insulin production, exercise sensibly, and eat adequate amounts of protein, you become more *insulin sensitive*. This means the receptor sites in your muscle cells can assimilate amino acids and glucose efficiently, which is the key to muscle building and recovery.

Reduced Disease Risk Factors: Ditching grains, sugars, other simple carbs, and processed foods, especially "bad fats" (trans and partially hydrogenated), will reduce your production of hormone-like messengers that instruct genes to make harmful pro-inflammatory protein agents. These agents increase your risk for arthritis, diabetes, cancer, heart disease, and many other inflammation-related health problems.

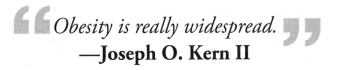
Obesity is really widespread.
—Joseph O. Kern II

A Separate Shelf for the Blueprint

You may be familiar with the decades-old Atkins diet program, named after Dr. Robert Atkins, the original proponent of "low-carb" dieting. Over the years, numerous other programs (e.g., South Beach and the Zone) have battled for shelf space supremacy. Diet best-sellers have varied from mostly credible to completely ridiculous. Followers of Atkins and other low-carb diets will indeed lose fat by strictly limiting carbohydrates and thus insulin production. However, an obsessive ultra-low-carb strategy can be unhealthy over an extended time period, because it limits your intake of some of the most nutritional foods known to humans—vegetables and fruits.

While the Primal Blueprint also advocates eliminating the extremely harmful processed carbohydrates and sugars from your diet, vegetables and fruits are a central component of the Primal Blueprint eating strategy. Vegetables and fruits (which consist mainly of carbohydrates) are nutrient-dense yet calorically sparse, so even generous portions of these foods will usually prompt minimal insulin production.

I should really say "seasonal fruits" and add a caveat that some moderation of fruit intake is warranted today. If you wish to reduce excess body fat, be advised that fructose (the carbohydrate form found in fruit) is more easily converted to fat in the liver than other carbohydrate sources such as simple sugar. This is particularly true if you are not exercising much and your glycogen stores are routinely full. Furthermore, we have only recently enjoyed year-round access to heavily cultivated modern fruits that are sweeter than the wild stuff Grok encountered during narrow ripening seasons. Bottoms up on the locally grown berries in the summer time, but ease off on that daily bowl of mangoes and pineapples as you strive to transform into a fat-burning beast.

One of the online Primal Blueprint appendices at Marks Daily Apple compares and contrasts the Primal Blueprint with popular diets such as Atkins, Low Fat (e.g., Ornish, MacDougall, Pritikin), Metabolic and Blood Typing, paleo-themed diets, South Beach, Vegetarian, and the Zone. Of all these mentioned, the paleo eating approach is the most similar to the Primal Blueprint. However, I refrain from even calling the Primal Blueprint a "diet" due to its comprehensive nature. The Primal Blueprint is a lifestyle—with some important but extremely flexible eating guidelines. I prefer to apply the eating laws in conjunction with the other eight Primal Blueprint lifestyle laws for best results.

80 Percent of Your Body Composition Success Is Determined by How You Eat

The Primal Blueprint eating philosophy might seem a little unusual at first for those trying to do the right thing by Conventional Wisdom. After all, here's a plan that suggests that most fats are not bad at all. In fact, pundits might describe the Primal Blueprint as a high-fat, moderate protein, fairly low-carb diet—particularly in comparison to the exceedingly high-carbohydrate diet that has been recommended for years by the USDA Food Pyramid and Food Plate visuals, the American Heart Association, and the American Medical Association.

We now know that these outdated and unwarranted suggestions to eat 300 or more grams of carbohydrates each day has contributed greatly to the destruction of human health. It's not unusual for an average American now to consume 500 or 600 grams of insulin-generating, fat-storing carbohydrates daily. Keep in mind that Grok and his clan probably worked hard to gather an average daily intake of only 80 to 100 grams of carbs, most of which was contained inside slow-burning fibrous wild plants—much harder to overeat even if they were lucky to find enough. By averaging between 100 and 150 daily grams (certain extremely active folks may adjust this upward, which I'll discuss later) of vegetable- or fruit-sourced carbs, and incidental carbs from nuts, seeds, and moderation foods such as high-fat dairy and dark chocolate, you can achieve optimally low levels of insulin, enjoy stable energy levels, and easily reduce excess body fat and keep it off. If you want to accelerate your fat loss for a period of time, lowering your average carb intake to 50 to 100 grams or less per day will allow you to easily drop an average of one to two pounds (one-half to one kilogram) of body fat per week. We will discuss this strategy in detail in Chapter 8. And you can do all this while eating until you're satisfied—no suffering!

Sitting down again? Here's another zinger that will blow your mind and set you straight about the secret to weight loss and long-term body composition success.…*Eighty percent of your ability to reduce excess body fat is determined by how you eat, with the other 20 percent depending on proper exercise, other healthy lifestyle habits, and genetic factors.*

It's as simple as this: if you have excess body fat, it's directly reflective of the amount of insulin you produce from your diet combined with your familial genetic predisposition to store fat. In plain-speak, if you eat like crap and have bad (genetic) luck, you'll get fat and sick and you'll probably die early. On the other hand, bad diet and good luck (having the "skinny gene") might allow you to avoid a plump figure, but also might result in a physique that I call "skinny fat"—having minimal subcutaneous fat, minimal lean body mass, and poor muscle definition, but with dangerous amounts of visceral fat surrounding the organs.

Furthermore, skinny fat folks can and do get heart disease, hypoglycemia, arthritis, sarcopenia (loss of muscle mass), chronic fatigue, compromised immune function, exhausted stress-management mechanism, and a host of other adverse health consequences heavily attributed to diet. A slender type 2 diabetic can experience an even greater risk for serious disease, because he or she is less able to activate the so-called thrifty genes that efficiently store excess dietary glucose in fat cells, and as a result, that glucose floats around in the bloodstream causing intense cellular damage. While the outward visibility and overall impact of poor lifestyle habits vary widely due to luck of the draw, we all share an evolutionary genetic predisposition to suffer chronic disease when we eat foods that are misaligned with our genes.

On the positive side, if you eat right, you can look your absolute best even if you have bad genetic luck. Your ability to reduce excess body fat and maintain desirable body composition is directly related to your ability to moderate insulin production with healthy dietary habits and, to a lesser extent, your willingness to follow a sensible exercise program that combines extensive low-level cardio, frequent brief, intense strength-training sessions, and occasional all-out sprints. Even if you have struggled with excess body fat for your entire life, you can quickly and dramatically alter your destiny by following the simple laws of the Primal Blueprint.

I'm not talking about achieving "success" with a short-term crash program. The Primal Blueprint is based on eating as much as you want, whenever you want, from a long list of delicious foods—and simply avoiding eating from a different list. When I say you will notice results quickly and dramatically, I'm referring primarily to the immediate increase and stabilization of energy levels, less hunger and mood swings related to "bonking" (running low on blood glucose), improved immune function, and a reduction in the symptoms of allergies, arthritis, and other inflammatory conditions exacerbated by the anti-nutrients in a grain-based diet.

Regarding weight loss, we must recognize that our minds are so messed up on this topic that it's hard to even have a sensible conversation about it. The stories of losing massive amounts of weight in a short time are so commonplace that we seem to expect nothing less when we pursue weight-loss goals. First, the Primal Blueprint is really about improving body composition, instead of just losing weight. This means a reduction in body fat percentage and an increase or maintenance of muscle or lean body mass.

Clearly, gaining muscle and losing fat produces more impressive appearance changes than dropping 20 quick pounds on a crash diet that depletes muscle mass and water. Lean body mass (muscle, skeleton, and all the rest of you that is not fat) is also directly correlated with "organ reserve"—the highly desirable ability of all your vital organs to function optimally beyond basal level (e.g., when your heart rate elevates during exercise). We'll discuss this critical longevity component further in Chapter 6.

When you trigger your genes to stop storing body fat and start burning it, as well as to build or maintain muscle mass, you can sensibly and realistically lose a pound or two of body fat per week. You can even do this with minimal exercise, but the fat loss (and the gaining, sculpting, or toning of lean muscle) will be accelerated significantly when you choose the right exercise regimen. Mostly, your success depends on how diligent you are in keeping dietary insulin levels low, thereby allowing your body to obtain more of your caloric needs from your stored body fat.

Not a day goes by without a friend, client, or MarksDailyApple.com commenter relating to me how he or she notices improvements within days of switching to the Primal Blueprint eating style. As I will detail in this chapter, you have the chance to alter your biochemistry at each meal—to stimulate a fat-burning metabolism and maintain consistent energy levels, or to do the opposite with poor food choices. The momentum you build with good choices will make it easier to discard old habits, while you gain instant gratification from satisfying meals and stable energy levels, as well as positive long-term health and metabolic consequences.

Insulin—The Master Hormone

The insulin story is perhaps the most health-critical concept in the book, so I want you to fully understand it on both a practical and a biochemical level. Like so many things in life, a moderate amount of insulin is good and a lot can be bad—very bad. By now you understand insulin's role as a storage hormone and that eating more carbs results in more insulin production. Insulin delivers nutrients to all cells, but for our purposes, we'll focus on insulin's role in delivering nutrients to liver, muscle, and fat cells. When the system works as designed by evolution, cell receptors use insulin as a key to unlock pores within the membrane of each cell. With the cell door open, nutrients can then be stored inside the cell. It's an elegant way for cells to gather the nutrients they need and also to eliminate excess glucose from the bloodstream (remember, excess glucose is highly toxic) and store it as fuel for a later date.

Unfortunately, when you produce too much insulin over a period of time, as happens when a modern diet is high in processed carbohydrates, several things go wrong. First, muscle and liver cells just aren't able to store a whole lot of glycogen (the stored form of glucose), so it's easy to exceed storage capacity. The average person can only store a total of about 400 grams (less than one pound) of glycogen in liver and muscle tissue (even a highly trained athlete can only store perhaps 600 total grams). When your liver and muscles become filled with glycogen, any glucose remaining in the bloodstream that isn't used in "real time" by your brain or muscles (such as during an intense workout) gets converted into triglycerides in the liver and sent to fat cells for storage.

When blood insulin levels are high, those same fat cells store not only the excess glucose but the fat you ate at your last meal. Moreover, high insulin signals the fat cells to hold on to the fat and not release it for energy. If the pattern of high insulin-generating meals continues, fat cells swell up and you gain weight. Eventually, especially among people who don't exercise much, muscle and liver cells start to become *insulin resistant,* which means their receptors become desensitized to insulin's nutrient storage signals (the aforementioned insulin key doesn't unlock the cell membrane to allow nutrients in). Inactive folks generally have plenty of muscle and liver glycogen stored at all times. Because they are unpracticed at burning energy and inefficient at restocking energy from dietary nutrients, insulin takes ingested carbohydrates and fats on an express train, passing right through the liver, to their ultimate destination in fat cells.

Continuing this process can lead to obesity and other metabolic syndrome symptoms. Eventually, even fat cells become resistant to further storage, because we only have a fixed amount of fat cells. At that point, the body's last line of defense against glucose (the complete gorging of a finite number of fat cells) has maxed out. Consequently, all hell breaks loose in terms of blood glucose toxicity and insulin damage—leading to even greater risk for diabetes, heart attack, blindness, the need for limb amputation, and other disasters.

Unless you are exercising incessantly to burn stored glycogen and fat, the more insulin your pancreas produces, the more resistant your muscle and liver cells can get. This happens because the genes responsible for these receptor sites turn themselves off or "down-regulate" in response to—and in defense against—the excessive insulin in your bloodstream. This is all part of the body's quest for balance and your genetic response to environmental signals.

This doesn't mean your daily PowerBar® is going to lead to limb amputation any time soon, but as you gain further understanding of the insulin story, it becomes clear how the shocking statistic of the average American gaining one and a half pounds of fat (two-thirds of a kilo) a year for 30 years is achieved. Conversely, when insulin levels are moderated (as happens with low carbohydrate eating and/or frequent exercise), your liver and muscle cell receptor sites become *insulin sensitive*—more effective at absorbing ingested nutrients transported by insulin. Furthermore, moderated insulin levels signal genes to make more receptor sites.

An insulin-resistant liver exacerbates the situation. The "no vacancy" sign hanging on the liver (due to insulin resistance) tricks some cells in your liver into believing they are starved for glucose. In response to the liver's storage cells refusing to accept glucose, your genes signal other specialized liver cells to commence gluconeogensis and dump more glucose into the bloodstream—despite the fact that there's already plenty in the bloodstream (talk about a communication breakdown!). Of course, your resistant muscle cells are deaf to insulin signaling as well, so the new, extra glucose your liver just made is also diverted to the eager fat cells—unless they too are over-gorged with fat. Here is a quick summary of some of the unpleasant consequences of becoming insulin resistant:

Fat cells can't release their stored energy into the bloodstream, where the fatty acids could be used as fuel, because insulin keeps the fat locked inside.

Fat cells get bigger (and fatter), so you gain weight.

More glucose stays in your bloodstream longer, causing damaging AGEs (advanced glycation end products). AGEs are chemical reactions that occur when blood-borne glucose molecules bind randomly with important proteins, rendering them useless. This can result in increased inflammation and risk of heart disease, as well as the circulation problems and neuropathies (nervous system disorders) that characterize type 2 diabetes.

Pancreatic beta cells, continually sensing high levels of sugar in the bloodstream, keep working harder and harder to pump out more and more insulin.

Eventually, the beta cells can become exhausted and stop working entirely—similar to the plight of insulin-dependent type 1 diabetics. All of this happens as a result of eating too many carbohydrates for too long and/or not exercising enough to maintain insulin sensitivity.

But wait, there's more! As bad as all that glucose remaining in the bloodstream is, chronically high levels of insulin are almost worse. Excessive insulin is very pro-inflammatory and can wreak havoc throughout the body. Scientists know that within any species, those that produce the least amount of insulin over a lifetime generally live the longest and remain the healthiest.

Excessive insulin is also now believed to be a central catalyst in the development of atherosclerosis. Insulin promotes platelet adhesiveness (sticky platelets clot more readily) and the conversion of macrophages (a type of white blood cell) into foam cells, which are the cells that fill with cholesterol and accumulate in arterial walls. Eventually, a cholesterol and fat-filled "tumor" blocks circulation in the artery, a situation further aggravated by increased platelet adhesiveness and thickness of the blood. In addition, insulin reduces blood levels of nitric oxide (a compound that relaxes the endothelium, the lining of your arteries), causing your artery walls to become more rigid. This drives up blood pressure and increases the sheer force of blood against the arterial wall, further exacerbating the atherosclerotic condition. I will further detail the chain of events causing atherosclerosis, and what you can do to prevent it, in the cholesterol section later in this chapter.

Once you understand the process, it's instructive to take a step back and realize how important exercise is to creating insulin sensitivity (along with low-insulin eating, of course). If you frequently empty your liver and muscle cells of glycogen with brief, intense workouts (you burn a little bit of glucose during the long, slow stuff, too), you become adept at not only burning calories, but also replenishing nutrients. Insulin will transport nutrients into your liver and muscle instead of just having them go straight to fat. If you are sedentary and eat a moderate or high-carbohydrate diet, there is no selection pressure (to borrow an apropos term from our evolution discussion) to be insulin sensitive. My foolproof prevention plan or, dare I say, cure—for those with type 2 diabetes, obesity, and heart disease, no matter how overwhelming their genetic predisposition is to these conditions—is to exercise according to the Primal Blueprint laws and to moderate dietary insulin production.

Levels of growth hormone and other important health-enhancing hormones are also adversely affected by insulin resistance. The pituitary gland makes growth hormone, which is then sent to the liver to signal the production of insulin-like growth factors (IGFs). Many of our cells have surface receptors for IGFs. Because of its similar structure, insulin binds to IGF receptors and prevents growth hormone-stimulated IGFs from doing their job.

Excessive insulin also interferes with thyroid function. The thyroid gland produces a hormone called T4, which is converted in the liver to T3, the primary hormone that controls energy metabolism. When your liver becomes insulin resistant, conversion of T4 to T3 declines drastically. This leads to a decrease in metabolic rate, increased fat storage, and diminished energy levels and brain function.

High insulin levels over long periods of time also hamper sex hormone synthesis, causing levels of testosterone, DHEA, and other sex hormones to decline steeply as we age. Hormone levels naturally decline over time, but this flagship premise of the multibillion-dollar anti-aging industry is very likely exacerbated by insulin resistance as opposed to the mere passing of the seasons. Remember, if Grok was lucky, he could enjoy dramatically better health and physical fitness into his 70s than most of today's baby boomers. Sex hormones are supposed to be transported through the bloodstream by globulin (a blood protein) to act upon target organs and tissues. When excessive insulin is present, these hormones can stay bound to globulin instead of getting dropped off at the target cells (e.g., the adrenal glands, sex organs, and brain) and doing their thing. Even an expensive anti-aging hormone regimen cannot override this undesirable condition caused by excessive insulin.

Clearly, the ideal strategy is to use only the insulin you need to restock muscle and liver glycogen stores, to rebuild muscle and other tissue with amino acids, and, finally, to transport fatty acids for a variety of essential metabolic functions (including energy storage). By maintaining an optimal balance between insulin and glucagon, you become like an ATM machine, always open for deposits and withdrawals based on your daily energy needs. Clearly, insulin is absolutely essential to life. It's just that chronic overproduction of insulin (also known as hyperinsulinemia) turns a good thing into a bad thing. It's as simple as this: when you eat the Primal Blueprint-style foods that fit your genes, you'll be able to fit into your jeans!

But a Little Bit Won't Hurt, Right?

If these clinical details about the long-term damage from a high insulin-producing diet are not sufficient to get you to change your breakfast order today, consider the short-term unpleasant effects of high-carbohydrate, insulin-producing meals and snacks (on otherwise healthy, nondiabetic folks).

Ingesting a high-carbohydrate food or meal (sugary foods and beverages, desserts, processed grains, etc.) generates an immediate increase in blood glucose levels, which has the short-term effect of elevating your mood, energy level, and alertness. In a matter of minutes, however, your pancreas secretes a requisite amount of insulin to quickly remove glucose from the bloodstream before it becomes toxic. Depending on the type and amount of carbs you consumed and your degree of insulin sensitivity, this insulin rush can eventually cause your blood glucose levels to decline so much that your glucose-dependent brain soon becomes low on fuel. As a result, you may feel sluggish, foggy, and cranky and have trouble focusing. While this explains the familiar post-lunch afternoon blues, extensive data also suggest a strong link between attention deficit/hyperactivity disorder (ADHD) and processed carbohydrate consumption/insulin production.

The ingestion of lots of carbohydrates, followed by the secretion of lots of insulin causing low blood glucose levels, is perceived as a stressful event by the hypothalamic-pituitary-adrenal (HPA) axis. This homeostasis-monitoring part of your endocrine system triggers the fight-or-flight response, causing your adrenal glands to release epinephrine (adrenaline) and cortisol into your bloodstream. Cortisol breaks down precious muscle tissue into amino acids, some of which are sent to the liver and converted into glucose through gluconeogenesis. The ensuing blood glucose rush gives you the boost your brain thinks you need—commonly at the expense of your muscle tissue!

Depending on your individual sensitivity to glucose and insulin, the stress response to this seesaw process may make you feel amped, jittery, edgy, and hyper, and you may have a racing heartbeat. Others may not experience any stress hormone buzz, likely because years of abusing this delicate life-or-death energy boosting mechanism (high-carbohydrate eating, excessive artificial light/insufficient sleep, and high-stress lifestyle) have exhausted your adrenal glands and pancreas. Instead, they'll just feel like taking a nap after high-carb meals. Consequently, your roller coaster ride will consist of a brief glucose high after meals, followed by sugar cravings (to repeat the cycle) and/or a desire for a nap once insulin starts going to work. However the particulars of your daily energy level and appetite fluctuations play out, all roads in this saga lead to burnout and elevated risk of disease and dysfunction.

Besides the unsettling energy swings and added stress, sugar also seriously hampers immune function as soon as it's ingested. We know that excessive and/or prolonged production of cortisol is a potent immune suppressor (the fight-or-flight mechanism diverts resources to provide an immediate energy boost). Research also shows that sugar itself can impair the function of immunity-related phagocytes (immune system cells that remove bacteria or viruses from the bloodstream) for at least five hours after ingestion.

This impairment happens through a process known as *competitive inhibition*, when excess glucose prevents all-important vitamin C from being transported inside certain immune cells. Because both molecules use the same mechanism and entry point to gain access to the inside of the immune cells, the presence of excessive glucose can overwhelm the transporter site and block vitamin C from entering. With your guard down, oxidative stress on your body increases as free radicals are allowed to run wild. Furthermore, your blood thickens as a response to these immune stressors, which is why heart attacks (in people predisposed to them) tend to occur after a meal.

Note that the chain of events described here happens routinely in a normal, healthy person who overdoes carbohydrate or sugar intake. Experiencing these high-low cycles from sugar ingestion is no fun, but it does mean you still have some sensitivity to the negative effects of sugar ingestion and insulin production. If you don't experience significant noticeable symptoms from eating lots of carbohydrates (particularly sugar), you are likely well on your way, or have already developed, the extremely problematic condition of insulin resistance. The analogy of a smoker feeling minimal ill effects from his or her habit applies here. I'd argue that a vast majority of the population is somewhere on this continuum, far outside of the healthy ideal of a diet that moderates carb intake and insulin production in line with our genetic requirements for health.

Naturally, grain or sugar products will jack up blood glucose levels quickly and produce a greater insulin response than consuming a similar amount of calories from vegetables and fruits or combining a few carbs with slower burning protein or fat calories. While it's obviously preferable to mute the immediate insulin spike, your diet's *total insulin production* is the most important element to consider. If you are routinely eating 150 to 300 grams (or more) of carbs per day, you will likely gain weight insidiously (unless you exercise like crazy) and still increase your risk of developing other associated health problems, including the "oxidation and inflammation" syndrome that is the major culprit behind heart disease.

Cholester-ALL: The Whole Story

The debate over the theory known as the lipid hypothesis of heart disease has raged on for years. Big Pharma and your helpful friends at the FDA, the AMA, and other reputed health agencies have done a great job of vilifying cholesterol and saturated fat as the major causes of atherosclerosis and heart disease. You know their story by now. Your arteries are like pipes. Cholesterol is the fatty, sticky gunk that clogs them up if you eat too many high-cholesterol animal products (meat, eggs) or saturated fats in general. According to Conventional Wisdom, you should eat a low-fat, low-cholesterol, high-complex-carbohydrate diet. If your diet or genetic "bad luck" results in a total cholesterol level of over 200, you simply take cholesterol-lowering statin medicines to safely reduce your risk.

In recent years, many elements of Conventional Wisdom's stance on cholesterol have been called into question. While there is significant dispute and uncertainty on the issue among respected experts, there is compelling evidence that freely dispensing powerful statin medications to reduce all forms of cholesterol offers minimal to no protection from heart disease and stroke. Furthermore, it's almost universally agreed that lifestyle modifications such as losing weight, reducing intake of processed carbs and fats, consuming omega-3 oils, exercising, and managing stress levels, can do a much better job than statins at eliminating the major heart disease risk factors.

Because I highly respect the valiant battle medical professionals are fighting with today's heart disease pandemic (after all, they often have little or nothing to do with patients until they show up in the waiting room with clogged pipes), I'd like to assert here that this is not a "Mark versus your doctor" battle of the egos. Rather, I believe this is an unbiased interpretation of cutting-edge data that extends beyond the narrow and dated "eating fat drives cholesterol drives heart disease" story that most of us are familiar with, including physicians. Remember, physicians don't necessarily have any specialized knowledge about the link between diet and heart disease from their medical training. Or if they do, it might be very outdated information. Like your plumber, their expertise is in dealing with already clogged pipes.

This discussion will give you a deeper understanding of exactly what causes heart disease (hint: it's oxidation and inflammation, driven primarily by poor food choices, excessive insulin production, and all forms of stress in excess, including overexercising) and help you do a better job minimizing heart disease risk than just following the party line of "Don't eat cholesterol—and take drugs if your numbers are high."

> *Using total cholesterol level—or even your LDL cholesterol value—is irrelevant in the absence of further context, such as Metabolic Syndrome and other accomplices to heart disease.*

Among the most notable research refuting the cholesterol story is the highly respected Framingham Heart Study. The study (which I reference often at MarksDailyApple.com) has followed the dietary habits of 15,000 participants (residents of Framingham, Massachusetts) over three generations. It is widely regarded as the longest (it began in 1948 and is still going strong!), most comprehensive study of health and illness factors on a population in medical history. It has led to the publication of more than 1,200 research articles in leading journals. Study director Dr. William Castelli summarized the issue unequivocally when he said, "Serum cholesterol is not a strong risk factor for coronary heart disease." Among the study's highlights are these:

There is no correlation between dietary cholesterol and blood cholesterol levels.

Framingham residents who ate the most cholesterol, saturated fat, and total calories actually weighed the least and were the most physically active.

Luckily for us, over the past decade, hundreds of bright, clear-thinking researchers have reexamined this data, conducted new research, and written extensively on how and why the Conventional Wisdom lipid hypothesis of heart disease is deeply flawed. (Google the term cholesterol skeptics and you'll discover an organized group called the International Network of Cholesterol Skeptics, populated by dozens of leading M.D.s and Ph.D.s in the field from across the globe.) Their research now shows that atherosclerosis is caused mainly by the excessive oxidation (and the ensuing inflammation) of a certain type of cholesterol that constitutes a small fraction of the mostly good stuff flowing through your bloodstream.

Ironically, in many cases, it appears that this oxidation might be made worse by consuming the very cholesterol-free polyunsaturated fats in vegetable and grain oils that the medical establishment led us to believe were healthier than animal fats! Furthermore, the drugs to lower cholesterol have done little or nothing to improve the health of most of the people taking them, while the side effects and expense have been devastating to millions more.

The Lowdown on Lipoproteins

Cholesterol is a little waxy lipid (fat) molecule that happens to be one of the most important substances in the human body. Every cell membrane has cholesterol as a critical structural and functional component. Brain cells need cholesterol to make synapses (connections) with other brain cells. Cholesterol is the precursor molecule for important hormones such as testosterone, estrogen, DHEA, cortisol, and pregnenolone. Cholesterol is needed for making the bile acids that allow us to digest and absorb fats. Cholesterol interacts with sunlight to convert into the all-important vitamin D. Bottom line is that you can't live without cholesterol, which is why your liver actually makes up to 1,400 milligrams a day regardless of how much food-borne cholesterol you consume—or how much you avoid it like the plague—in your diet.

Because cholesterol is fat-soluble (it does not dissolve in water—think balsamic vinegar staying intact in a dish of olive oil) but must travel to and from cells in the watery environment of the bloodstream, it needs to be carried by special spherical particles called lipoproteins (the name means "part protein and part lipid"). There are several varieties of lipoproteins with different transporting functions—chylomicrons, LDLs, IDLs, HDLs, and VLDLs (as well as subfractions of those)—but the three we are concerned with here are VLDLs, LDLs, and HDLs (very low-density, low-density, and high-density lipoproteins, respectively). Each of these lipoproteins carries a certain percentage of cholesterol, triglycerides, and other minor fats. Your blood test values for triglycerides and HDL, LDL, and VLDL cholesterol represent the combined total in your bloodstream of what all the lipoproteins are transporting.

VLDLs, the largest of these cholesterol complexes, are manufactured in the liver in the presence of high levels of triglycerides. Hence, VLDLs comprise 80 percent triglyceride and a little cholesterol. After leaving their birthplace in the liver, these lipoproteins deliver their cargo to fat and muscle cells for energy. Once these VLDLs have deposited their triglyceride load inside a fat or muscle cell, their size decreases substantially and they convert into either large, fluffy LDLs or small, dense LDLs—in both cases bearing mostly cholesterol and a little bit of remaining triglyceride. Large, fluffy, or "buoyant" LDLs are generally harmless, even at relatively high levels (this has a strong genetic component), as they go about their assigned task of delivering cholesterol to the cells that need it.

The real trouble starts when triglycerides are unusually high in the bloodstream, causing your body to convert VLDL into small, dense LDL. This condition can occur routinely when you eat a high-carb diet (even if it's a low-fat diet), because excessive insulin production drives the conversion of ingested carbohydrate into fat (triglycerides). Obviously, the condition can also occur when you eat a moderate-carb, high-fat diet, because insulin will see to it that both excess carbs and fat get circulated in the bloodstream and stored in fat cells.

Dr. Dean Ornish and other proponents of low-fat eating will tell you that reducing fat intake quickly reduces cholesterol and triglyceride levels. This is absolutely true, as confirmed by numerous best-selling books as well as newspaper and magazine feature stories touting quick and dramatic results (lowered cholesterol and triglyceride levels) from fat-restrictive diets. But the reason is this: your liver makes cholesterol as a raw material for the bile salts that help you digest fat, so if you aren't eating much fat, your genes will be given the signal to down-regulate cholesterol production.

> *Low-fat eating requires you to consume excessive carbs, by default, to obtain your daily energy requirements*

However, low-fat eating requires you to consume excessive carbs, by default, to obtain your daily energy requirements. This leads to excessive insulin production and, as you recall, kick-starts the cycle that eventually leads to heart disease. Any way you slice it, consuming too many carbs leads to high triglycerides (not to mention the other risk factors detailed in the forthcoming sidebar "How to Sneeze at Heart Disease").

With high triglycerides in your blood, VLDL production skyrockets to handle the extra load, and these particles can be altered into the small, dense LDLs that have been shown to be a major factor in atherosclerosis and heart disease. Being small and dense, these small, dense LDLs (why can't all medical nomenclature be this easy?) can become stuck in the spaces between cells lining the artery and then become oxidized. This oxidative damage causes inflammation and begins a process of destruction that I will detail shortly.

Research has shown that people with Metabolic Syndrome or type 2 diabetes all have elevated levels of both triglycerides and these small, dense LDL particles. Of course, these same people have substantially increased risks for heart disease and stroke.

The remaining cholesterol complex with which you might be familiar is the high-density lipoprotein (HDL), which takes cholesterol back to the liver for recycling. HDLs also clean up any damaged or oxidized cholesterol that might cause problems later, including removing the small, dense LDL particles and oxidized cholesterol that have become stuck in the artery wall. These tiny but powerful cholesterol complexes are often called the "good cholesterol" or "nature's garbage trucks." Scientists generally agree that the more HDL you have, the lower your risk for heart disease. As you might have imagined, people with Metabolic Syndrome and type 2 diabetes also typically have low levels of beneficial HDL. Exercise is one of the cheapest, easiest, and most effective ways to raise HDL. Consuming saturated fat is another!

Murder Mystery Dinner—Oxidation and Small, Dense LDL Are Guilty!

As mentioned earlier, because lipoproteins have a lipid surface, they are subject to oxidation. Like oils left open in your kitchen, they can go rancid when they come in contact with oxygen. When this happens lipoproteins—and the cholesterol inside—can become damaged. Of course, oxidation happens all the time throughout the body, and we have evolved some effective antioxidant systems (namely catalase, superoxide dismutase, and glutathione) to prevent too much of this damage from getting out of control. Furthermore, consuming ample levels of high-antioxidant foods (vegetables, fruits, nuts and seeds, dark chocolate, red wine) and antioxidant supplements (such as vitamin E, CoQ10, beta-carotene, and lycopene) can help mitigate some of the damage. It's also extremely convenient that HDLs can remove some of the damaged cholesterol and take it back to the liver for recycling.

Your cholesterol processing system has evolved to expect a certain range and quality of dietary fat, protein, carbohydrate, and antioxidants, as well as a certain level of exercise (to help promote insulin sensitivity in the muscles and maintain high levels of HDL) to provide appropriate gene signals and avoid artery disease. And because HDL particles are very small, they can get into the spaces between arterial wall cells and clean up the oxidized cholesterol. That's why Big Pharma has tried—so far unsuccessfully—to create an effective drug to raise HDL and address existing atherosclerosis (some physicians prescribe the combination of prescription fibrates and over-the-counter niacin to raise HDL, but this treatment can be problematic and is not widely used).

The cholesterol processing system has served humans and most other mammals well for millions of years—until recently. As mentioned previously, oxidized small, dense LDLs are small enough that they can get trapped in the spaces between endothelial cells lining the artery (sometimes called gap junctions). Even if they are not oxidized to begin with, once trapped, LDLs can oxidize in place because they are sitting there continually exposed to oxygen passing by that's attached to hemoglobin in the red blood cells. Either way, this oxidation eventually causes injury and inflammation to the arterial wall, prompting the body's immune system to send macrophages (scavenging white blood cells) to gobble up the oxidized LDLs at the site where the first particles were trapped.

The immune system tries hard to do its job, but the macrophages are overwhelmed by absorbing so much oxidized LDL. The consumption of oxidized LDL causes certain genes to convert these macrophages into foam cells that attach to the arterial lining, laying the foundation for future trouble. The lesion prompts more macrophages to come to the rescue. They try to gobble up more and more oxidized LDLs floating by, increasing the severity of the lesion over time. This is the familiar saga of plaque accumulation on the arterial wall. The plaque grows and eventually compromises the inner diameter of the artery. If allowed to continue, this process can eventually occlude blood flow or break off as a clot, preventing blood—and oxygen—from reaching a vital organ. This describes your classic heart attack or stroke.

The oxidation of these small, dense LDLs most likely happens for a variety of reasons that have to do with modern dietary habits more than anything else: a high intake of unstable polyunsaturated fats (PUFAs) from vegetable oils in the diet (PUFAs incorporated into the lipid layer are much more prone to oxidation than are saturated fats); a reduced intake of natural antioxidants in the diet, which would otherwise mitigate oxidation; the presence of fewer HDL particles to remove oxidized lipids (low HDL cholesterol readings may be partly caused by high-carb diets); and the fact that small, dense LDL particles do not bind as easily to the LDL receptors on muscle and fat cells. Unable to release their cholesterol load and with typically fewer HDL particles to gobble them up, these small, dense particles linger longer in the oxygen-rich bloodstream until they oxidize. By the way, atherosclerosis occurs in the arteries and not the veins because venous blood has very little oxygen.

Note that the oxidation and inflammation process described has little or nothing to do with your total cholesterol or even your total LDL cholesterol levels. In most cases, atherosclerosis is a result of the oxidation of a small fraction of the total amount of LDL in your blood—the small, dense LDL particles. If you have little or none of these in your blood, your risk for heart disease drops dramatically. Also, if your HDL is high, it's very unlikely that you'll encounter a problem, because HDL does a great job of scavenging the oxidized cholesterol from LDL in the bloodstream.

Unfortunately for some of us, poor diet, lack of exercise, stress, certain drug therapies, and, yes, family genetic history can all contribute to the increased production of the dangerous small, dense LDL particles. Your doctor can test for them if you ask, but most common blood tests don't yet distinguish between the benign "fluffy" forms of LDL, sometimes called pattern A, and the small, dense particles, called pattern B. A comprehensive lipid blood panel such as the Berkeley HeartLab test will typically provide values for total cholesterol, HDL, LDL, VLDL, and triglycerides and indicate relative particle sizes.

A physician will generally dispense medication if your total LDL levels exceed a certain figure (this varies by doctor and individual patient profile), knowing your body will respond to the statins with a quick overall reduction regardless of particle size. This will indeed lower all forms of LDL (including both the good and bad kind), but it's a much more sensible—and safe—option to simply alter dietary and exercise habits and minimize insulin production, thereby preventing excess accumulation of triglycerides in the blood and allowing the cholesterol system to work as intended. In fact, the combination of low carbs and good fats in Primal foods will generally raise HDL and lower both triglycerides and small, dense LDL. Meanwhile, compelling evidence suggests that Primal Blueprint-style eating and exercising will allow you, regardless of your genetic predisposition, to essentially have no participation in this heart disease saga whatsoever. If you feel any hesitation here, go get a "before" blood panel, eat Primally for 21 days, and then get another panel. It's virtually certain you will see an impressive alteration of unfavorable numbers, giving you the motivation and clarity you need to plunge wholeheartedly into Primal eating.

Statin Stats Stink!

Isn't it ironic, then, to discover that statins and other cholesterol-lowering meds do not have any ability to influence LDL particle size and can only lower total LDL by reducing both the good and the bad versions? The fact that some people taking statins experience a dramatic reduction in total cholesterol or in LDL means very little in the context of the true oxidation and inflammation nature of heart disease. To be clear, statins do slightly reduce the risk of heart attacks among men under the age of 65 who have had a prior heart attack. However, many doctors now believe that these benefits are independent of their "cholesterol-lowering" properties, and instead come from an anti-inflammatory effect that addresses the more proximate cause of heart disease. A cheaper and more effective anti-inflammatory effect can be achieved by eating foods high in omega-3 or taking fish oil supplements, exercising sensibly instead of chronically, or getting more sleep if you are deprived.

> ❝ HDL does a great job of scavenging the oxidized cholesterol from LDL in the bloodstream... if your HDL is high, it's much less likely you'll encounter a [heart disease] problem. ❞

By simply adopting the Primal Blueprint laws, you can enjoy superior results without the perilous side effects and huge expense of drug therapy. In the case of statins, known side effects include muscle pain, weakness and numbness, chronic fatigue, tendon problems, cognitive problems, impotence, and blood glucose elevations. These side effects are believed to be due in large part to statins' interference with the normal production of a critical micro-nutrient known as coenzyme Q10 (CoQ10). CoQ10 is essential to healthy mitochondrial function (energy production) and defending your cells against free radical damage. Statin therapy is believed to lower CoQ10 levels by up to 50 percent. Ironically, CoQ10 plays a particularly important role in the healthy function of the cardiovascular system, and heart attack patients show depressed levels of CoQ10! Some researchers suggest that statins' depletion of CoQ10 may nullify any potential benefits of statin therapy.

So why are millions being misguided to take dangerous, powerful drugs when lifestyle intervention is more effective and less expensive and has no side effects? Perhaps we like to search for easy answers with quick results, and statins produce a graphic and quick decline in blood cholesterol levels. Like other elements of Conventional Wisdom, there are billions of dollars invested and powerful market forces pushing us in the direction of swallowing drugs and their side effects, while the full story is lost amidst the hype of "lower your numbers quick!"

If you are currently taking statins or other medications, I realize that asking you to reject Conventional Wisdom and the specific recommendations of your trusted physician can put you in a very uncomfortable position. I strongly urge you to engage in lifestyle modification (after all, there are no side effects or potential compromises to your drug regimen when you improve your diet), while concurrently addressing the possibility with your doctor of gradually reducing your dependence on medication based on the ensuing favorable blood test results.

How to Sneeze at Heart Disease

The catchall term Metabolic Syndrome is used to describe an assortment of heart disease risk factors widely attributed to today's prevailing poor dietary and exercise habits. The highly respected Cleveland Clinic states that "the exact cause of Metabolic Syndrome is not known…[but] many features are associated with insulin resistance." Five markers are universally used as reliable indicators of *Metabolic Syndrome.* If you have three or more of these markers, you are diagnosed as having the condition. Here are the five markers:

1. Elevated fasting blood glucose of **100 mg/dl** or greater.
2. Blood pressure of **130/85 mm Hg** or greater.
3. Waistline measurement of **40 inches** or more for men and **35 inches** or more for women.
4. HDL of less than **40 mg/dl** for men and less than **50 mg/dl** for women.
5. Triglycerides of **150 mg/dl** or greater.

The U.S. government and other sources report that some 47 million Americans have Metabolic Syndrome—about one in five Americans. It's a chronic condition that develops and worsens over time (with no discernable physical symptoms, except that expanding waistline…) unless you take dramatic steps to alter your lifestyle. The Cleveland Clinic and *Journal of the American Medical Association* report that more than 40 percent of Americans in their 60s and 70s have the condition. Dr. Richard Feinman, one of the most often-published and highly regarded researchers in the fields of nutrition and metabolism, has suggested that "Metabolic Syndrome may be defined by the response to carbohydrate restriction" (that is, if you restrict carbs, the symptoms subside).

A routine physical exam and blood panel will give you an indication of your Metabolic Syndrome status. Many experts recommend a few additional blood tests to assess overall health and risk factors, including:

C-Reactive Protein: High sensitivity C-reactive protein (hs-CRP) is produced by your liver as part of an immune system response to injury or infection. In the absence of other acute infections, high levels of hs-CRP in your blood are associated with an increased risk of heart attack, stroke, and sudden cardiac death. Because atherosclerosis is primarily a disease of inflammation, some researchers contend that hs-CRP is a strong predictor of your heart disease risk. Given that cholesterol tests have become less reliable in predicting risk, especially among those with normal or low cholesterol levels, hs-CRP seems to be a good alternative.

Lp2A: Another key inflammation marker associated with small, dense LDL particles.

How to Sneeze at Heart Disease (continued)

A1c (estimated average glucose): A1c measures how much glucose is attached to a hemoglobin molecule, a reliable marker for the dangers of elevated blood glucose levels over an extended time period. This is a superior test to the more common blood glucose readings (something commonly tracked by diabetics with a portable machine) that vary throughout the day and are strongly influenced by meals.

Fasting Blood Insulin Levels: High fasting insulin levels are indicative of prediabetic conditions.

How to Sneeze at Heart Disease: Diet and Exercise Prevention Tips

If you are diagnosed with or on the borderline of Metabolic Syndrome, following the Primal Blueprint for 21 days can turn four of the five Metabolic Syndrome markers around (it might take a bit longer to get your waistline back in the safe zone) and cause your heart disease risk to plummet—even if you have a family history of obesity, high cholesterol, and heart disease. Here are some specific recommendations and corresponding benefits of following the Primal Blueprint:

Balance Omega-6:Omega-3 Ratios: Minimizing consumption of omega-6 polyunsaturated fats gives you a greater surface area of saturated (and therefore protected) fats in lipoprotein lipid layers and fatty membranes. Increased consumption of omega-3 oils helps control the inflammation that is the precursor for atherosclerosis and virtually all other metabolic diseases.

Exercise Primal Blueprint Style: Regular exercise helps lower LDL and raise HDL.

Increase Antioxidant Intake: If your antioxidant intake is appreciable (eating your vegetables?), it's likely that you'll help your natural defenses against oxidation. Supplements are a great idea if you lead a stressful life (who doesn't?), your diet falls short from time to time, or you are at an increased risk of heart disease.

Reduce Carb Intake: This will help lower your production of triglycerides, raise HDL, lower LDL, and dramatically lower the small, dense LDL (because it's high levels of triglycerides that prompt small, dense LDL production).

Put Inflammation at Ease with Omega-3s

A major feature of Primal Blueprint eating is that it provides high levels of healthy saturated and unsaturated fats. While Conventional Wisdom generally positions saturated fats as something to diligently restrict, they are an excellent energy source and offer a variety of nutrients critical to health. Consuming ample amounts of saturated fat helps prevent oxidative damage to your cells (saturated fat is an integral part of cell membranes). While your eyes might bug out at this statement, it's virtually irrefutable and proven by many respected long-term studies:

" Eat (healthy) fat to help prevent cancer and heart disease. Avoid fat and increase your risk of cancer, heart disease, and even obesity. "

Fortunately, omega-3 polyunsaturated fatty acids don't have an image problem and are universally regarded as healthy. Adequate omega-3 consumption supports healthy cardiovascular, brain, skin, and immune function. By turning on genes that improve blood circulation, reducing inflammation, and supporting healthy cholesterol and triglyceride levels, omega-3s help reduce the risk of high blood pressure, blood clots that cause heart attacks, arthritis, autoimmune disorders, and cognitive problems such as depression, Alzheimer's, and even ADHD. The important role of omega-3s in supporting cognitive function is made even more evident by the fact that half the brain consists of fat, including concentrated levels of the omega-3 docosahexanoic acid, DHA.

The benefits of adequate omega-3 intake and optimum fatty acid balance are strikingly evident from data on cultures that consume substantial amounts of fat but have markedly reduced heart disease rates compared to Westerners, such as the traditional Japanese diet (i.e., for those who frequent sushi bars instead of the 3,598 McDonald's in Japan) centered around fish and vegetables.

Another form of polyunsaturated fats called omega-6s plays a vital role in our health as well, but their extreme prevalence in the Standard American Diet

diet—from vegetable oils, animal fats, bakery items (donuts, cookies), and processed snacks (the highly offensive trans and partially hydrogenated fats are classified as omega-6)—leads to a dangerous imbalance of excessive omega-6 and deficient omega-3. The ideal omega-6:omega-3 balance (O6:O3) is 1:1 or 2:1, ratios that Grok likely met with ease. Even 4:1 is okay today, but the typical modern eater has an O6:O3 ratio of 20:1, or even 50:1! It's also interesting to note that imbalanced fatty acid intake can exacerbate the insulin resistance problem discussed earlier. Omega-6 fats (particularly arachidonic acid) suppress expression of the insulin receptor gene GLUT4 (promoting more fat storage), while omega-3 fats increase expression of GLUT4 (promoting insulin sensitivity and less fat storage).

Once again, your genes are only doing what they are told to do according to the signals you give them. The imbalance of fatty acids in the typical modern diet triggers a genetically programmed inflammation response throughout the body. Under normal circumstances, inflammation is your body's highly desirable first line of defense against pain, injury, and infection. Inflammation processes detect and destroy toxic material in damaged tissue before it can spread to the rest of the body. Consider examples like a bee sting, taking an elbow to the face, or turning an ankle on a hiking trail—the reddened skin, black eye, and ballooned ankle help your body quarantine the damage from the trauma to the inflamed areas, instead of letting toxins run wild through the bloodstream. Unfortunately, an out-of-control inflammation response (also known as systemic inflammation)—resulting from stress and imbalanced dietary and/or exercise habits—confuses your body into thinking it's under assault from destructive, infectious foreign agents or that a major trauma has just occurred. That's when the disease process begins.

In my own athletic example, the extreme stress of my Chronic Cardio training regimen and my highly inflammatory grain-based diet led to excessive and prolonged inflammation throughout my body. What I should have been seeking was a more desirable temporary state of moderate inflammation (pumped muscles, elevated heart rate, oxygenated lungs), from a Primal Blueprint-aligned training regimen and plenty of recovery time for my body to return to homeostasis. The systemic inflammation I experienced from overtraining tore down my muscles, joints, and immune system.

Interestingly, after extreme endurance events like a marathon or ironman race, blood levels of CPK (creatine phosphokinase; it leaks into the bloodstream when muscle, heart, or brain tissue is traumatized) can be elevated for weeks afterward. In fact, if you ran a marathon and then—just for kicks—

immediately headed over to a hospital emergency room, a doctor might think you were suffering from a heart attack! In my case, when I adjusted my diet and training habits, virtually all my inflammatory and immune-suppressing conditions vanished.

We know that most forms of systemic inflammation have a strong dietary component and can usually be resolved with a few dietary modifications. Nevertheless, Conventional Wisdom within the medical community has recommended fighting our widespread inflammation-related health problems with corticosteroids, COX-2 inhibitors such as Vioxx and Celebrex, and other nonsteroidal anti-inflammatories (asthma meds work on a similar chemical pathway).

I have a nonscientific name for this approach: *digging a hole to install a ladder to wash the basement windows.* As you might imagine, because these medications interfere with normal hormone pathways and gene expression, they almost never address the underlying cause of inflammation. They simply mask the pain in the short term—if they mask it at all. Dietary modification (and exercise modification if you are overdoing it) is almost always a superior method of treatment and protection against pain and serious diseases triggered by systemic inflammation.

> *I have a nonscientific name for treating lifestyle-related health problems with pharmaceuticals:* **digging a hole to install a ladder to wash the basement windows.**

The *Primal Blueprint* eating style, with its emphasis on high omega-3 foods (such as oily, cold water fish, pasture-raised animal meats and eggs; and leafy green vegetables) and its aversion to processed foods and excessive omega-6 oils, provides an ideal dietary fatty acid balance without you really having to worry about it. When you combine healthy eating with the other Primal Blueprint laws, you can naturally avoid the systemic inflammation that is now believed to be the root cause of the major health problems affecting modern humans.

Context In, Calories Out— Understanding the Macro Nutrients

While you likely have a basic understanding of what carbohydrate, protein, and fat do in the body, it's important to examine the role of each nutrient further in the context of how they support the Primal Blueprint. This is particularly true in light of the massive misinformation, distortion, and confusion presented by opposing camps on this issue.

Most popular daily diets (and fitness programs) follow the "calories in, calories out" Conventional Wisdom method of weight loss, failing to understand the importance of context when making this otherwise literally accurate edict. Your body uses macronutrients for a variety of different functions, some of which are to provide structure and some of which are to provide energy (as calories), immediately or well into the future. Moreover, the body acts as either a fuel storage depot (and as a toxic "waist" site) or a supplier of energy (calories), depending largely on the hormonal signals it gets from your lifestyle behaviors. Because your body always seeks to achieve homeostasis (balance), the notion of you trying to zero in on a precise day-to-day or meal-to-meal eating plan is generally fruitless, not to mention practically impossible and incredibly frustrating.

To figure your true structural and functional fuel needs (and, hence, to achieve your body composition goals), it's important to understand how the three major macronutrients work in the body—or should work when you eat in a manner aligned with optimal gene expression.

Protein

Most nutrition researchers are in agreement that protein is essential for building and repairing body tissues and for overall healthy function. Intake recommendations among doctors and nutritionists vary, with most falling in the range of 0.5 to 1 gram of protein per pound of lean body mass per day. There were days when Grok and his family probably obtained two or three times that amount, so if you happen to overdo your protein significantly on any given day or aren't the type to obsess about such things, you'll almost certainly be well within safe guidelines.

To calculate or estimate lean body mass, you must first determine your total weight and percentage of body fat. You can do this using any of numerous methods ranging from costly water tank tests to the easier fat scales, skinfold calipers, or online calculators using certain body measurements. Most good gyms can help you with this, or you can just estimate roughly for these purposes, knowing that the average moderately fit male and female carry about 15 percent and 22 percent, respectively. Multiply your total weight by your percent body fat to attain your "fat" weight, and then subtract that figure from your total body weight to obtain your lean body mass. For example, a 155-pound woman with 25 percent body fat (39 lbs) has a lean body mass of 116 pounds (155–39=116).

At a minimum you need 0.5 gram of protein per pound of lean mass per day to maintain your "structure" and healthy body composition. If you are moderately active, you need closer to 0.7 gram, and if you are an active athlete (or under a fair amount of stress), you need as much as one gram of protein per pound of lean mass. That's at a minimum, but it's on a daily average. So, our 155-pound moderately active woman with 116 pounds of lean mass (25 percent body fat) needs an average of 82 grams of protein per day (116 x 0.7). If she gets 60 or 70 some days and 110 on others, she'll still be in a healthy average range. She could even fast a day or two occasionally and, provided she has been regularly eating Primally and doesn't overexercise on fasting days, easily preserve her muscle using the body's tendency to burn fat and retain protein stores in the short term. On the other hand, if she exceeds the 110 grams, it's also no problem if she's eating Primally, because the excess protein will convert to glucose, which will reduce her dietary carbohydrate needs (see next section). At 4 calories per gram, her daily average of 82 grams is only 328 calories per day in protein.

This formula works with kilograms as well. The minimum protein requirement would be around 1.1 grams of protein per kilo of lean mass; moderately active persons would require around 1.5, and very active folks around 2.2 grams per kilo. Again, I'm not concerned with you counting or even meeting this requirement every single day. You'll find yourself intuitively arriving at a comfortable number or range of protein grams within a week of Primal Blueprint-style eating. You will discover that it's quite easy to eat one gram of protein per pound of lean body mass without a lot of planning, and pretty difficult to eat much more than two grams per pound without forcing yourself to. You simply aren't as hungry when you moderate processed carb intake and avoid insulin crashes and sugar cravings.

If you have ample stored glycogen in your muscle tissues and liver (not a problem for most people unless you are engaged in high-volume, high-stress endurance training or severely restrict your carbs a la the Atkins Diet) and your body is getting the rest of its energy efficiently from fats, it's likely that the protein you consume will go first toward the repair or building of cells or enzymes. Proponents of the "a calorie is a calorie" Conventional Wisdom will pipe in here that excess calories are always converted or stored as fat, regardless of their original ingested state. This is true, of course (remember, the Primal Blueprint doesn't like to piss off scientists!), and when we eat a high-carb, high-insulin producing diet, those excess calories indeed are stored as fat. But we must then ask what excess fat calories do when there is not a lot of insulin in the bloodstream (given that they cannot easily be stored as fat without insulin giving them a ride). No problem; the body will respond by raising metabolic rate (to burn more calories at rest) and by increasing the production of ketones, which may be burned or excreted (more on this shortly).

In summary, if you are the type to enjoy and observe details in your macronutrient intake, I suggest you strive to obtain your protein requirements first, in the activity level-influenced range discussed previously. Focus on quality sources of protein such as the pasture-raised or organic animal products that are detailed in the next chapter.

Carbohydrates

If you've forgotten everything you ever learned in biology, just remember this and own it: *carbohydrate controls insulin; insulin controls fat storage*. Carbohydrates are not used as structural components in the body; instead, they are used only as a form of fuel, whether burned immediately while passing by different organs and muscles, or stored for later use. All forms of carbohydrates you eat, whether simple or complex, are eventually converted into glucose, which the brain, red blood cells, and nerve cells generally prefer as a primary fuel. For reference, a little less than one teaspoon of glucose dissolved in the entire blood pool in your body (about five quarts in the case of a 160-pound male) represents an optimal level of blood glucose.

In most healthy people, glucose that is not burned immediately (exercising muscles prefer glucose, if it is available, but don't absolutely require it unless they are working at high intensity for long periods) will first be stored as glycogen in muscle and liver cells. When these sites are full, glucose is converted into fatty acids and stored in fat cells. It's insulin's job to take glucose out of the bloodstream and put it somewhere fast.

Unless you deplete lots of muscle glycogen every day, there is no physiological reason for you to consume high levels of carbohydrates. In fact, carbohydrates are not required in the human diet for survival the way fat and protein are. The body has several backup mechanisms for generating glucose internally: from dietary fat and protein, as well as from proteins stripped from muscle tissue (all done via gluconeogenesis). Some researchers have estimated that the body manufactures up to 200 grams of glucose every day from the fat and protein in our diet or in our muscles. Good thing, because entire civilizations have lived for thousands of years on 50 or fewer grams of carbohydrates a day.

> *There is no biological requirement for dietary carbohydrate in the human diet. The Primal Blueprint is an 'eliminate bad carbs' diet.*

That said, the Primal Blueprint is not designed to be an extremely low-carb diet, because this strategy would restrict your intake of some of the most nutrient-dense foods on the planet—vegetables and fruits. I don't even characterize the Primal Blueprint as a "low-carb" diet, as much as it is an "eliminate bad carbs" diet. I don't advocate portion control or even diligently counting your macronutrient intake. You may want to journal now and then to establish benchmarks and reference points (visit paleotrack.com or FitDay.com, input a day or two of foods you eat, and it will generate a breakdown of macronutrients and calories), but you don't need to. It's really easy to stay in the optimum range of 100 to 150 grams per day of carbs, even when you eat a ton of colorful vegetables and fairly liberal servings of fruit, as long as you stay Primal and consume no grains or legumes. For example, a huge salad, two cups of Brussels sprouts, a banana, an apple, a cup of blueberries, and a cup of cherries totals only 139 grams of carbs.

Note: Perhaps you are familiar with the concept of "net carbs" when measuring macronutrient intake. This is a calculation that subtracts fiber, because fiber is usually not digested and moderates the blood glucose impact of a carbohydrate food. For the sake of simplicity (and to assert the Primal Blueprint philosophy that you don't need many carbs, nor any additional fiber from grain foods), all the calculations and zones in this book represent *gross* total carbohydrate grams.

The Carbohydrate Curve—What'll It Be? The "Sweet Spot" or the "Death Spiral"?

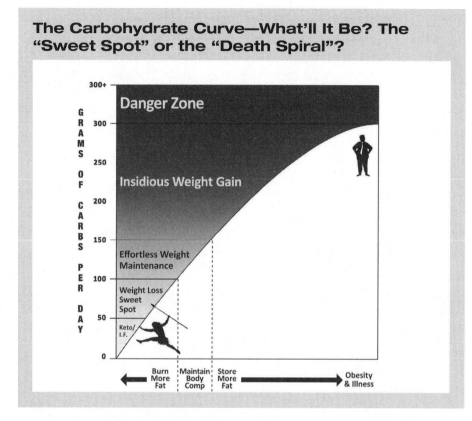

The Primal Blueprint Carbohydrate Curve illustrates how carbohydrates impact the human body and the degree to which we need them, or don't need them, in our diet. Carb intake is the decisive factor in your weight-loss success or failure, and excessive carb consumption is arguably the most destructive modern lifestyle behavior. Eliminating grains and sugars from your diet could be the number one most beneficial thing you ever do for your health!

0 to 50 grams per day: *Ketosis and Accelerated Fat Burning*

Acceptable for occasional one- to two-day Intermittent Fasting efforts toward aggressive weight loss (or longer term, for medically supervised weight-loss programs for the obese and/or type 2 diabetics), provided adequate protein, fat, and supplements are consumed. Excellent catalyst for quick, relatively comfortable weight loss and not at all dangerous. (Grok relied heavily on fat metabolism and ketosis to account for the difficulty in obtaining appreciable amounts of carbs in daily life.) Not recommended as a long-term practice for most people due to likely deprivation of high-nutrient-value vegetables and fruits.

50 to 100 grams per day: *Primal Sweet Spot for Effortless Weight Loss*

Minimizes insulin production and accelerates fat metabolism. By meeting average daily protein requirements, eating nutritious vegetables and fruits, and staying satisfied with delicious high-fat foods (meat, fish, eggs, nuts, seeds), you can lose one to two pounds of body fat per week in the "sweet spot." Delicious menu options that land in the sweet spot are detailed in Chapter 8.

100 to 150 grams per day: *Primal Blueprint Maintenance Range*

Allows for genetically optimal fat burning, muscle development, and effortless weight maintenance. Rationale supported by humans eating and evolving in this range or below for millions of years. Dietary emphasis on vegetables, fruits, nuts, seeds, and animal foods, with grains and processed sugars eliminated.

A prior history of heavy carb intake may result in a brief period of discomfort during the transition to Primal Blueprint eating. Adequate consumption of satisfying foods (high-water-content fruits and vegetables, high-fat snacks like nuts and seeds, and meals emphasizing animal foods) helps protect against feeling deprived or depleted.

150 to 300 grams per day: *Steady, Insidious Weight Gain*

Continuous insulin-stimulating effects prevent efficient fat metabolism and contribute to widespread health conditions. This zone is the de facto recommendation of many popular diets and health authorities (including the USDA Food Pyramid!) despite the clear danger of developing Metabolic Syndrome. Chronic exercisers, active, growing youth, and those with physically strenuous jobs may eat at this level for an extended period without gaining fat, but eventually fat storage and/or metabolic problems are highly probable.

This "insidious" zone is easy to drift into, even by health-conscious eaters, when grains are a dietary centerpiece, sweetened beverages or snacks leak into the picture here and there, and obligatory fruits and vegetables are added to the total. Recall that Wendy Korg's trip to Jamba Juice for a healthy afternoon snack resulted in 187 grams of carbs ingested at one sitting. Starting your day off with a bowl of muesli cereal, a slice of whole wheat toast, and a glass of fresh orange juice might seem right off the "heart-healthy" menu at the luxury spa—but the numbers start racking up (that's 97 grams right there!), and the disastrous insulin-spike/sugar-craving cycle is set in motion. Despite trying to do the right thing by cutting fat and calories, many frustrated people still gain a pound or two of fat per year for decades as a result of the carb intake in the insidious range.

300 or more grams per day: *Danger Zone!*

Zone of the average American's diet, and in excess of official USDA dietary guidelines (which suggest you eat 45 percent to 65 percent of calories from carbs), thanks to stuff like soda tipping the scales over. Extended time in the danger zone results in almost certain weight gain and Metabolic Syndrome. The danger zone is the primary catalyst for the obesity and type 2 diabetes epidemics, as well as numerous other significant health problems. Immediate and dramatic reduction of grains and other processed carbs is critical.

Carb Curve Variables: The 50-gram/200-calorie variation within each range on the curve attempts to account for individual energy disparities: a light, moderately active female will observe the low end of the range, while a heavy, active male will subscribe to the high end. If you insistent upon doing Chronic Cardio, you will likely have to increase carb intake to account for regular depletion of stored liver and muscle glycogen and an elevated metabolic rate. You can experiment with consuming 100 additional grams of carbs for every hour of vigorous exercise and notice how your body responds. However, I'd prefer that you simply adjust your training program to conform to Primal Blueprint guidelines and thus reduce your need for dietary carbohydrate.

Fat

I've already discussed how the common admonition to keep dietary fats low is truly unfounded in most credible research. Consuming healthy fats from animal and plant sources supports optimal function of all the systems in your body. Furthermore, ingesting fat helps you feel full and satisfied in a way that ingesting carbohydrates cannot. Because fat has little or no impact on blood glucose levels or insulin production and takes far longer to metabolize than carbohydrates, you will feel a deep and long-lasting satisfaction from consuming ample amounts of fat in your diet.

I understand that this is a controversial topic that will be met with some opposition. Please take it upon yourself to gain a clear understanding of the issue, learn to distinguish healthy fats from unhealthy, and sort out misleading Conventional Wisdom that frowns upon food staples that drove human evolution. The highly respected Nurses' Health Study tracked the dietary habits of 90,000 nurses over two decades. It is the largest epidemiological study of women in history, leading to the publication of 265 published scientific papers in leading journals. The study showed no statistically significant association between total fat intake (or cholesterol intake) and heart disease. Many other studies have attempted to establish a firm connection, yet none have demonstrated that a high-fat diet by itself causes heart disease. So how can it be that low-fat eating became the Conventional Wisdom? I believe that the otherwise well-meaning, well-educated folks in the low-fat camp are influenced by a few factors that lead them to the party line conclusion that a high-fat diet is unhealthy.

> *The Nurses' Health Study (90,000 nurses, two decades) showed no statistically significant association between total fat intake (or cholesterol intake) and heart disease.*

1. Failure to distinguish between good fats and bad fats: The skyrocketing rates of obesity, heart disease, and cancer from eating a diet high in both processed carbs and chemically-altered fats have unfairly implicated all fats as dangerous. As I discussed earlier and will cover further in the next chapter, the typical modern diet is grossly imbalanced between omega-6 fats and omega-3 fats. We ingest way too much of the former (from processed foods, polyunsaturated oils, and grain-fed animal products) and way too little of the latter (from oily, cold water fish, pastured eggs and meat, and omega-3 capsules).

Furthermore, we consume excessive amounts of the highly toxic partially hydrogenated fats and trans-fats (they are not quite the same but are closely related and both evil). These "Franken-fats" are created by heating and chemically treating vegetable and seed oils to become solid. Solidifying fats effectively extends shelf life and improves the flavor of processed foods. These fats are easily oxidized to form free radical chain reactions that damage cell membranes, body tissue, and immune function. Because your brain, nervous system, and vascular system are primarily composed of membranes, any dysfunction in these critical areas can be devastating. Research confirms that consumption of trans-fatty acids and partially hydrogenated fats may promote inflammation, aging, and cancer. *The New England Journal of*

Medicine reviewed numerous studies and reported a strong link between trans-fat consumption and heart disease.

2. Carbs making fat look bad: Fat is calorically dense at nine calories per gram. If you consume excessive carbs (150 to 300 grams or more per day), produce a high level of insulin, and eat any appreciable amount of fat along with your high-carb diet, your fat intake will contribute directly to making you fat. You know the saying "Which came first, the chicken or the egg?" Well, in this case, it's neither the chicken nor the egg making you fat—it's the carbs! The carbs cause high levels of insulin which steer both carbs and fat (and protein) into your fat cells.

> *Which came first, the chicken or the egg? In this case, neither. It's the carbs that make you fat!*

3. Propaganda and flawed science manipulated into Conventional Wisdom: The machinations of public policy bureaucracy often leave rational thinking in the dust in favor of protecting and promoting corporate interests and the reputations of politicians. While I am all in favor of capitalism, it's unsettling how much decision-making power is controlled by corporations that spend billions of marketing dollars molding and shaping Conventional Dietary Wisdom in the direction of profits, with little regard for health.

The story of how saturated fat came to be vilified begs mention of the work of American scientist Ancel Keys. Keys was an eloquent and dynamic early promoter of the link between saturated fat intake, cholesterol levels, and heart disease. Keys received notoriety in the 1960s for his efforts to transition the public away from saturated fats to replacements such as polyunsaturated oils or low-fat eating in general. It has taken decades, at a dawdling pace, to recognize the folly of his health suggestions. For example, Keys didn't even connect obesity to heart disease risk, and the foundation of his work was compromised when he was criticized for hand-picking examples (comparisons of fat intake and heart disease rates among different cultures) that supported his hypotheses. In fairness, Keys also did some great work helping to popularize the Mediterranean diet (highlighted by the liberal intake of healthy fats), even spending his last few decades living in a small town in Italy and studying the residents' dietary habits.

On a bureaucratic level, the U.S. government has time and again shown a penchant for doggedly defending the status quo and vigorously squashing voices opposing Conventional Wisdom. A shining example of the influence of power and money on the development of public policy is found in the FDA's so-called imitation policy, passed in 1973 (without Congressional approval, thanks to some clever legal maneuvering). The legislation relieved food manufacturers from having to use that pesky "imitation" designation on labels of foods created with artificial ingredients (coffee creamers, egg mixes, processed cheeses, whip cream, and hundreds more), as long as manufacturers added synthetic vitamins to their concoctions to approximate the benefits of similar whole foods.

Mary Enig, Ph.D., a renowned nutritionist, lipid biochemistry expert, and author of *Know Your Fats*, from the University of Maryland, has spent a career battling Conventional Wisdom's take on fat intake and heart disease. In the 1970s she was a central figure in challenging the corruption and misinformation dispensed by the USDA and the U.S. Senate's McGovern Committee (headed by former presidential candidate George McGovern). Influenced by highly questionable and lobby-influenced testimony, the committee published its report (many believe McGovern was hoodwinked by subordinates to buy into flawed conclusions) directing Americans to replace saturated fat with polyunsaturated fatty acids and to limit fat intake in general, which was then disastrously replaced with excessive carbohydrates.

On the heels of these cultural turning points, ensuing government-funded research tends to fall in line with the committee recommendations. The notion that fats are bad gained momentum, became adopted into Conventional Wisdom, and is still going strong! The discussion of the food propaganda topic is compelling enough to fill entire books (check out *Fast Food Nation*, *Food Politics*, *Appetite for Profit*, and *Good Calories, Bad Calories* for fascinating and detailed examinations of the topic), so I'll wrap here by asserting the point that it's unwise to blindly trust Conventional Wisdom when it comes to fat and to dietary habits in general.

Ketones—The Fourth Fuel

By now you know that we evolved to burn primarily fats and a little glucose. We can also burn protein, when certain amino acids enter the energy pathways through a part of the glucose cycle (as happens when we run out of glucose or glycogen during a long workout or during starvation). Protein can also be converted to glucose in the liver. While most cells in our body can easily burn both fats and glucose, there are a few select cells that function only on glucose (some brain cells, red blood cells, and kidney cells, for example). Without glucose, those cells would cease to function and we would not last very long. The minimum daily glucose requirement to keep those systems running has been estimated at between 150 and 200 grams per day, but recent research shows that after a little adaptation, some of these cells can operate effectively on a fuel known as ketones, dramatically reducing your overall glucose requirement.

Ketones were crucial to our evolution. As we have already discussed here, our ancestors rarely had steady access to carbohydrates like we do today. In fact, they may have gone weeks or months without appreciable carbs, so they had to evolve a system whereby the liver could take protein either from the muscles or directly from the diet and convert it into glucose through gluconeogenesis. This system worked to keep Grok alive during short periods of starvation or longer periods when meat (protein and fats) was plentiful but plants (carbs) were not. Today we can tap into this same system and prompt our genes to speed up the process of fat loss when we cut carbs while still consuming adequate dietary protein. In this scenario, we never have to sacrifice lean muscle in pursuit of fat loss (the unfortunate story of traditional calorie-restriction weight loss) if we eat Primally.

Manufacturing glucose from protein requires its own source of energy, so liver cells happen to use fats (fatty acids, really) to fuel this conversion. When liver cells are involved in gluconeogenesis, they are unable to completely burn off those fats to the final end products of carbon dioxide and water. Consequently, they produce an energy-rich by-product known as a ketone (also called a ketone body). Ketones are safe, desirable, energy-efficient forms of fuel. They are quite literally the fourth fuel. In fact, when you become well adapted to burning fats on the Primal Blueprint, one of the side benefits is that you will also become keto-adapted. That means that over a few weeks of reducing carbs (and, hence, decreasing insulin) and increasing the relative amounts of healthy fats in your diet, you will send signals to your genes that result in an increased production (an up-regulation) of the metabolic "machinery" used to effectively burn ketones throughout your body.

Many cells actually prefer ketones over glucose, given the choice between the two. Cardiac muscle, skeletal muscle, and even certain brain cells thrive on the four and a half calories per gram delivered by ketones. After a little keto-adaptation, the brain can do very well getting 75 percent of its energy from ketones. The fact that we can so easily convert to this alternative energy plan may be the best proof that Grok didn't always have access to lots of carbs. A 2004 article in the *Journal of the International Society of Sports Nutrition* referred to numerous studies suggesting that a low-carbohydrate intake and the resulting mild ketosis may offer many benefits, including reduction of body fat, minimized damage from insulin resistance and free radicals (caused by metabolizing a high-carbohydrate diet), and a reduction of LDL cholesterol.

So what exactly is ketosis then? Ketones can't be stored conveniently the way fats (and excess glucose) can be stored in fat cells or the way glucose can be stored as glycogen. Ketones simply circulate in the bloodstream where they are available to be picked up by any cells that want and need the energy they provide. Ketosis is the scientific name for a relative condition in the body where ketones start to accumulate in the bloodstream to a point beyond which they can all be picked up for energy. There is nothing wrong with being in ketosis. It is a natural, normal part of human energy production and metabolism. You have probably been in mild ketosis any time you have fasted or skipped a couple of meals in a row.

If you haven't yet become keto-adapted, as is the case with most people who eat a moderate to high-carb diet and then decide to fast, the ketones aren't yet able to be burned as efficiently. Ketones happen to be somewhat acidic, and because the body works hard to maintain a slightly alkaline (non-acidic) state, unused ketones are excreted in urine, stool, or even breath. Some describe the smell of ketone breath as that of overly ripe apples or acetone. If you are new to Primal eating, you will require a few weeks to reprogram your genes to become more efficient at burning ketones. As your body adapts to a genetically optimal low carbohydrate eating pattern, you will burn ketones effectively and excrete less, thereby further reducing your glucose requirements.

Some people—including some misinformed doctors—maintain an unnecessarily dim view of ketones and ketosis. I believe these criticisms arise because the diets in question allow for only 20 grams or less of carbs per day, a level that does not allow for the plentiful intake of nutrient-rich vegetables. While we are not meant to run predominantly on carbohydrate energy, we do depend heavily on the nutrients offered by vegetables and most fruits. Other people may be mistaking ketosis for *ketoacidosis*, a much different (and potentially deadly) condition that affects insulin-dependent diabetics and alcoholics.

In the Primal Blueprint maintenance zone, you rarely even get to a state of ketosis. (But you will still burn lots more fat and produce more ketones than high-carb people.) Because 100 carb grams a day seems to be the cutoff point above which ketosis is reduced, the recommended range of 100 to 150 grams per day of vegetable- and fruit-based carbs is plenty to fuel the glucose and glycogen-dependent systems while the majority of our energy comes from fat.

On the Primal Blueprint accelerated fat-loss program (detailed in Chapter 8), you will eat in what I call the sweet spot—a level of mild ketosis—by consuming 50 to 100 grams of carbs per day. Here, the protein needed for gluconeogenesis comes from your diet (not your muscles) and you will have plenty of fat to meet your daily fuel requirements.

By understanding how the metabolic processes work for protein, fat, carbohydrates, and ketones, and knowing that you can control the rates at which each one burns by improving your diet and exercise habits, you needn't agonize over day-to-day calorie counting. As long as you are eating Primal foods, you will be able to maintain your personal ideal body composition and mitigate your risk of diet-related health conditions and diseases.

> " *My doctor told me to stop having intimate dinners for four. Unless there are three other people.* "
> —**Orson Welles**

Eating Well

The Primal Blueprint is about enjoying a healthy, happy, balanced lifestyle. As Dr. Andrew Weil said in describing the title of his book *Eating Well for Optimum Health*, "eating well" refers not only to choosing natural, nutritious foods, but also to enjoying the experience as one of the great pleasures of life. It's likely that Grok appreciated food much more than we do today, because he had to work so hard for his meals and was never assured of success. Throughout history, food has represented a centerpiece of cultural celebration—let's not kill the momentum now! The key to eating well is to eliminate distractions and negative influences while you are eating, which will allow the physical sensations of hunger and the simple pursuit of pleasure to have predominant influence on your dietary habits.

The "Oh, Positive" Diet

If you wish to succeed with healthy dietary habits, it's important that you discard any negative emotions you have toward eating and embrace each meal as an opportunity to enjoy yourself. I strongly recommend that you give yourself permission to eat as much as you want, whenever you want, for the rest of your life. While this suggestion might scare the heck out of you, releasing yourself from restriction and deprivation enables you to become more connected with your physical nutritional needs rather than being driven by emotional triggers.

Take notice of that point in every meal where you have attained satisfaction and feel comfortable stopping—not the point at which you are full, but the point at which you are no longer hungry for the next bite—knowing that you can eat again whenever you like. If you wish to enjoy a treat once in a while (hopefully Primal-approved, but hey—maybe not!), do so with full attention and awareness to the pleasure that every single savored bite gives you. Reject feelings of anxiety, guilt, or rebellion connected to your food choices, and replace them with the idea that you deserve to eat the most delicious, nutritious foods possible.

When it comes to specific meal choices, I prefer to let my taste buds guide me to the most enjoyable and nourishing diet within the broad guidelines of the Primal Blueprint. Forget the scientifically unproven admonitions to eat certain food-type combinations at certain times, or to align your food choices with your racial heritage, body shape, or blood type (I can't remember if my blood is O positive or O negative, but when I eat my Primal Salad most after-noons, my brain always thinks, "Oh, positive!").

Humans have evolved on widely differing diets from settlements all over the globe. While there are certain genetic predispositions to grain or dairy allergies, for example, Primal Blueprint foods satisfy and nourish everyone, regardless of where the last 5 or 500 generations in your bloodline lived or what they ate. Essentially, my goal is for you to become a modern forager with a keen sense of what you need to do (or not do) to thrive day in and day out. When you eat Primal Blueprint style, there is no city you can't travel to, no restaurant you can't negotiate with, no grocery store you can't shop in, and no family holiday you can't endure!

Eating on Grok's Clock

Ever notice how some people freak out if they miss a meal or can't find exactly what they want on a menu? They become irritable and start complaining about being light-headed—as if their world might stop if they don't inhale some calories right away. Ironically, other than a lifetime of cultural socialization and a metabolism they've built to depend on ingested carbs instead of fat, there is no reason skipping a meal should be a big deal. Our ancestors ate sporadically—with continually varied mealtimes and food choices. Given the variables of the seasons and hunting success or failure, they didn't always have enough food or a varied diet. Our genes thrive on intermittent scarcity and can even handle occasional excess. In fact, they expect it.

Our genetic ability to thrive on intermittent eating habits is an important concept to retain, because it unburdens you of having to eat every meal on a set schedule, to balance food groups (meat with starch, grains with protein, etc.), or to align your foods with time-of-day traditions (cereal for breakfast, sandwich for lunch, etc.). Skipping meals, fasting briefly, and simply freeing yourself from an obsessive need to eat three squares or six small meals a day when the clock strikes a particular hour might actually benefit your body. Doing so will align you more closely with your historic genetic experience. Unburdened by the strict and ill-advised "rules" of Conventional Wisdom, eating becomes much simpler and more enjoyable.

On this topic, it's interesting to note that your need to consume calories on a regular schedule will diminish substantially when blood glucose levels are moderated and you start burning fat and ketones more efficiently through low-insulin Primal Blueprint dietary choices. By contrast, if you eat the typical Western diet of 300 to 500 grams of carbohydrates per day (instead of the 100 to 150 from plant sources as suggested by the Primal Blueprint), you are going to experience significant blood glucose fluctuations and corresponding cravings for quick-energy, high-carbohydrate foods. This is perhaps the single quickest and most exciting revelation for converts to the Primal Blueprint eating style. By eliminating sugars, grains, and legumes from your diet and emphasizing Primal foods, you will experience more consistent energy levels and a comfortably diminished appetite. You'll become a fat-burning beast!

> *By eliminating sugars, grains, and legumes from your diet and emphasizing Primal foods, you will experience more consistent energy levels and a comfortably diminished appetite.*

These benefits will be long lasting, but they might take a bit of time to realize. Every once in a while, people commenting on MarksDailyApple.com mention difficulties with energy level swings during the first three weeks of their transition to a Primal eating style. During this transition period, your body expects sugar as fuel (which it's getting less of) but hasn't rediscovered yet how to get the most out of your fat reserves. Don't worry, it will. By limiting carbs (and, hence, lowering insulin) you are sending a new series of hormonal signals to your genes. In turn, they are down-regulating their sugar-burning systems and up-regulating their fat- and keto-burning machinery.

While you may experience a few episodes of light-headedness during the transition, rest assured that the shift will be complete in a few weeks and energy levels will dramatically improve. Meanwhile, grab a handful of macadamia nuts or a cold drumstick to munch on if you get hungry for a snack (I'll detail some of my favorite snack choices in Chapter 4). You should always satisfy your cravings with abundant amounts of approved foods instead of suffering through them with willpower and other flimsy, short-duration weapons. Don't worry, these Primal food choices will totally satisfy you without bringing about a sugar crash later, as will happen when you reach for a bagel. This is due to the high caloric density and slow burn rate of foods high in fat and/or protein (such as meat, fish, fowl, eggs, avocados, butter, coconut products, nuts and seeds, olives, and high-fat dairy products) and the high water and fiber content of vegetables and fruits.

Because modern life is all about schedules, we often find it convenient and enjoyable to eat regular meals. This is fine. I'm simply suggesting you pay more attention to your hunger levels than to the clock. For example, I eat breakfast on most days, but in a wide range of food choices and total calories—based on my appetite, activity level, and the day's schedule. Frequently I will have a huge omelet with four to five eggs, cheese, chopped mushrooms, peppers, onions, and tomatoes, and topped with some bacon and avocado. On other days I will grab some macadamia nuts or make a Primal smoothie to have on the go. Then again, on some days I simply skip breakfast altogether, with no accompanying guilt, hunger pangs, or low blood glucose. As long as you are eating Primally most of the time, it all works well.

When your food choices and meal times are flexible, you feel less stress and more pleasure from your diet. The key is to make informed choices that minimize your exposure to toxic foods and, when you indulge or get off track, allow your body to return quickly to balance. If you enjoy a decadent dessert or a weekend away from healthy food options, simply eat a few low-insulin producing meals in a row and return to regulated energy levels and optimal metabolic function. Even a short walk after a big meal and rich dessert can mitigate the insulin response by diverting glucose from the bloodstream into working muscles.

One Small Scoop for Mankind

When you eat Primal Blueprint style, the consequences of your food choices become crystal clear. Eat right and you have discernibly more energy and health. Stick with it and your body composition goals happen effortlessly. Slide a little bit and you might get halfway to your goal (or less, owing to the vicious cycle of insulin-driven sugar crashes and cravings), have a little less energy, and maybe catch an extra cold or two due to compromised immune function.

Every once in a while, I'll have a lapse in judgment and indulge in something like a small scoop of gourmet ice cream. It tastes delicious for the four minutes it takes to eat it (but not quite up to par with a bowl of fresh blueberries and raspberries with whipped cream), but invariably I experience bloating and gas in the ensuing hour as well as a bit of a sugar crash. Because these lapses are out of my normal habit pattern, I am highly sensitive to the consequences of choices like these.

Understand that I enjoy the taste of ice cream as much as anyone, but I will assert my position that after eating Primally for some time, even the occasional treat that's not Primal Blueprint approved—for me—is just not worth it. I don't mean to come off as a food Nazi. I assure you that I'm tempted frequently, and in the future will certainly indulge, in a non-Primal manner again (and again after that…). I'm merely trying to illustrate how, once you're sensitized to the negative effects of unhealthy choices, it gets easier to turn down what used to seem impossible to resist. This is especially true when you clearly understand the consequences of each and every food choice that you make, whether they are aligned with your primal genes or not.

When you use defense mechanisms like "everything in moderation," "you only live once," and the like, you disguise the fact that over years and decades, those little ice cream outings can add up literally to hundreds of pounds of ingested substances that are toxic to your body. Furthermore, as unhealthy food choices ingrain themselves (pun intended) into your daily life, I believe you become desensitized to the negative effects they have on your health. This concept is illustrated by heavy tobacco or caffeine users who are able to function somewhat normally (that's not saying much) with volumes of chemicals in their bloodstream that would floor the casual user or teetotaler.

The complete lack of regimentation or caloric deprivation in the Primal Blueprint eating style (I refuse to use the word diet because it implies regimentation) is the secret to its long-term success. You don't have to force yourself to go hungry or to feel deprived or negative about eating. Simply make sensible choices by welcoming the abundant selection of delicious foods whenever you want, and transition out of habitually consuming foods that may taste great for a brief moment but make your body feel bad or create long-term metabolic stress.

Dealing with the (Maybe Radical) Change to Primal Blueprint Eating

If you argue that life will never be the same without your bowl of Raisin Bran® or a heaping plate of pasta and garlic bread, try these suggestions:

80 Percent Rule: Do the best you can, taking your transition step-by-step at a comfortable pace and relieving yourself from the pressure of perfection. Be sure that your indulgences are sensible, as I detail in Chapter 4. Over time, you will naturally and comfortably become more compliant, particularly with the restriction and elimination of grains, sugars, and legumes.

Build Momentum: As you continue to make progress eating the way you were designed to eat, you will notice a heightened sensitivity to how food affects your body, both positively and negatively. During my years as an athlete, I thought my recurrent digestive bloating and post-meal fatigue were due to hard training or simply the end of a long day—not from subclinical allergic reactions to excessive processed carbohydrates and/or dairy products.

Can you relate to that hyper, racing heart sensation that comes after consuming a sugary dessert? It's probably something that we've been aware of since childhood—a little annoying but no big deal, right? It was only when I started to aggressively clean up my diet a decade ago that my sensitivity went to the next level. What a pleasure it was to leave the dinner table feeling totally satisfied, yet alert and energetic—and not having to unbuckle the belt a notch or two! Passing on dessert took a little getting used to, but I noticed that the sacrifice of a few moments of instant gratification paled in comparison to not having to deal with sugar highs and sugar crashes. Plus, as you cut out simple carbs, you begin to lose your craving for them. Hence, you escape the vicious cycle that befalls even those with tremendous willpower trying to do the right thing but eating the wrong stuff.

Five Favorite Meals Strategy: Pick your five favorite Primal Blueprint-approved meals and rotate them for the first three weeks of your transition to Primal Blueprint eating. Maybe it's broiled salmon and steamed broccoli. Lamb chops with grilled zucchini and summer squash. Rotisserie chicken (with the skin—preferably organic) and a large steamed vegetable. As much colorful, creative salad as you want. Liberal snacking on Primal Blueprint-approved snacks. Yes, you are removing the baked potato, corn on the cob, Cheerios®, baguettes, and other beige staples from the picture, but the discomfort of a habit change can be greatly assuaged when you can look forward to as much as you want of your favorite Primal foods during the crucial transition period to the Primal Blueprint eating style.

Never Struggle, Suffer, or Go Hungry: Surround yourself with Primal Blueprint-approved foods and enjoy them as much and as often as you like. Always have a Primal snack nearby to help you through the transition period. That said, pay close attention to your hunger levels and eliminate emotional triggers that negatively influence healthy eating. Stop eating not when you are full—by then you've had too much—but when you are no longer hungry.

Substitute: Consider whether you can switch out some of your old favorite meals, snacks, and even treats for interesting new Primal Blueprint options. I used to be a big blueberry pancakes and granola guy, but whatever deprivation I might have felt at first in eliminating the "stack" from my life was more than made up for by a dozen bites of a delicious Primal omelet. Consider the overall impact of your current favorite foods on your body and if they are all truly worth it. A fine Italian meal of pasta and gelato will please most any palate, but if you feel bloated, gassy, and sleepy in the hours afterward, a better strategy might be to consider some of the many other delicious, Primal Blueprint-approved items on the menu (or off it, from a polite request) at the same restaurant.

Chapter Summary

1. Primal Blueprint Foods: Eat nutritious plants and animal products (the meat, fish, fowl, eggs, nuts, seeds, vegetables, and fruit that have driven human evolution for two million years) and avoid processed foods (sugars, grains) to create a metabolically efficient, nutrient-dense diet. Benefits of Primal Blueprint eating include enhanced cellular function, improved immune and antioxidant function, optimal development and repair of muscle tissue, enhanced fat metabolism and weight management, a reduction in disease risk factors, and a stabilization of daily appetite and energy levels. While Primal eating is low-carb in comparison to the Standard American Diet, it advocates abundant consumption of nutritious carbs such as all vegetables and certain fruits.

2. Insulin is the Master Hormone: Perhaps the most important health benefit of eating Primally is moderating the wildly excessive insulin production of the Standard American Diet. Eighty percent of your ability to achieve body composition success is determined by your diet. When you moderate insulin production, you access and burn stored body fat for energy, preserve or build muscle, and minimize disease risk factors.

When the delicate insulin balance is abused by consuming too many carbs for too long, havoc ensues: cells become insulin resistant, excess glucose is present in the bloodstream, more fat is stored, and it becomes increasingly difficult to mobilize that fat for an energy source. This sets the stage for the development of serious conditions such as Metabolic Syndrome, type 2 diabetes, and heart disease. Synthesis of important hormones, including thyroid hormones, testosterone, and human growth hormone is also hindered by excessive insulin production, creating an accelerated "aging" effect that has more to do with your breakfast choices than chronology. While the long-term effects of excess insulin production are dire, there are also serious immediate drawbacks to consuming high-carb snacks or meals. The sugar high/insulin release/stress response cycle causes problems with fatigue, mental focus, mood swings, and jitters, resulting in burnout.

3. Cholesterol: Cholesterol is critical to healthy cell structure and numerous metabolic functions. Conventional Wisdom's lipid hypothesis of heart disease is a flawed and narrow perspective on the actual chain of events and risk factors that contribute to heart disease. The lipid hypothesis has been refuted in recent years by the Framingham Heart Study and many other respected studies and experts. The true risk factors are best characterized by the common health condition of Metabolic Syndrome. In many cases, only small, dense LDL causes problems in the arteries, and only when triglycerides are high and systemic inflammation is present. These risk factors are typically a consequence of excessive insulin production, a poor omega-6:omega-3 ratio, and poor exercise habits (either sedentary or too stressful). Furthermore, sufficient levels of HDL, generated by healthy eating and exercise habits, can often mitigate any potential threats from small, dense LDL. Conversely, the primary function of statin drugs—lowering cholesterol levels—does not directly address these risk factors. Statin's purported anti-inflammatory benefits can be easily achieved through diet, exercise, and supplementation, saving the expense and harmful side effects of prescription statin therapy.

4. Healthy Fats: Primal foods provide high levels of the highly touted omega-3 fatty acids, which support healthy cardiovascular, brain, skin, and immune function, and of saturated fats, which promote cellular health and dietary satiety. The optimum ratio of omega-6:omega-3 intake is dangerously out of balance in the modern diet. Efforts should be made to minimize omega-6 intake and bump up omega-3 intake. This helps keep the inflammation response under control and protects against serious disease conditions resulting from uncontrolled inflammation.

5. Macronutrients: Understand the "context of calories" beyond the "calories in, calories out" concept of weight loss maxim. Obtain between 0.7 and 1 gram of protein per pound of lean body weight (range based on activity level) per day to ensure healthy metabolic function and to preserve lean muscle mass. Limit carbohydrate intake to an average of 100 to 150 grams per day (or 50 to 100 grams per day if you seek accelerated fat loss), which will happen automatically when you enjoy plenty of vegetables and fruits and avoid grains, sugars, legumes, and other processed carbs. The Carbohydrate Curve summarizes how various levels of carbs impact your health and weight management success.

With protein and carb intake dialed, fat becomes your main caloric energy variable. Deeply satisfying high-fat foods are a great source of energy and unlikely to make you fat when you moderate insulin production. Conventional Wisdom's prejudice against fat comes from mistakenly attributing the negative effects of processed fats to all fats. Ketones are known as the fourth fuel because they provide an efficient energy source when carbohydrate intake is low. They are a by-product of gluconeogenesis in the liver. Dipping into ketosis now and then is a safe strategy to reduce excess body fat.

6. Eating Well: Enjoy your meals without deprivation, restriction, emotional stress, or other negativity. Choose your favorite foods from the broad list of Primal Blueprint-approved choices and don't obsess about calories, nutrient ratios, regimented mealtimes, or food combinations. Eat

(continued)

Chapter Summary (continued)

until you feel satisfied instead of habitually stuffing yourself until you are full. Realize that your genes evolved to easily handle sporadic eating habits without energy lulls or metabolic slowdowns and can do so after 21 days of reprogramming, allowing you to become a fat- and keto-burning beast!

7. Transitioning to the Primal Blueprint: When adjusting to the Primal Blueprint eating style, discover desirable substitutes (you can rotate them over and over if you like) to avoid feelings of deprivation from discarding old meal choices. Have plenty of Primal Blueprint foods available for snacks and meals so you don't suffer or feel depleted. Follow the 80 Percent Rule by being compliant 80 percent of the time and not stressing about perfection. Notice your heightened sensitivity to how foods affect your body, and leverage that awareness to stay on the path of high-energy, effortless weight management and optimal gene expression with Primal Blueprint foods.

CHAPTER 4

Primal Blueprint Law #1: Eat Plants and Animals

(Insects Optional)

In This Chapter

I detail the health benefits of eating Primal Blueprint style and how to choose the best products in the food categories of animal foods (meat, fish, fowl, and eggs), vegetables, fruits, macadamia nuts, herbs and spices, moderation foods (coffee; high-fat dairy; other nuts, seeds, and nut butters; supplemental carbs, water), sensible indulgences (red wine, dark chocolate), and certain high-quality nutritional supplements (multivitamin/mineral/antioxidant formula, omega-3 oil, probiotics, protein powder, and vitamin D).

Locally grown, pesticide-free, or certified organic vegetables and fruits are the most nutritious and safest. They are packed with antioxidants and micronutrients that support health and help prevent disease. Some moderation is warranted with fruit to emphasize locally grown, in-season, high antioxidant fruits, such as berries, and avoid excessive year-round consumption. Local, pasture-raised, or certified organic animal foods are healthy and nutritious and will help you reduce excess body fat and build lean muscle. They are free from the offensive ingredients (hormones, pesticides, and antibiotics) and processing methods found with mass-produced foods. Eggs are healthy and nutritious. They have been mistakenly maligned due to the flawed assumption that their high-cholesterol content is a heart disease risk factor. The budget increase for buying local or organic plant and animal products pales in comparison to the importance of leading a healthy life and avoiding disease risk factors.

If we're not supposed to eat animals, how come they're made out of meat?
—Tom Snyder

If you are trying to memorize the most important, life-changing sound bites from the Primal Blueprint, here's another one: animals (meat, fish, fowl, and eggs) and plants (vegetables, fruits, nuts, seeds, and herbs and spices) should represent the entire composition of your diet. While vegetables, fruits, and herbs and spices don't provide a ton of calories, they should represent your main source of healthy carbohydrates and micronutrients (vitamins, minerals, antioxidants, anti-inflammatory agents, and thousands of other phytonutrients). Animal foods are calorically dense, stimulate minimal insulin production, offer the best forms of healthy protein and fat, and should represent the bulk of your caloric intake.

In Grok's time, the bulk of calories in the human diet (estimates range from 45 to 85 percent, depending on geography) came from eating a variety of animal life, including insects, grubs, amphibians, birds, eggs, fish and shellfish, small mammals, and some larger mammals. In general, those living closer to the equator consumed more plants and less animal food, while those at colder latitudes with fewer plant options consumed more meat.

These meat sources provided significant amounts of protein and all types of essential fatty acids and vitamins. Grok often ate as much as 300 or 400 grams of protein and up to 200 or more grams of fat in a day during times of plenty—and yet maintained a svelte physique. Of course, he also ate very limited amounts of carbohydrates, produced moderate levels of insulin, and excelled at using stored fat as fuel. These macronutrient breakdowns allowed him to build or preserve muscle and provided ample fuel for both long treks and short bursts of speed.

Animal foods are healthy and nutritious and will help you reduce excess body fat, build lean muscle, and generally promote peak performance. While I highly respect those who have philosophical objections to consuming animal flesh, it must be asserted that the Conventional Wisdom suggesting animal foods are directly correlated with obesity and heart disease, or that vegetarianism is somehow healthier, is grossly inaccurate. Like it or not, our bodies have evolved for two million years on animal foods, ever since meat eating became a survival factor and a trigger to population expansion on earth (our ability to migrate to the higher latitudes depended on us developing "meat-adaptive" genes).

Primal Blueprint Food Pyramid

for effortless weight loss, vibrant health, and maximum longevity

Herbs, Spices, Extracts
High-antioxidant/nutritional value

Sensible Indulgences
Dark chocolate, red wine

Supplements
Multi, omega-3, probiotics, protein/meal powder, vitamin D

Moderation Foods

Fruits - Locally grown, in-season, high-antioxidant (berries, pitted fruit)
High-Fat Dairy - Raw, fermented, unpasteurized
Starchy Tubers, Quinoa, Wild Rice - Athlete's carb option
Other Nuts, Seeds and Nut Butters - Great snack option

Healthy Fats

Animal fats, butter & coconut oil (cooking)
Avocados, coconut products, olives & olive oil, macadamias (eating)

Vegetables

Locally grown and/or organic. Abundant servings for flavor, nutrition and antioxidants.

Meat • Fish • Fowl • Eggs

Bulk of dietary calories: saturated fat (energy, satiety, cell & hormone function)
and protein (building blocks, lean mass). Emphasize local, pasture-raised or certified organic.

Revisions to pyramid since 2009 hardcover:

Macadamia nuts: Elevated above other nuts and seeds due to concerns about moderating omega-6 intake. Other nuts and seeds have unfavorable O6:O3 ratios.

Meat, Fish, Fowl, Eggs: Moved to base as primary calorie source. "Emphasize local, pasture raised": Local is superior to organic since organic animals likely have grain-supplemented diets (more popularity, more mass production elements), lowering nutritional value, versus the diets of pastured animals.

Vitamin D: Added to supplements to respect the challenges of obtaining adequate sunlight year-round outside the tropics.

Other: Quinoa added as supplemental carb (it's a chenopod, not a grain; good nutritional value, no anti-nutrients). More attention to avocado, coconut, and olives. Less emphasis on fruit (easy to overdo, especially when trying to reduce fat).

The fact remains that no culture or society has ever survived for an extended period of time on a meatless diet. While it would seem to be much easier to live and evolve without having to run around and kill animals, the truth is that we need the concentrated, nutrient-rich energy source of meat to support accelerated brain development—our distinguishing feature that brought us to the top of the food chain.

Remarkably, about 500 calories a day are required just to fuel the human brain (both primitive and modern brains). Anthropological evidence strongly suggests that it was saturated fats, protein, and omega-3 fatty acids from animal foods that provided both the raw materials and energy necessary for the human brain to grow larger and more sophisticated over the course of evolution. Our ability to catch and cook meat (cooking makes meat easier to chew, swallow, and digest) was critical in our branching up and away from our mostly vegetarian ape cousins.

At this point in our discussion, it's important to acknowledge that over the past decade, some studies about red meat consumption have prompted alarming headlines that "excessive" consumption of red meat may be associated with a slightly increased risk for cancer and heart disease. In all such studies to date, however, there has been no distinction or separation between groups that consumed local, pasture-raised, or certified organic red meat and the vast majority of participants who ate the standard hormone-laden, grain-fed, antibiotic-laced meats mass-produced by Concentrated Animal Feeding Operations (CAFO). Nor has there been any evaluation of the negative effects of excessive carbohydrate intake in the Standard American Diet when it comes to how we metabolize meat (remember that carbs and fats consumed together increase triglyceride production in the liver). Furthermore, most of these studies (in which participants self-report their dietary intake) include in the general red meat category all manner of popular processed meats (hot dogs, breakfast sausage, chemically-treated jerkys, bacon, bologna, salami, etc.), which generally contain nitrosamines and other potential carcinogens. These agents have been shown to accelerate the formation and growth of cancer cells throughout the body. Of course, the Primal Blueprint suggests that you avoid those meats entirely.

Authors of these studies also offer another possible explanation for the increase risks: overcooking of meat. You may have heard that some forms of seared, burned, or overcooked meat may contain heat-altered chemical by-products called heterocyclic amines (or HCAs) that may be carcinogenic if consumed frequently over long periods of time. Since mankind has been cooking with fire for hundreds of thousands of years, it's apparent that we have developed a host of natural genetic adaptations to allow us to eat most properly cooked foods without problems. Furthermore, some studies indicate that consuming antioxidant-rich foods (such as vegetables, fruits; herbs and spices, and even red wine and dark chocolate) along with cooked meats can essentially neutralize any potentially harmful by-products of overcooking. Of course, the Primal Blueprint would argue that eating only "clean" meats, avoiding nitrosamine-laden processed meats, using appropriate cooking techniques (like slow-roasting, undercooking, or using crock pots or sous-vide cookers), enjoying a variety of different forms of animal foods, eschewing deep-fried or high-heat barbequed meats, or eating certain forms of meat raw (sushi, tartar, etc.), will likely eliminate any possible risk altogether.

While it's indisputable that our bodies thrive on the rich and unique nutrients provided by animal foods, it is possible—albeit pretty darn difficult—to be healthy and enjoy a nutritious diet without consuming meat. However, it will be a real challenge to obtain sufficient protein and fat—or simply enough calories—to fuel an active lifestyle while also avoiding grains, sugars, and legumes, foods that by choice or default constitute a high percentage of calories for vegetarians and vegans. If you shoot for moderate or high grain consumption in an effort to make up for the absence of meat, you are probably going to encounter a host of possible health challenges.

> *Animals (meat, fish, fowl, and eggs)
> and plants (vegetables, fruits, nuts, seeds,
> and herbs and spices) should represent
> the entire composition of your diet.*

Animal fats used in cooking (butter, chicken fat, lard, tallow) have long been maligned by Conventional Wisdom in the movement toward polyunsaturated fatty acids (PUFAs) that has spanned the last few generations. However, saturated fats (solid at room temperature, unlike PUFAs) are the most beneficial fats with which to cook. While they are not teeming with micronutrients, and you may wish to limit them somewhat in favor of more densely nutritious calorie sources (such as the meat or vegetables you might be cooking!), they are not at all bad for you, as we've been conditioned to believe.

In contrast, PUFAs become easily oxidized when heated, contain too much omega-6, and are a strong contributor to the oxidation and inflammation conditions detailed in Chapter 3. The sidebar "Primal-Approved Fats and Oils" later in this chapter lists my favorite fats and oils, as well as which ones to avoid.

Brightly colored vegetables and fruits supply high levels of antioxidants that are critical to good health. The flavonoids, carotenoids, and myriad other important phytonutrients found in these foods can serve as a powerful first line of defense against oxidative damage from aging, stress, and inflammation. Moreover, antioxidants and other phytonutrients appear to contain cancer-fighting properties, support immune function, aid in digestion, and help preserve muscle mass, a critical longevity component for those of advanced age.

While leading a healthy, balanced lifestyle will activate the genes that make our built-in antioxidant systems (catalase, superoxide dismutase, and glutathione) fight hard against cellular and DNA breakdown, research suggests that we may require additional antioxidant support from foods and supplements. Of course, most processed foods, meats, and starchy carbohydrates are devoid of antioxidants, while vegetables, fruits, and nuts are the best sources of these natural antioxidants.

Remember the discussion of oxidation as a central heart disease component? Well, antioxidants protect against oxidative damage in the body. It follows that if you want to be healthy and prevent disease, vegetables (and fruits, with a bit of moderation and selectivity) must play a prominent role in your diet. It is also apparent that modern food-processing methods, which include growing produce in soil bereft of important minerals, and the widespread use of pesticides, may further hamper our efforts to get enough antioxidants. Consequently, many people may benefit from a prudent supplement program.

For a quick primer, red plants (pomegranates, cherries, watermelon) have been shown to help reduce the risk of prostate cancer as well as some tumors. Green fruit and vegetables (avocados, limes, bell peppers, zucchini) are high in carotenoids that have a powerful antiaging effect and are especially helpful for vision. Yellow and orange fruits and vegetables (bananas, papayas, carrots, butternut squash, pineapple) offer beta-carotene for immune support as well as bromelain, which has been shown to aid in digestion, joint health, and the reduction of inflammatory conditions. Cruciferous ("cross"-shaped, with a branch and leaves) vegetables, including broccoli, Brussels sprouts, kale, arugula, turnips, bok choy, horseradish, and cauliflower, have demonstrated specific anticancer, antiaging, and antimicrobial properties. Nuts and seeds provide high levels of beneficial unsaturated fatty acids, fiber, phytonutrients, antioxidants (e.g., vitamin E and selenium), and a host of essential nutrients (e.g., manganese, magnesium, zinc, iron, chromium, phosphorous, and folate).

Plant foods also naturally promote a beneficial balance between acidity and alkalinity (also known as "base" or non-acidic balance) in your bloodstream. Almost all cells prefer a slightly alkaline environment to function properly, but many metabolic processes, including the normal production of cellular energy, result in the release of acidic waste products. The buildup of acidic waste is toxic to your body, so it works very hard at all times to preserve a slightly alkaline environment, measured by the familiar "pH" levels. While we have evolved several highly refined buffering systems to balance our pH, ingesting too many acid-producing foods and not enough alkaline-forming foods makes it that much more difficult to achieve pH homeostasis.

As you might guess, heavily processed foods, sugars, grains, deep-fried foods, alcohol, caffeine, cigarettes, carbonated drinks, artificial sweeteners, and many recreational and prescription drugs are acid-forming in the body, a precursor to many health problems and diseases. In contrast, by eating sufficient amounts of alkaline-forming foods—vegetables, fruits, nuts, and seeds—you optimize your acid/base balance and improve metabolism to burn fat, build muscle, and reduce your susceptibility to environmental and dietary toxins. Meat and dairy products also happen to be acid-forming, making it essential to balance the intake of these foods with sufficient vegetables and fruits that support alkalinity.

Meat and Fowl

Many of the Conventional Wisdom health objections to eating animal foods can easily be countered by eating local, pasture-raised, 100 percent grass-fed, or certified organic sources of meat. This suggestion is highly recommended due to the generally poor quality of much of today's mass-produced feedlot animals, which typically contain hormones (to grow them bigger quickly and therefore increase profits), pesticides (ingested from their own inferior food sources; vegetarian advocates claim that 80 to 90 percent of your total dietary pesticide exposure comes from eating meat, although that's disputed by the EPA), and antibiotics (to prevent widespread illness resulting from consuming immune-suppressing feed and living in filthy, cramped feedlots and coops). Hormones, pesticides, and antibiotics: these three stooges can really mess up your efforts to eat in a healthy manner.

Furthermore, today's feedlot cattle, chickens, and other animals are usually fed a diet of fortified grains, which have a similar effect on their bodies as on a human's! Purchase your meats at a chain grocer or big-box store, and there's a good chance you'll end up eating a malnourished, insulin-resistant, and quite possibly diseased animal whose meat is higher in omega-6 fats—a far cry nutritionally from Grok's fresh, lean, wild kills. Finally, humane reasons compel many to avoid meat. The animals we typically dine on consume half of our crop harvest; their waste pollutes air, rivers, and streams; and many claim they are subjected to horrifying treatment at unsanitary production facilities (as detailed in such books as *Fast Food Nation, The Omnivore's Dilemma, Diet for a New America*, and even *Skinny Bitch*).

> " *My favorite animal is steak.* "
> —**Fran Lebowitz**

For these reasons, I strongly urge you to look for local sources of pasture-raised meat whenever possible—typically found at farmer's markets. If local, pasture-raised meats are not available, the next best alternative is USDA certified organic. Clearly, there is a continuum here where you can find options that are various degrees away from ideal. While the ultimate meat would be a wild animal with lots of lean mass, and a nutritious, high omega-3 natural diet, there aren't many of them running around the continent these days. Beyond local, pasture-raised animals from small farms or USDA certified organic animals, there is minimal regulation in this industry, and assorted other descriptors such as "free-range" and "all-natural" have only minimal significance (more details in the "Meet and Greet For Your Meat" Sidebar).

Fortunately, the popularity of eating locally and/or organic is skyrocketing, so you should have good luck finding healthier animal products in your area. If not, you can utilize some of the excellent resources on the Internet, such as americangrassfedbeef.com and eatwild.com. Besides being free of hormones, pesticides, and antibiotics, pasture-raised animals offer two to six times more omega-3 and monounsaturated fats than feedlot animals do. If, for reasons of budget or availability, you find yourself eating a less-than-ideal source of meat, always choose the leanest possible cuts and simply trim the excess fat. This will significantly limit your potential exposure to these toxins. Of course, you can add back some delicious fat by cooking the now leaner meat in butter!

A Little Meet and Greet for Your Meat

Following are brief descriptions of common labels on meat products to help you make informed purchasing decisions. Many of the terms have no official designation or are not regulated in a meaningful manner.

Local, Pasture-Raised: The premier choice for meat; the ultimate in sustainability and minimal carbon footprint. A locally raised chicken, cow, or lamb grazing in the open pasture consumes a variety of grass, grubs, worms, and bugs that are rich in nutrients such as omega-3 fatty acids and assorted vitamins and minerals that are deficient in CAFO animals.

Certified Organic: Raised on grass or grain feed without antibiotics, hormones, genetic engineering, irradiation, sewage sludge, or artificial ingredients and afforded "conditions which allow for exercise, freedom of movement, and reduction of stress appropriate to the species." Suppliers are subject to regular inspection by USDA-approved third parties. Animals may not be locally raised (and in fact may have traveled a great distance to your market) and have possibly received grain-based feed to supplement calories obtained on the free range. This results in a slightly-to-significantly less optimal nutritional profile than a 100 percent pasture-raised/grass-fed animal.

Certified: USDA evaluated the meat for class, grade, or other quality characteristics (e.g., Certified Angus Beef).

Chemical-Free: This vague term is not defined or recognized by the USDA and has virtually no significant meaning on a package.

Conventional: Absent any special label designations, you are likely buying a mass-produced animal raised on feedlot grains with pesticide residues, growth hormones, and antibiotics. Such animals are often treated inhumanely.

Country of Origin Labeled (COOL): Specifies where the animal was raised, slaughtered, and processed—sometimes including multiple locations (USDA regulated). As with produce, local products are preferred.

Free Range: Applies to poultry only, indicating animal was given "access" to outdoors. Has no legal definition or third-party verification and is often abused by growers. "Access" can refer to a large indoor facility (where animals have been conditioned to remain) with a door to a small outdoor area. No guarantee that meat is free from hormones and antibiotics.

Fresh: Implies that the meat has not been frozen (internal temperature dropping below 26 degrees Fahrenheit) prior to sale; no relevance to how animal was raised, fed, or slaughtered, and not third-party verified.

Grass-Fed, Grass-Finished, Pasture-Raised, Pasture-Finished, etc.: Animals afforded access to grass, but no guarantee of grain-free diet unless a "100 percent" qualifier appears on label. Even then, no guarantee that meat is free from hormones or antibiotics. Terms are not regulated or third-party verified and are thus inferior to USDA certified organic.

Hormone/Antibiotic Free: No legal definition or third party verification. Suggests an improvement from conventional products, but inferior to USDA certified organic.

Humane Designations: Animal Welfare Approved, American Humane Certified, Certified Humane Raised & Handled, or Free Farmed are common terms. The first designation, from the Animal Welfare Institute, certifies that animals were treated humanely throughout all life stages. Their designation (and the others) has strict standards for outdoor access; diets free of hormones, pesticides, or antibiotics; and freedom from overcrowded conditions. Furthermore, the terms are third-party verified. Humane certified animals are probably a suitable choice in the absence of local or USDA-certified organic meat.

Kosher: Meats prepared under rabbinical supervision and guidelines. The designation relates more to slaughtering methods, segregation of implements and production facilities (meat cannot be mixed with dairy products, etc.), and other factors that may or may not be related to health quality.

Natural: Meat free of artificial flavors, colorings, and preservatives. No relevance to how animal was raised, fed, or slaughtered, and not third-party verified.

Vegetarian Diet: This pertains to the animal's diet only and does not guarantee that the animal had access to pasture or humane treatment.

Fish

Fish offer a rich source of omega-3 fatty acids (particularly the important omega-3 fractions known as DHA and EPA that are not present in most other foods), complete protein, B complex vitamins, selenium, vitamin D, vitamin E, zinc, iron, magnesium, phosphorous, antioxidants, and other nutrients. A 2006 study by the Harvard School of Public Health indicated that regular consumption of fish helps dramatically reduce the risk of heart disease and that the benefits (particularly the omega-3 content) outweigh the potential risks of ingesting toxins from polluted waters.

Regular consumption of fish has been shown to exert a strong anti-inflammatory effect, reduce risk for heart disease, help protect against asthma in children, moderate chronic lung disease, reduce the risk of breast and other cancers by stunting tumor growth, and ease the symptoms of rheumatoid arthritis and certain bone and joint diseases. Nursing and pregnant women enjoy a host of benefits from fish consumption, including support for fetal and early childhood brain and retinal development and a lowered risk of premature birth.

While the benefits of eating fish are substantial, you should learn to choose wisely to avoid fish possibly tainted with environmental toxins, and to steer clear of certain farmed species that you should never eat (some farmed species are fine; we'll cover the particulars shortly). The risk of ingesting fish tainted by environmental contaminants (heavy metals such as mercury, polychlorinated biphenyls [PCBs], dioxins, and other toxins) can be countered by emphasizing fish caught by domestic operations in remote, pollution-free ocean waters. The healthiest sources of fish are small, oily cold water fish, such as wild-caught Alaskan salmon, sardines, herring, anchovies, and mackerel.

Certain fish at the top of the marine food chain, such as swordfish and shark, should be limited or avoided due to their tendency to accumulate concentrated contaminants. However, the popular refrain to limit fish intake due to mercury poisoning concerns has been exaggerated. The Western Pacific Regional Fishery Management Council, based in Hawaii, asserts that most every Pacific Ocean fish except sword and shark contain substantially high enough levels of selenium (a potent antioxidant) to negate concerns about mercury toxicity. "Our favorite fish are more likely to protect against mercury toxicity than cause it," according to the Council.

The reason to avoid some species of farmed fish is that they are often raised under unsanitary conditions similar to those of ranch animals, and exposed to high levels of dangerous chemicals, such as dioxins, dieldrin, toxaphene, and other pesticides or toxic residue. These chemicals (from contaminated sediments in their fish meal) are easily absorbed into fat cells. Farmed fish may be routinely exposed to their own waste and are often fed artificial dyes (to match color with wild varieties; e.g., wild salmon derive their pink color from the healthy carotene astaxanthin in their natural diet) and antibiotics to ward off the high risk of infection and disease from living in cramped farms. The waste from a large salmon farm is estimated to equal the sewage from a city of 10,000 people. A 2004 report in the popular journal *Science* warned that farmed salmon contained 10 times the amount of toxins of wild salmon and should be eaten rarely—once every five months—due to their high cancer risk. Hey, *Science*—how about never?

While wild salmon offers 19 to 27 percent of its total fat in omega 3s, farmed Atlantic salmon (by far the most common farmed species) contains significantly less omega-3s, less protein, and much higher levels of omega-6 fats (obtained from their commercial feed, unlike the omega-3-rich algae that nourishes wild fish). Of additional concern is the estimated three million salmon that escape from their pens into the ocean each year, contaminating and genetically diluting nearby wild salmon (farmers' daughters sneaking out to fool around with wild boys from out of town—what else is new?).

Use discretion and look for wild Alaskan salmon, even if your budget requires that you choose less expensive frozen fish at times. You can also look for farmed coho salmon as a healthy, budget-friendly alternative, especially from fresh water tanks. Avoid Atlantic farmed salmon (ask your waiter; sorry, it's probably Atlantic) due to concerns about industrial and environmental contamination and inferior nutritional value.

Having warned you of the risks of some types of farmed fish, I can also assert that there are certain other categories of farmed fish with minimal toxin levels and superior nutritional profiles that make them acceptable to consume. You just have to do a little homework. If you do choose to eat farmed fish, insist on domestic sources to alleviate the risk posed by polluted waters and lax chemical regulations in high-producing countries such as China. Barramundi, catfish, crayfish, and tilapia from domestic farms have impressive nutritional profiles and minimal toxin risks. Farmed trout from the United States or Canada is nutritionally comparable with wild trout, with minimal contaminant concerns, making it another sensible choice. Farmed shellfish are okay because they don't eat artificial foods and have similar living circumstances as wild shellfish—i.e., they are attached to a fixed object. However, make a strong effort to eat fresh over frozen shellfish.

If you are wild about salmon and willing to endure the trade-off of a big carbon footprint and substantial expense to get a quality product, you can do your shopping online at such Web sites as wildpacificsalmon.com, seabeef. com, jdockseafood.com, or vitalchoice.com. The first site, wildpacificsalmon. com, offers a choice of a half-dozen different species, all caught in Alaska and shipped across the United States via FedEx next-day in vacuum-packed, cold-insulated containers. This site also features extensive details about the benefits of eating wild salmon and the dangers of eating farmed salmon.

For smart shopping, cultivate a relationship with a local dedicated fish market or farmer's market vendor. Fish from a specialty vendor is more likely to be fresh than grocery store fare. Take aggressive, close-up sniffs of the offerings. Odor should be nonexistent for fresh water fish and perhaps a faint ocean smell for salt water fish. Bad fish will have the unmistakable smell of, well, bad fish. Inquire about the source of the fish and stay away from Chinese or Asian imports, both farmed and wild-caught.

Finally, be advised that the safety, quality, and sustainability of fish are in constant flux. Check resources such as the Marine Stewardship Council, Monterey Bay Aquarium Seafood Watch (montereybayaquarium.org) and the Environmental Defense Fund (edf.com) for up-to-date information.

> *"Most farmed fish should be avoided because they are raised in unsanitary, waste-infested waters; have dangerous chemical additives in their diets; and offer much lower levels of omega-3s than their wild counterparts."*

Eggs

Eggs can be freely enjoyed as an excellent source of healthy protein, fat, B complex vitamins, and folate. Be sure to obtain local, pasture-raised, or organic chicken eggs, which contain up to 20 times more omega-3s than factory-produced, grain-fed chicken eggs. The popular Conventional Wisdom "heart-healthy" concept of discarding the yolk to avoid cholesterol is misguided, as the yolk is one of the most nutrient-rich foods you can find—laden with omega-3s and the other aforementioned nutrients. In contrast, egg whites, besides being a good source of complete protein, have otherwise a rather low nutrient content. Furthermore, and contrary to Conventional Wisdom, there is no proof that eggs have anything to do with blood cholesterol or your risk for heart disease.

A Harvard Medical School study of 115,000 subjects over the span of 8 to 14 years demonstrated no correlation between egg consumption and heart disease or stroke. A 2008 study published in the *International Journal of Obesity* suggests that eating two eggs for breakfast (not just the whites—the whole deal) is healthier than eating a bagel. Your local farmer's market should be teeming with pasture-raised eggs. Otherwise, most quality grocers, health food stores, co-ops, and national chains (e.g., Trader Joe's and Whole Foods Market) stock abundant sources of organic eggs. If you have trouble finding organic eggs near you, visit localharvest.org and perform a zip code search.

" Eliminating processed or packaged foods and bottled beverages and growing your own fruits and vegetables can reduce your budget and improve your dietary quality. "

Going Primal on a Dime

I understand that buying organic animal products can be cost-prohibitive. I will accept—proudly—criticism of the Primal Blueprint as an "elitist" diet, and elaborate on this philosophical issue in Chapter 9. For now, I'll stand as a strong advocate for healthy living and getting your priorities straight, including budgeting for the best foods you can afford—even if this means your diet potentially (but not necessarily, if you do a little legwork) becomes more expensive and cumbersome.

If you sharply cut back or eliminate processed carbohydrates from your diet, you avoid the vast majority of the high-cost (and high-profit), low-nutritional-value products in the store. Shifting from bottled waters, juices, and all manner of sweetened beverages to a simple water-filtration system in your home can save money and improve dietary quality. Switching from designer foods such as synthetic energy bars and meal replacements (Kelly Korg spends about 70 bucks a month on her twice-daily Slim-Fast shakes) to such basics as trail mix, jerky, or farm-fresh eggs can also reduce your budget while improving dietary quality.

Consider growing your own fruits and vegetables in your backyard garden or renting a patch in an urban community garden. Perhaps there is even a co-op or farmers' market in your area where you can trade time for food? "Cowpooling" (divvying up a butchered local animal amongst friends) can also be economical. Ultimately, clever Primal purchasing strategies can get you close to break even with your "before" Primal Blueprint grocery expenses.

Even the most vocal complainers about high-priced local or organic food might benefit from examining their discretionary purchases and moving healthy food up the priority list. You have the right and also the obligation—to yourself and your loved ones—to pursue the absolute highest dietary quality possible. Yes, it may require more time, energy, and even expense, but the payoff is arguably greater than that of any other lifestyle change you ponder (new TV, new car, new clothes, vacation, etc.). And not to sound trite, but an investment in your health today pays dividends far greater and far longer than you might ever see in your 401(k).

Now that I've climbed down off my soapbox, let's admit that real-world concerns may have you falling short here and there of the ideal spelled out in these pages. It's important to default back to the big-picture view that the Primal Blueprint is a way of life, not a boot camp. If you are agonizing over which fruit stimulates less insulin or you find yourself eating conventional hamburger at the company picnic, yet are diligent enough to toss the buns in the garbage before you dig in, congratulations are in order for the momentum and awareness you have already created. Every step you take toward living Primally puts you that much closer to your health and fitness goals—and makes you that much more adept at righting the course when the inevitable deviations happen.

Vegetables

It is preferable to select locally grown, in-season, organic vegetables whenever possible. The shiny, buffed-up vegetables on display in our local supermarkets are typically cultivated in an objectionable manner—sprayed with pesticides, picked too early (and then artificially ripened by exposure to ethylene gas), jet-lagged from their distant origins (thumbs-down from a green perspective), and even genetically modified to grow bigger and more colorful, albeit at the cost of being less nutritious.

It may take some acclimation to center your diet around vegetables, as we are so accustomed to reaching for packaged, high-carbohydrate snacks as a first option. Don't follow the example of restaurants that serve skimpy vegetable portions seemingly just for decoration; serve yourself heaping portions that crowd everything else on your plate! Enjoy vegetables raw, steamed, baked, or grilled—even slathered in butter if you like. Cook or slice up extra portions for easy preparation or snacking the following day. Reject your attachment to cultural meal traditions centered on starches or grains and get wild and colorful with your meals. Have some steamed carrots and beets with your eggs for breakfast or kale, squash, and chicken for lunch. Try some of the many delicious vegetable-focused recipes at MarksDailyApple.com, *The Primal Blueprint Cookbook*, or the *Primal Blueprint Quick and Easy Meals*. Grab some stuff you've never tried before and ask your grocer about the best preparation methods.

While virtually all vegetables offer excellent nutritional value, some offer particularly high levels of antioxidants. One of the best objective resources to determine the antioxidant power of any vegetable, fruit, herb, or other food is the USDA's ORAC (Oxygen Radical Absorbance Capacity) report. I like to aim for at least 10,000 ORAC units a day, which is easily obtained from a few servings of the top fruits and vegetables (the USDA recommends a much lower number, between 3,000 and 5,000 per day). Here (in alphabetical order, not rank order. Don't worry—they're all gold medal winners) is a list of some of the highest antioxidant vegetables. Make a special effort to include these regularly in your meals:

1. Avocado
2. Beets
3. Broccoli
4. Brussels sprouts
5. Carrots
6. Cauliflower
7. Eggplant
8. Garlic
9. Kale
10. Onion
11. Red bell pepper
12. Spinach
13. Yellow squash

If, for reasons of budget or availability, you decide to eat conventionally grown produce, note the varying levels of residue exposure depending on the item. Be particularly careful to avoid conventional sources of vegetables that have a large surface area (leafy greens, including spinach and lettuce, are treated with some of the most potent pesticides) or a skin that is consumed (bell peppers are perhaps the most pesticide-tainted vegetable; also avoid conventional celery, cucumbers, green beans, winter squash, and carrots). If you do find yourself purchasing these, be sure to soak and/or rinse them with soap or a fruit/vegetable wash solution, which you can find in any health food store.

Macadamia Nuts

Macadamia nuts earn a distinction above other nuts and seeds because of their superior nutritional value. They are predominantly monounsaturated fat (84 percent—more than any other nut or seed), which is less likely to be stored as fat, and helps raise HDL and lower LDL. They have the most favorable O6:O3 ratio of any nut (actually with minimal amounts of both). Since they are mostly monounsaturated fat, macadamias contain minimal amounts of the omega-6 fatty acids that we are looking to minimize.

Macadamias contain all the essential amino acids, various forms of healthy fiber, high levels of vitamins, minerals, and plant nutrients, and only trace amounts of carbohydrate. The flavenoids and tocopherols in macadamia nuts offer excellent antioxidant properties. They have a rich and satisfying taste, making them a great snack. Macadamia nut butter is hard to find, but worth the effort and additional expense. Check out ArtisanaFoods.com for 100-percent raw, organic macadamia/cashew nut butter, and many other nut butters and natural products that are delicious.

Coconut Products

Integrating coconut products (oil, milk, butter, water, flakes, and other derivatives) into your diet provides a variety of health benefits and can conveniently replace SAD foods such as milk, flour, and polyunsaturated cooking oils that can compromise your health. Coconut is an excellent source of a special type of fat—medium-chain fatty acids—that are difficult to find even in a healthy diet. While all vegetable oils comprise some ratio of monounsaturated, polyunsaturated, or saturated fatty acids, there is another classification based on molecular size or length of the carbon chain within each fatty acid. Nearly all oils we consume are classified as long-chain fatty acids. Coconut's distinctive medium-chain composition has been shown to offer protection from heart disease, cancer, diabetes, and many other degenerative illnesses, to improve immune function and fat metabolism, and to protect against liver damage from alcohol and other toxins, and deliver anti-inflammatory and immune-supporting properties.

Nearly one-third of the global population has had coconut as a dietary centerpiece of their traditional diets for centuries. Of particular note are Polynesian cultures that are remarkably free of heart disease despite (or should I say in large part because of) heavy coconut intake and high saturated fat diets. Asia Pacific cultures love the healing properties of coconut and use coconut extensively in their traditional medicine, particularly for skin and digestive conditions since it offers potent antimicrobial properties.

Due to its high saturated fat content, coconut oil is especially resilient to oxidation and free radical formation, even when heated to high temperatures during cooking. Unfortunately, coconut has been maligned along with other saturated fats for several decades, beginning with the Standard American Diet's migration to polyunsaturated oils in the 1960s. Coconut is indeed the most saturated of all vegetable oils; 92 percent saturated, it's solid at room temperature but will liquefy in hot weather. While it may seem like a minor issue, cooking and preparing recipes with coconut oil instead of polyunsaturated oils can be one of the healthiest dietary changes you can make. *The Primal Blueprint Cookbook* and *Primal Blueprint Quick & Easy Meals* have extensive recipes featuring coconut or substituting familiar ingredients (flour, milk, PUFAs) with coconut products.

To get started on the coconut bandwagon, grab a jar of coconut oil at a health food store or elite market and use it for pan frying. Get some coconut milk and use it as a liquid base for smoothies or for replacing dairy milk. Get some coconut flakes and enjoy them in smoothies, sprinkled on salads, or with nuts as a trail mix. On those special occasions when you need a carbohydrate beverage during or after exercise, coconut water is a great choice. Try some coconut manna as a delicious spread on vegetables or dabbed onto some squares of dark chocolate (find at a health food store or elite grocer). Visit MarksDailyApple.com and review the many posts on coconut (including some amazing desserts) as you explore this wonderful new dietary centerpiece.

Mark's Favorite Primal Snacks

Beef Jerky: How Primal can you get? Branch out and try buffalo, turkey, and venison. Choose natural products, not the gas station fare with unhealthy additives.

Celery: Enjoy with cream cheese or macadamia nut butter.

Cottage Cheese: Enjoy with nuts, berries, balsamic vinegar, or other creative toppings.

Dark Chocolate: Any lingering sweet tooth issues relating to your transition to Primal eating can be assuaged with a couple squares of dark chocolate (look for 75 percent or greater cacao content).

Fish: Canned tuna or sardines (yes, packed in oil) can easily replace a full meal for nutrient intake and satiety.

Fresh Berries: Raspberries, blueberries, blackberries, strawberries—all are Grok-like, nutritious, and very satisfying. Add some heavy cream for a good dessert option.

Hard-Boiled Eggs: Sprinkle some salt, spices, and a little olive oil in a ziplock bag and then roll the peeled egg around in the bag for a tasty snack.

Macadamia Nuts: Best Primal health value due to high monounsaturated content (and great taste!)

Other Nuts and Seeds: Almonds, pecans, walnuts; pumpkin, sunflower, sesame seeds; nut butters except peanut butter. Enjoy with some moderation due to O6:O3 ratio goals.

Olives: Great source of monounsaturated fatty acids and a central reason for the compliments lavished on the Mediterranean diet.

Trail Mix: Emphasize nuts and seeds. A little dried fruit or even some dark chocolate chips are okay, but avoid yogurt-covered raisins, M&M's and other high-carb ingredients, and peanuts.

Web Site: MarksDailyApple.com has hundreds of postings for snack and recipe ideas, including some creative make-your-own Primal snacks. We also have dozens of our ever-popular "top 10 lists" for everything you can think of relating to meat, vegetables, fruits, seasonal favorites, recipes, foods to avoid, and healthy dietary habits.

Fruits

While fruits are outstanding sources of fiber, vitamins, minerals, phenols, antioxidants, and other micronutrients, some moderation is warranted for a few reasons. First, modern cultivation and chemical treatments have resulted in fruits that are large, brightly colored, uniformly shaped, and extra sweet, with much less micro-nutrition than the small, varied, highly fibrous, deep-colored, less sugary, and less insulin-stimulating fruits that Grok foraged for. Second, these overly sweetened beauty queens are available year-round thanks to modern growing and transportation methods. Third, fructose, the predominant carbohydrate form contained in fruit, can cause significant metabolic problems when consumed in excess—as can easily happen with year-round availability. This is particularly true when combined with the wildly excessive intake of grains and sugars in the Standard American Diet.

When fructose (the carbohydrate form contained in fruit) is consumed, it's converted in the liver into not only usable carbohydrate in the form of glucose, but also into triglycerides (fat). For heavy exercisers who regularly deplete muscle glycogen, fruit is a great choice to efficiently reload their liver glycogen. On the other hand, if your glycogen stores are already full, as happens when you don't engage in regular short bouts of intense exercise, that Sunday brunch strawberry could just as easily convert into fat in the liver, and then get dumped into the bloodstream.

High blood triglycerides interfere with the function of the hormone leptin, causing you to want to overeat rather than to rely on your stored body fat for energy. Possibly one-third of the population is fructose intolerant to some degree, evidenced by digestive symptoms such as flatulence, cramps, bloating, irritable bowel syndrome, and diarrhea. Excessive fructose consumption is also linked to fatigue, insulin resistance, diabetes, and high blood pressure.

Yep, eating too much fruit can make you fat...even more so than eating too much fat, since at least fat will make you feel full! It's not my desire to scare you away from eating fruit, but simply to help you recognize that fruit is a source of sugar and should generally be consumed in moderation. The most simple and sensible approach is to try and emulate Grok by eating fruits grown locally during their natural local ripening seasons (exceptions granted if you live in a fruit-challenged climate), especially if you are trying to shed excess body fat.

Choosing the Best Fruits

Three major categories that affect fruit quality are growing methods, nutritional value (antioxidant levels as well as how much the sugar content affects your metabolism), and risk of pesticide exposure. The "Fruit Power Rankings" chart in this section details which types of fruits to enjoy in abundance, which to eat in moderation, and which to strictly avoid. Regarding growing methods, organic fruit (or fruit grown locally without the use of pesticides) offers vastly superior nutritional value to conventionally grown fruits. Some experts estimate that organic fruits are 10 times richer in key micronutrients than their conventional counterparts! Organic fruits must manufacture high levels of antioxidants to defend themselves against pests—something conventional fruits don't have to worry about, thanks to their treatment with synthetic herbicides and pesticides.

Organic is not always the be-all and end-all, however. Organic fruits from distant lands are less tasty and nutritious because of their premature picking and long transit time to market. Even if local fruit is not certified organic, your local farmer likely uses less offensive growing methods than do large commercial operations, and the optimum picking time means the fruit has matured to be bursting with great nutrition and taste. Those living in progressive areas with thriving farmer's markets and food co-ops might even encounter fruits designated as wild. As the term conveys, these fruits are as good as it gets…if you can find them. If you are so inclined, you may want to visit seedsavers.org or seedsofchange.com to purchase seeds and plant your own wild-variety fruit trees, berry bushes, and vegetable plants.

> *Year-round availability of overly sweetened fruit can lead to excessive intake and rapid conversion of fructose (the carbohydrate form in fruit) into fat.*

Be strict (particularly with children, due to their substantially higher risk of harm from pesticides) about avoiding conventionally grown fruits with soft, edible skins that are difficult to wash, such as berries. You can be less strict about fruits with tough, inedible skins that peel; they offer a protective barrier against chemical ingestion. If you must eat conventional fruits, wash your fruit thoroughly with soap or a special solution. Avoid genetically modified fruit, a concept that elicits serious health and philosophical concerns and is about as far away from Grok as you can get. Genetically modified organisms (GMOs) have not been subject to sufficient research to guarantee their health and safe ingestion.

Most all fruits offer a host of nutritional benefits, but some (detailed on the chart) are relatively low in antioxidant values while having a high impact on your blood glucose/insulin production. *Paleo Diet* author Loren Cordain, Ph.D., ranks common fruits according to a "Total Metabolic Fructose" (TMF) to take this factor into consideration. Fruits with high TMF scores (sometimes referred to as "high-sugar" or "high glycemic" fruits) warrant moderation, particularly if you are trying to reduce excess body fat.

In light of the popularity of juicing, it's important to note that whole fruits are vastly superior to juice—even the most nutritious, freshly squeezed glass. Juice is generally higher in sugar and lower in many other micronutrients than its produce sources, because juicing eliminates the nutrient-rich skin and fiber and provides a more concentrated, less filling source of carbohydrates than whole foods do. Recall that Kelly Korg's 24-ounce Strawberry Surf Rider smoothie contained 71 grams of sugar. That's like eating 51 large strawberries! (Can you say, *Cool Hand Luke*?) I strongly suggest passing on juice in favor of whole foods.

If your eyes are bouncing up and down the page sorting out which fruits are good and bad, relax! If you've junked sugars, grains, legumes, and PUFAs to become preoccupied with prioritizing your fruit choices, you're progressing nicely. I'm certainly not advocating sitting forlornly off to the side at the Fourth of July picnic, watching others eat the hot dogs, corn on the cob, and watermelon. By all means enjoy the watermelon guilt-free (just forget the former two and smuggle in your own smoked wild salmon for a main course!). Simply use a bit of restraint for certain fruits, particularly if you are pursuing ambitious fat-reduction goals.

Fruit Power Rankings

You can be more selective by considering a fruit's growing methods, pesticide risk, and glycemic/antioxidant values (high-antioxidant, low-glycemic fruits being the best), and TMF scores. Each list is ranked in order of best to worst.

Growing Methods

1. Wild: Hard to find—plant your own or hit the farmer's market!

2. Local organic or pesticide-free: Superior choice for nutritional value, taste, and safety.

3. Local conventional: Superior to remote organic due to freshness and ideal picking time. Wash thoroughly with soap or vegetable solution.

4. Remote organic: Ranks below local conventional due to negative effects of transportation and premature picking.

5. Remote conventional: Avoid due to diminished nutritional value and pesticide risk. (Hint: if it's out of season in your area, don't eat it!)

6. GMO fruit: Don't even think about it. Instead, ask yourself, "What would Grok do?" 'Nuff said.

Nutritional Value:

This list comes from my unscientific blending of antioxidant values, glycemic index values, and total metabolic fructose values. You may find it useful but please default to the big picture—enjoy local, seasonal fruit and ditch grains!

1. Outstanding: High-antioxidant, low-glycemic, low-TMF fruits, including all berries, most stone (pitted) fruits (cherries, peaches, apricots), avocado, casaba melon, lime, lemon, tomato, and guava.

2. Good: Lower-antioxidant, higher-glycemic, medium-TMF fruits, including apples, bananas, cantaloupe, cherries, grapefruit, kiwi, and pomegranates.

3. Moderate or Restrict: Low antioxidant, high-glycemic, higher-TMF fruits, including dates, dried fruits (all), grapes, mangoes, melons, nectarines, oranges, papayas, pineapples, plums, and tangerines.

Pesticide Risk

1. Low risk: Fruit with tough, inedible skin, including bananas, avocados, melons, oranges, tangerines, mandarins, pineapples, kiwis, mangoes, and papayas.

2. High risk: Fruit with soft, edible skin, including apples, apricots, cherries, concentrated juices, grapes, nectarines, peaches, pears, raisins, raspberries, strawberries, and tomatoes.

Mark's Top 10 Favorite Fruits

Naturally, everything on this list assumes a locally grown, pesticide-free, or organic variety. Consult the three previous sections to ensure your pesticide risk is minimized and you otherwise choose the most nutritious fruit possible—and avoid problematic fruits. These are in my personal rank order, but again, anything on this list is great.

1. Blueberries, strawberries, raspberries, blackberries, cranberries, and nearly all other berries
2. Avocados
3. Cherries
4. Apples
5. Peaches
6. Pears
7. Figs
8. Grapefruit
9. Kiwis
10. Apricots

Herbs and Spices

No discussion of healthy eating would be complete without the inclusion of herbs and spices. Although these tasty additions provide minimal calories, they are packed with significant amounts of important micronutrients. Extensive evidence suggests that herbs and spices support cardiovascular and metabolic health, may help prevent cancer and other diseases, and improve mental health and cognition. Some of the highest antioxidant values (from ORAC scores) among all foods can be found in herbs and spices. Certain marinades and herbal preparations are so powerful in their antioxidant capacity that they have been shown to mitigate or eliminate potential issues that may arise from overcooking meat.

Herbs are generally green plants or plant parts used to add flavor to foods. Herbal extracts have been used for thousands of years in Eastern medicine and continue to enjoy widespread popularity today for their powerful immune and health-supporting properties. Spices, on the other hand, are typically dried seeds, fruits, and plant parts. Spices are used to enhance flavor, add color, or help prevent bacterial growth on food.

You can bet that Grok partook of the many varieties of plants he encountered. Throughout history, herbs and spices have played a large role in the human diet and even in culture as a whole. During the Middle Ages, spices were a currency with substantial economic value. Their popularity to enhance flavor and preserve food was the catalyst for the fervent exploration of the globe by such explorers as Marco Polo, Columbus, and Magellan.

The specific health properties of individual herbs and spices could fill an entire book. A couple of headliners that are easy to integrate into everyday meals include curcumin (offers potent anti-inflammatory effects and high antioxidant value) and cinnamon (regulates blood sugar and demonstrates high antibacterial, anti-inflammatory, and antioxidant values). Visit MarksDailyApple.com for extensive coverage of numerous herb and spice benefits.

Moderation Foods

While they may not be exactly what our ancestors ate, moderate consumption of the following foods can add some nutritional benefit to your diet without negative consequences, provided they are not overemphasized. Furthermore, I want to make the Primal Blueprint as accessible and enjoyable to as many people as possible. If you are pursuing ambitious fat-reduction goals, you will probably want to eliminate some of these from the picture.

Coffee

Coffee is fine in moderation, as long as you avoid using caffeine as a crutch to raise energy levels. Proper diet and exercise should enable you to wake up feeling refreshed and energized each morning, and to avoid afternoon blues caused primarily by high-carbohydrate eating habits. Make an effort to drink organic coffee, as many big coffee-producing countries don't regulate chemical and pesticide use.

Research is mixed on the effects of caffeine on the body. Some studies suggest that caffeine can actually reduce risk of heart disease and cancer and enhance fat metabolism, particularly during exercise. Other studies are inconclusive, while still others suggest that caffeine is harmful to the cardiovascular system, does not enhance fat metabolism, and stresses the adrenal glands as an artificial central nervous system stimulant.

It seems reasonable that it's unhealthy to ingest a beverage that can keep you cranking at warp speed when what you really need is a nap. However, it appears that a cup or two a day won't hurt. I myself enjoy coffee, especially after adding heavy cream and a pinch of sugar (yes, a pinch won't hurt). It's a warm and comforting element to my morning routine, especially on those freezing cold winter mornings in Malibu…

High-Fat Dairy Products

Some purists in the paleo-diet world totally eschew dairy of any kind, but I have concluded from extensive research that certain forms of dairy are suitable for some people and not for others. Truth is, Grok probably did not consume much in the way of dairy products. He certainly didn't go around milking wild beasts; that phase of agriculture didn't start until about 10,000 years ago at the earliest. On the other hand, since he ate most parts of the animals he killed, Grok also very likely consumed the milk in mammary glands he ate on occasion (along with kidney, liver, heart, lung, intestines, bone marrow, and brain), so it's not accurate to say he completely avoided dairy.

Dairy does not need to be an essential part of anyone's diet (the "Got Milk?" advertising campaign notwithstanding) and many of us might be well served never having dairy again. But if you are one who exhibits no acute problems (lactose intolerance or casein sensitivity) and have a desire to keep some dairy in your diet, certain dairy products can offer a decent source of nutrition and be acceptable under the Primal Blueprint. Just be sure to select carefully to minimize potential problems and obtain maximum nutrient benefit.

The best dairy choices are raw, fermented, unpasteurized, unsweetened, and high-fat options such as ghee, butter, full cream, aged cheese, cottage cheese, cream cheese, Greek-style full fat yogurt, half and half, kefir, and raw whole milk. Stick to pasture-raised/grass-fed or organic dairy products to avoid the hormones, pesticides, and antibiotics common in commercial dairy products. Eliminate fruit-sweetened yogurt, frozen desserts, and other high-carb dairy offerings. Stay completely away from regular pasteurized, homogenized, two-percent and skim milk.

Fermented dairy products may help you avoid the immune system issues and allergenic reactions that many have toward the lactose and casein in cow's milk. They also offer a good source of probiotics (healthy bacteria for your intestines). Raw dairy products undergo the least processing, increasing their nutritional value. High-fat dairy products have low levels of the objectionable casein protein, which I will discuss shortly. And how can you not love an eating style that lets you have butter and heavy cream (both of which are almost entirely comprised of healthy saturated animal fat)? Choosing organic dairy offerings protects you from the dangers of the hormones, pesticides, and antibiotics prevalent in commercial dairy products.

Cheese does have broad appeal and can play a minor role in a healthy diet. Play it snooty and go for the high-quality, aged stuff—not the industrialized ooze found in mini-mart nacho machines. Aged cheese is a fermented food, so it contains little to no lactose. Cheese offers high-quality fats and proteins, as well as many other essential nutrients, with a satisfaction level that's just as important as the aforementioned health benefits. For a change of pace, try some raw, non-pasteurized cheese that is loaded with good nutrition.

Having offered possible options of what might constitute acceptable dairy, let's now look at why milk doesn't necessarily "do a body good." Lactose is a carbohydrate in milk that is difficult to digest for many who stop producing lactase (the enzyme that helps digest lactose) after age three or four. This is in alignment with our genetically programmed transition away from breast-feeding in early childhood (breast milk contains significant lactose).

The incidence of lactose intolerance varies wildly by ancestral heritage—something that is believed to be a rare example of recent genetic change through selection pressure in the manner of evolution (I discuss this topic at length in the Q&A Appendix at MarksDailyApple.com). People of herder ancestry (and hence high dairy consumption)—such as the Swedes and Dutch—are generally quite tolerant. Other ethnic groups—such as those of African or Asian descent (i.e., the majority of the global population)—

have high rates of lactose intolerance. If you carefully examine your dietary habits, you may discover incidences of bloating, gas, cramping, or diarrhea in conjunction with consuming milk products—all indications that you have some level of lactose intolerance and should avoid milk and other lactose-heavy dairy products, including ice cream.

> **"Milk doesn't necessarily "do a body good."**
> **At least the usual storebought kind. The**
> **calcium benefits are overstated, and it often**
> **contains agents such as lactose, casein,**
> **hormones, pesticides, and antibiotics."**

Casein is a protein that can have autoimmune-stimulating properties and can initiate very serious allergic reactions in some people, particularly those who have experienced "leaky gut" syndrome as a result of a concurrent intolerance to grains. Casein is believed to contribute to or exacerbate conditions such as celiac disease, Crohn's disease, irritable bowel syndrome, asthma, and possibly autism in some people. Success has been reported treating these conditions holistically with a wheat- and dairy-free diet. *Paleo Diet* author Loren Cordain notes that a substance known as epidermal growth factor (EGF) in milk and other dairy products can increase cancer risk and tumor progression and also suggests that milk and other dairy products worsen acne cases.

These negatives do not even address the consequences of consuming the hormones, pesticides, and antibiotics contained in commercial milk and dairy products. Fortunately, the dangers and objections of the commonly used recombinant bovine growth hormone (rBGH—an agent given to cows to increase their milk production) are well publicized, leading some forward-thinking nations to ban its use and sophisticated consumers to steer clear of milk made with rBGH.

Milk's modern processing methods also present health objections. Milk that is homogenized and pasteurized is certainly free of dangerous bacteria, but it is also devoid of beneficial bacteria, vitamins, and enzymes due to the heating process. Furthermore, the homogenization process alters the otherwise healthy milk fats by reducing the size of the fat globules, interfering with their digestibility. Bottom line: even if you don't have any acute symptoms, it's sensible to conclude that during the first couple years of life, milk consumption should be limited to mother's milk. From there, it's a matter of choosing your dairy wisely and not making it the foundation of your diet.

For those who recoil at the suggestion to limit intake of milk, let's examine further some of the Conventional Wisdom about dairy that is flawed. Yes, most dairy is an excellent source of calcium, but we don't need nearly as much calcium as we have been led to believe. The United States and other Western nations with high dairy intake nevertheless have high rates of osteoporosis, suggesting that calcium is not the be-all and end-all for bone health. Experts are in agreement that magnesium, vitamin D, vitamin K, potassium, and other agents are also extremely important. Furthermore, just like with omega-3 and omega-6 fatty acids, these agents need to be obtained in proper balance to provide optimal bone health benefits, an area where the average Western diet falls short. Today, we generally consume too much calcium (largely from heavy use of dairy products). This hampers our ability to absorb magnesium because the two nutrients compete on the same absorption pathways.

To make matters worse, many of us don't consume enough magnesium (found in leafy greens, nuts, seeds, and fish) or synthesize enough vitamin D (from sun exposure, as I will detail in Chapter 7). Many experts believe that vitamin D intake might be more critical than calcium to bone health. Furthermore, chronic stress may play a huge role in osteoporosis, since the stress hormone cortisol inhibits calcium uptake by bones, rendering ingested calcium less effective. How about that? Taking a break from your busy day to bag some rays in your lounge chair might be better for your bones than drinking a glass of milk or swallowing a bunch of pills!

Since we've discussed the importance of promoting an alkaline environment in the body, it should be noted that dairy foods are acid forming—a reality that actually hampers calcium absorption. For your calcium needs, you are better off consuming easily assimilated, high-calcium, alkaline foods, such as leafy greens, nuts, oranges, broccoli, and sweet potatoes, or calcium-rich fish, including wild salmon and sardines. All told, it would be preferable to push dairy aside in favor of the Primal Blueprint stalwarts of meat, vegetables, fruits, nuts, and seeds. That said, when you look at the spectrum of foods from best to worst, the previous list of allowable dairy is still a preferred choice over grains, if you are going to depart from the Primal Blueprint now and then.

Approved Fats and Oils

Many fats and oils offer significant health benefits, but they are generally high in calories with minimal vitamin and mineral values. Obviously, Grok didn't press oils in his day, but his omega-3 intake was quite high from animal and plant sources. Today, we need all the help we can get toward optimum essential fatty acid balance. Many oils offer a way to boost your intake of omega-3s and other healthy monounsaturated and saturated fats. I'd advise moderation in this category because I'd rather enjoy the delicious taste of fatty whole foods, such as avocados, coconut, macadamia nuts, oily, cold water fish, olives, meat, and eggs to obtain my fat calories.

For cooking, animal fats (butter, ghee, lard, recycled bacon grease, and tallow and coconut oil) are great choices, because they are temperature-stable, even under high heat. The best oil to consume with meals is domestically grown, extra-virgin, first cold press only olive oil (yes, a mouthful; I'll explain the importance of these distinctions shortly). Olive oil, the most monounsaturated oil, offers proven cardiovascular benefits (raises HDL and lowers LDL cholesterol) and has powerful anti-inflammatory and antioxidant properties. It's very good for cooking at low heat, but be careful because excessive time at high temperatures can compromise the health benefits of olive oil.

As you probably know, various processing methods dramatically affect the health quality of olive oil, with extra virgin designated as the purest form. The use of the "extra-virgin" moniker is loosely regulated, and there is a tremendous disparity in quality between local extra-virgin olive oil and imports from Greece, Italy, or Spain (which comprise the vast majority of products on the market). As with fruit, you should strive for oil produced locally or at least domestically for maximum freshness. The additional distinction "first cold press only" suggests that the olives have been pressed only once and bottled immediately, instead of being repeatedly pressed for maximum crop yield (this is the most common method, particularly with the large bottle–low price imports). You may have to contact the manufacturer to determine whether your bottle is indeed first cold press only.

You'll notice the difference with a single taste of a locally grown, first cold-pressed extra virgin olive oil in comparison with a much blander, duller-tasting extra virgin import. The aroma and taste are incredibly powerful—the high level of tocopherols (a potent antioxidant) may actually sting the back of your throat! In my estimation, nothing beats a Primal Big Ass salad with a generous drizzling of olive oil. Visit lucerooliveoil.com to learn more about superior growing and harvesting methods used by this small family business in Northern California.

High omega-3 oils are a good way to bump up your omega-3 intake if you don't eat a lot of oily, cold water fish. Omega-3 fish oil capsules are a convenient daily supplement, or you can get bottled omega-3 oils at a health food store or fine market. These oils are extremely delicate and easily suffer damage from exposure to heat, light, oxygen, and time. Thus, you'll often find them refrigerated and in small containers.

Look for something other than flax oil. While flax is the most common offering and is high in omega-3, recent research suggests that the predominant type of omega-3 found in flax oil, alpha-linoleic acid (ALA), is difficult to assimilate in the body. It must be enzymatically converted into the more useful omega-3 fractions: docosahexanoic acid (DHA) and eicosapentanoic acid (EPA). Even then, there's still no guarantee that your body will handle that conversion efficiently. Some alternative offerings you might find are borage, cod liver, krill, salmon, and hemp seed. Always compare the expiration dates on a few bottles within the same brand and buy the one with the most amount of time left on it.

It's best to store all oils (all kinds, but especially high omega-3s) in the refrigerator and to use them quickly—usually within six weeks of opening. Remember, while omega-3 oils are healthy, they are still subject to rancidity and, when exposed to air, they will oxidize a bit. If you detect a slightly rancid smell in any oil or if it's been on the shelf for more than six months, discard the product immediately.

Primal-Approved Fats and Oils

The list of approved oils (in alphabetical order) contains a variety of saturated and unsaturated types, with different ideal uses. Review the list carefully, stockpile your fridge, and be sure to stick to the best intended use for each.

1. Animal Fats: Chicken, duck, or goose fat; lard (aka pork fat), beef, or lamb tallow; and other animal fats are excellent for cooking because their saturated composition makes them temperature stable; they won't oxidize under high heat.

2. Butter: An excellent choice for cooking or enhancing the taste of steamed vegetables, butter is a good source of vitamins A and E as well as selenium.

3. Coconut Oil: Temperature stability and numerous health and immune-supporting benefits make it an excellent choice for cooking. Find an organic brand and try it in the Primal Energy Bar or Primal Chocolate Mousse recipes at MarksDailyApple.com!

Primal-Approved Fats and Oils (continued)

4. Dark Roasted Sesame Oil: This oil's intense flavor makes it a great choice for wok vegetables, meat, or salads. Some alternative healers promote its antibacterial properties to heal wounds and prevent infection.

5. High Omega-3 Oils: These delicate oils are a great addition to salads or protein shakes for an omega-3 boost. Choose borage, cod-liver, krill, salmon, hemp seed, or hi-oleic sunflower or safflower seed oils (not to be confused with their unhealthy polyunsaturated derivatives) as alternatives to flax.

6. Marine Oils: Typically delivered in capsule or soft-gel supplement form, these fish or krill oils are an excellent source of omega-3s.

7. Olive Oil: Choose locally or domestically grown, first cold press only, extra-virgin, and savor the flavor! Best not to cook with olive oil due to temperature fragility. If you must, use the lowest heat practical.

8. Palm Oil: The unprocessed variety (not to be confused with widely used partially hydrogenated palm oil) is great for cooking.

Other Nuts and Seeds and Their Derivative Butters

Nuts and seeds are concentrated foods that represent an energy source (some might call it a "life force") for future generations of their plant—packed with protein, fatty acids, enzymes, antioxidants, and abundant vitamins and minerals. You can conveniently carry and eat nuts and seeds anytime, anywhere. They stimulate minimal insulin production and will keep you satisfied for hours until your next meal. Numerous respected studies (Iowa Women's Health Study of 40,000 women, Harvard School of Public Health's Nurses' Health Study of 127,000 women, and Physicians' Health Study of 22,000 men are among the most prominent) suggest that regular consumption of nuts significantly reduces the risk of heart disease and diabetes.

Nevertheless, some moderation is warranted with nuts due to concerns about O6:O3 ratios and caloric density. Most nuts except macadamia contain multiple more omega-6 than omega-3 fatty acids. For example, walnuts are lauded for being a great source of omega-3s—the highest of any nut or seed—but they are five times higher in omega-6 than omega-3. What's more, some people who transition to a Primal eating style tend to overdo nuts as they try to fill the void left by ditching grains, sugars, and legumes. If you are used to frequent, perhaps even absent-minded, snacking to get through the day, and you switch from carbs to nuts, you may eat enough extra calories over the short term to compromise fat loss efforts. Understand that with nuts and other high-fat foods, a little goes a long way. A handful of nuts will satisfy hunger and provide fatty acids to burn for hours afterwards. Unlike carbohydrate snacking, you don't experience the insulin crash leading to cravings for more snacks in the ensuing hours.

Almonds, hazelnuts, pecans, pine nuts, pistachios, walnuts, flaxseeds, chia seeds, pumpkin seeds (best O6:O3 ratio among seeds—"only" 2:1), and sunflower seeds are all nutritious and satisfying—great for salads or as snack fodder. The ever-popular peanuts should be avoided. Peanuts are technically a legume, not a nut. They are highly allergenic and also can contain dangerous molds that produce aflatoxin, a potent carcinogen. Obviously, avoid nuts that have been processed with sugary or oily coatings or other offensive ingredients.

Use a mini food processor to grind nuts and sprinkle onto salads, over baked vegetables, or even into omelets. Whole nuts (in the shell) will last up to a year without spoiling. Shelled nuts have less shelf life, and sliced nuts less again. Store nuts in the refrigerator (or freezer, if longer than six months) to prolong freshness. If your nuts have a rancid, oily smell or any discoloration, fleckings, or signs of mold, discard them. Concerns about pesticide exposure from nuts is minimal due to protection offered by shells. Don't worry about looking for organic nuts; less than one percent of US tree nut farmland is certified organic anyway.

Nut and seed butters offer a versatile and great-tasting way to spread your intake of nuts and seeds over different meals and snacks. Take care to choose cold-processed butters that are simply ground up (at low temperatures and free of added ingredients—except salt, which is fine), and refrigerate them at all times. Many health proponents claim raw nuts, seeds, and butters have superior nutritional value to those that have been roasted, so by all means choose raw products if you can find them. Almond butter is believed by many to be the best butter choice besides macadamia. Almonds have the highest protein content of any nut (20 percent of total calories) and are high in antioxidants, phytonutrients, vitamins, minerals, and plant sterols that support health and lower disease risk.

Supplemental Carbs

Sweet potatoes (the orange variety are typically called yams), quinoa, and wild rice are the best choices for heavy exercisers who require additional dietary carbohydrates to replenish frequently depleted muscle glycogen. These select few folks who fall into the "need supplemental carbs" category are effortlessly maintaining ideal body fat levels, and train so heavily that bonking (a sudden and severe drop in energy) and delayed recovery are occasionally concerns—think Tour de France cyclists, NBA basketball players, or high school cross country runners.

If you decide that you need supplemental carbs, sweet potatoes and yams are superior to the more starchy white, russet, red, or new potatoes. Quinoa is technically not a grain, but a chenopod—closely related to beets, spinach, and tumbleweeds. Vegetarians or Primal enthusiasts looking for a grain-like taste or recipe base laud quinoa for being a complete protein (containing all nine essential amino acids, with 12-18 percent of total calories as protein) and free from gluten. Wild rice is also not a true grain but an aquatic grass. It offers a better nutritional value than grains, a nearly complete profile of essential amino acids (14 percent protein calories), and is gluten-free. Categorize these supplemental carbohydrate foods as an indulgence. They may be enjoyable, but are likely unnecessary—especially if you are trying to reduce excess body fat.

Water: Obey Your Thirst, It's Not Too Late

"Drink eight glasses of water a day to ensure good health." "By the time you're thirsty, it's too late." We've heard these adages our entire lives as part of Conventional Wisdom's 10 (or 20, or whatever) commandments to be healthy—right up there with "drink milk to get your calcium," "eat your grains for fiber," "stay out of the sun to prevent skin cancer," "cut down on fat to lose weight," and other fables. While adequate hydration is paramount to good health, there is absolutely no scientific evidence to support the misguided rule of thumb that you should drink eight glasses of water per day.

After conducting research for 11 months with the assistance of a professional librarian, Dr. Heinz Valtin, former chair of physiology at Dartmouth Medical School and one of the world's foremost experts on kidney function, discovered no conclusive studies about drinking eight glasses of water per day. Valtin believes that the myth originated in the 1940s when the National Institute of Medicine first issued recommendations for dietary nutrient intake, including water. Their suggestion to consume about two liters of water per day (this equals about eight 8-ounce glasses) for optimum hydration contained the long-forgotten comment that "much of this can be gained from the solid food we eat."

Indeed, raw milk is 90 percent water, chicken 54 percent, ground beef 53 percent, pizza 50 percent, white bread 30 percent (but, of course, we wouldn't be eating any pizza or bread, right?), and so on. Caffeine and alcohol, which constitute a significant portion of total fluid intake for many adults, have long been thought of as diuretics that dehydrate you by increasing urine flow. While this is true when you drink in excess, your daily cup of coffee, bottle of beer, or glass or two of wine will actually contribute to hydration levels and not lead to any appreciable fluid loss.

When you experience such variables as hot weather and increased activity levels, your thirst mechanism works wonderfully to dictate how much you need to drink each day. This is a mechanism that has evolved over millennia to prevent dehydration, which is one of the quickest ways you can die. To date, there is no archaeological evidence that Grok wore a CamelBak during his extremely active life (or even a leather bota bag, for that matter!), but he did just fine scooping water out of streams, licking the dew off of leaves, and maintaining adequate hydration incidentally through his diet.

Even when your water intake fluctuates significantly, your kidneys and endocrine system work very efficiently to promote optimum fluid levels in your bloodstream. When you experience even a slightly higher than normal concentration of your blood volume, an agent known as antidiuretic hormone goes to work increasing the absorption of water from the kidneys and returning it to the bloodstream. According to Dr. Valtin and other experts, if your blood becomes concentrated by about two percent, your thirst mechanism will kick in big time, telling you to consume additional fluids. It is only when your blood becomes concentrated by five percent that the medical concerns regarding dehydration present themselves. Dr. Valtin further asserts that while dark urine indicates a need to drink perhaps a glass of water, there is no validity to the idea that your urine needs to be clear to indicate that you are adequately hydrated.

Even with a wide variation in water intake, our bodies do a great job at maintaining normal blood concentration. And yes, there is such a thing as too much water. Hyponatremia is a serious and occasionally fatal condition in which sodium levels become too diluted in the blood as a result of overconsumption of water. What's more, some believe that drinking too much fluid near or during meals can result in poor digestion and excretion due to the dilution of stomach acids that are critical to the digestive process.

As an alternative to the bottled water industry-influenced mantra, "drink, drink, drink!" without regard to your thirst, I recommend consuming a sensible amount of fluid each day, using your thirst as a guide to maintain optimum hydration. Sometimes this might be eight glasses of water, sometimes much less than half that. Heavy exercise, hot temperatures, body weight, and the water content of the foods you eat are obviously all significant variables.

When in doubt, obey your thirst! (Finally, a marketing slogan with a ring of truth to it!)

Sensible Indulgences

The following indulgences can actually promote health when you partake sensibly. Moderation is the key here. With that in mind, here are a few items that Grok rarely or never enjoyed, but which can be added to a Primal lifestyle with little or no downside.

Alcohol

Red wine is the superior alcoholic beverage choice for its impressive antioxidant benefits. Recent studies have shown so many health-enhancing benefits from the resveratrol in red wine that red wine extracts have become very popular supplements. Beer is marginal (after all, it's made from grain!), while hard liquor and mixed drinks using sweetened beverages are the most objectionable. Note that alcohol calories (at seven per gram) are devoid of nutritional value and are generally the first to burn when ingested, which means the burning of stored body fat is interrupted while you indulge.

Furthermore, studies have clearly shown that alcohol in excess of one or two glasses a day can increase the risk of cancer (as well as auto accidents, divorces, bar fights, and other tribulations), so let's be clear that I'm not advocating anything but extremely responsible alcohol consumption, with a clear preference for red wine.

> " *Forget love—I'd rather fall in chocolate!* "
> —*Sandra J. Dykes*

Dark Chocolate

Dark chocolate is rich in antioxidants and brain-stimulating compounds known as phenolic phytochemicals or flavonoids. The ORAC values of cacao powder and dark chocolate are higher than those of virtually any fruit or vegetable! Chocolate is the most craved food in the world for a reason—a chemical called phenylethylamine. Phenylethylamine has been found to trigger a feeling similar to falling in love. Choose dark chocolate, eat moderate portions, and enjoy with total awareness and absolutely no guilt.

Be sure to get the absolute highest quality chocolate you can find, because not all chocolates are created equal, from both a taste and a health perspective. Dark chocolate with a high percentage of cacao has far more health benefits and fewer health objections than milk chocolate does. Milk chocolate bars (Hershey's, etc.) are generally high in sugar and low in antioxidants, while the darker the chocolate, the less sugar and more antioxidant benefits you will enjoy. I recommend choosing chocolate that is 75 percent cacao or greater (anything with more than 50 percent cacao content is classified as bittersweet chocolate). However, as you get closer to 100 percent cacao, the lack of sweetness can make this indulgence tough to appreciate (85 percent is perfect for me). It may take a bit of time, but once you attune to the rich taste of high cacao content dark chocolate, you'll likely lose your affinity for milk chocolate, which will consequently seem too sweet. Read labels when choosing your brand, looking for more fat and fewer carbs. My favorite, Trader Joe's Dark Chocolate Lover's 85 percent cacao, contains 20 grams of fat, 13 grams of carbs, and 4 grams of protein. Other brands run closer to 50/50 on fat-to-carb grams.

Organic chocolate offers you the comfort of greater oversight of the growing, harvesting, and processing procedures—important due to the fact that conventional cacao beans have a high pesticide content and commonly arrive from countries with questionable growing regulations and safety standards.

Finally, a Word About Supplements

Given the lack of certain critical nutrients in even the healthiest diets (refer to the discussion on the drawbacks of conventional animal, vegetable, and fruit products) and the excessive stress levels of hectic modern life, using premium quality supplements in a few key categories can be quite effective to keep you Primal-aligned and support general health. The fact that Grok didn't use supplements doesn't mean we can't benefit from using small doses of certain concentrated natural substances to assist us in achieving optimal health. As you may know, I own and operate a supplement company called Primal Nutrition, so I'm hardly an impartial observer on this issue. If you object to me covering stuff that I sell in this book, I invite you to skip ahead to the next chapter on exercise!

While supplementation is a personal choice and sometimes a difficult budget expense to justify, I urge you to consider a bare minimum program to stay Primal-aligned and promote optimal gene expression. If you lead an extremely active life and/or have elevated stress factors, you may wish to investigate a more comprehensive regimen, with details available at primalblueprint.com. Following is an overview of some supplements that can address the major shortcomings in our modern eating and lifestyle habits.

Multivitamin/Mineral/Antioxidant Formula

Eating, exercising, and living according to the Primal Blueprint will help mitigate much of the oxidative damage modern humans sustain as a result of eating the Standard American Diet, performing chronic or insufficient exercise, getting inadequate sleep and sunlight, and coping with generally excessive life stress levels. Your internal antioxidant systems work quite well when you are healthy and stress-balanced. However, pushing the limits with sub-par meals, jet travel, emotional stress, or chronic exercise can quickly compromise your digestive, immune, and endocrine systems, and other aspects of general health.

We need a broad mix of antioxidants on a daily basis, because they work in different ways and in different parts of the cell. Too much of any single antioxidant (in the absence of others) has been shown to have potentially negative effects, as a few recent vitamin E-only studies delivering negative results have demonstrated. Unfortunately, many of the best sources of dietary vitamins, minerals, and antioxidants historically have all but disappeared or have been rendered impotent by today's aggressive factory farming techniques. In the fruit industry, for example, obtaining the highest possible sugar content has replaced nutritional value as the focus.

When you take a quality broad-spectrum antioxidant formula (containing hard-to-get nutrients such as full-spectrum vitamin E—not just alpha-tocopherol; mixed carotenoids—not just beta-carotene; tocotrienols, n-acetyl-cysteine, alpha-lipoic acid, curcumin, resveratrol, milk thistle, CoQ10, and quercetin, to name a few), the agents work synergistically to mitigate oxidative damage and recycle back to their potent antioxidant form. For that reason, I choose to take a high-potency multivitamin loaded with extra antioxidants every day.

Omega-3 Fish Oil

In Grok's day, virtually every animal he consumed was a decent source of vital omega-3 fatty acids. The fish he caught ate algae to produce omega-3 fatty acids rich in EPA and DHA (which helped build the larger human brain over a couple hundred thousand years). The animals he hunted grazed on plants that generated high levels of omega-3. Even the vegetation Grok consumed provided higher levels of omega-3s than the levels found in today's plants. In Grok's diet, the ratio of pro-inflammatory (bad) omega-6 to anti-inflammatory (good and healthful) omega-3 was close to 1:1.

Today, even a conscientious eater can fall short of ideal O6:O3 ratios and consequently exist in a constant state of mild systemic inflammation. Normalizing your ratio is a matter of strictly minimizing omega-6 intake and boosting omega-3 intake by eating lots of oily, cold water fish and/or taking a daily dose of highly purified omega-3 fish or krill oil supplements. The research on fish oils is extraordinarily positive, showing such benefits as decreased risk for heart disease and cancer, lowering of triglycerides, improvement in joint mobility, decreased insulin resistance, and improved brain function and mood. The drug companies are even starting to recognize the power of this "natural medicine" and have begun promoting prescription fish oil (at four times the price of a comparable supplement, of course!). As healthy as my own diet is, I rarely go a day without taking a few grams of an omega-3 fish oil supplement.

Probiotics

Grok ate dirt at pretty much every meal. Hey, when you never wash your hands, your food, or anything else, for that matter, you pretty much can't avoid it. But with all that soil came billions of soil-based organisms (mostly bacteria and yeast) that entered his mouth daily and populated his gut. Most were "friendly" bacteria that actually helped him better digest food and ward off infections. In fact, much of Grok's (and our) immune system evolved to depend on these healthy "flora" living in us symbiotically. Grok also ate the occasional unfriendly organisms that had the potential to cause illness, but as long as the healthy flora well outnumbered the bad guys, all was well. Several trillion bacteria live symbiotically in the human digestive tract—some good and some bad. Much of your health depends on which of the two is winning the flora war.

The problem today is that not only do we avoid dirt, but we also pursue sterility to the extent that we virtually eliminate all forms of bacteria—even the healthy stuff—from our diet. Of course, given the germs that prevail in the civilized world, it's probably best that we do thoroughly wash or cook everything we eat. For most healthy people, exposure to routine germs doesn't usually present a problem. As long as there are some healthy gut bacteria present (healthy, natural foods contain these probiotics inherently—even if we wash them); as long as we don't get too stressed out (stress hormones can kill off healthy flora) or too sick (diarrhea and vomiting are ways the body purges bad bacteria—but it purges good bacteria as well), eat too much processed food (sugar, grains, trans and partially hydrogenated fats, and chemical additives support the growth of unhealthy bacteria and yeast, while choking out healthy flora), or take antibiotics (antibiotics tend to kill most bacteria, good and bad—that's their job); and as long as we are eating well, those healthy bacteria can flourish and keep us healthy.

Of course, the healthy bacteria balance in our intestinal tract gets compromised regularly in all the ways mentioned (even with generally healthy people), creating an opportunity to benefit from supplementation. You don't necessarily need to take probiotics every day, because once these "seeds" have been planted in a healthy gut, they tend to multiply and flourish easily on their own. Rather, consider taking extra probiotics under times of great stress, when you have been sick or are taking (or have just taken) a course of antibiotics, when you are traveling (particularly to foreign countries, where unfamiliar bacteria—even good stuff from good foods—can overwhelm your digestive system), or when you detect any sign of compromised immune function (the digestive system is critical to immune function). The reversal of fortune from a few days of taking probiotics can be dramatic. "Better than eating dirt," I always say.

Protein Powder/Meal Replacement

Restricting your intake of processed carbs often means being at a loss for quick, convenient snacks or small meals. We are so conditioned to reach for a bagel, an energy bar, chips, crackers, and other grain-based products or sweets for snacks, we often run short on convenient, transportable, nonperishable options for an afternoon pickup snack or mini meal. While not exactly Primal, protein powders/meal replacements do combine the best of 21st-century technology with a true Primal intent: get me a fast, good-tasting source of nutrients without too many carbs or unhealthy fats. I prefer microfiltered whey protein to obtain an impressive profile of all the essential and nonessential amino acids, and coconut milk solids to provide healthy fats that can be delivered in a powdered formula.

I also recommend finding a product that tastes great when mixed only with water, so you don't have to add sugary juices or milk just to choke it down. That way you can always throw in a piece of fruit if you like for added calories or flavor. If I am in a hurry and want a quick, high-protein start to my day, my morning smoothie shake takes less than a minute to make and covers the bases I need covered. Adding some omega-3 oil covers you on two critical Primal areas. Micro-filtered whey, while derived from dairy, has insignificant amounts of lactose, so it's fine for most all lactose-intolerant folks.

Vitamin D

Vitamin D supplements can be useful when you are unable to obtain enough direct sunlight to manufacture abundant stores of this agent (which is technically a precursor hormone, not a vitamin). Sunlight is by far the most plentiful source of vitamin D; even an excellent diet provides for only a fraction of your vitamin D needs. Following the basic strategy outlined in Chapter 7 to get adequate sun exposure should enable you to maintain a sufficient blood level of vitamin D year-round, since vitamin D can be stored in your fat cells for winter use.

Unfortunately, many modern citizens are vitamin D-deficient for a variety of reasons: indoor-dominant lifestyles, minimal intake of oily, cold water fish (by far the most plentiful dietary source), consumption of high levels of phytates (nutrient depletion increases vitamin D requirements), obesity (excess body fat inhibits vitamin D absorption), or avoidance of the sun (or screening obsessively; listening preschool moms?) due to misguided fears about skin cancer. Getting enough vitamin D is especially challenging for those living at latitudes above 49 degrees (runs along Canada/US border, thru Paris, central Germany and near the Southern border of Russia; oh— almost forgot—and Southern Chile, Argentina, and New Zealand) or those with dark skin pigment living outside of tropical latitudes.

Beyond those in the aforementioned high-risk categories, many of us can benefit from routine vitamin D supplementation in the winter months, when the sun's rays are of insufficient intensity to facilitate vitamin D production. In the continental US, this is the case for three to four months per year. Those in the 50s latitudes and higher (Canada, Northern Europe, and Scandinavia) are inhibited for seven to eight months per year.

Expert vitamin D advocates recommend obtaining an average of 4,000 International Units (I.U.) per day of vitamin D. You can easily bag 5,000-10,000 I.U. during a single half-hour sunbathing session in the summertime. In the wintertime, I recommend supplementing with 2,000 I.U. of vitamin D per day. If you struggle to remember to take pills consistently, you can take a bunch of vitamin D at once with no ill effects. I am fair-skinned, live at 34 degrees latitude in Los Angeles, and get a ton of sun exposure during the summer, but I still supplement during the winter to be extra sure that my blood levels are adequate.

If you have even a hint of the aforementioned risk factors, consider obtaining a blood test for "25-vitamin D" or "serum 25(OH)D." Make sure you ask for these specific tests, since many doctors are uninformed about which tests are the most accurate. Your vitamin D goal range is 40-60 ng/ml. If your reading is under 40 ng/ml, take aggressive action to get more sunlight and/or supplement diligently. Even if you are not the pill-popping type, the recommendation to supplement with vitamin D should be strongly considered. Dietary sources for vitamin D are inadequate, supplements are inexpensive, and maintaining adequate vitamin D levels is critical to healthy cellular function and cancer prevention, including melanoma.

The aforementioned categories represent what I believe to be the most useful products to consider for supplementation, but there are numerous other product categories and individual supplements that address more specialized needs. Among them are phosphatidylserine (PS), which improves cognitive function and moderates cortisol spikes in the bloodstream; and buffering joint compounds (glucosamine, chondroitin, MSM, and enzyme cofactors), which support connective tissue and alleviate pain. A knowledgeable healthcare practitioner may recommend other products to address your particular needs.

Supplement Quality

Regardless of what brand of products you choose, you should be extremely vigilant in an industry that is minimally regulated by the FDA. Good manufacturers have a tightly controlled production environment where every single raw material that goes into the finished product is easily sourced and certified by the supplier. Contact your supplement manufacturers and ask if they obtain "Certificates of Assay" attesting to the source, potency, and purity of each ingredient. Ask if their products are produced in a pharmaceutical-grade manufacturing environment. Ask whether they adhere to the "Good Manufacturing Practices" (GMP) that is overseen by the Food and Drug Administration. Notice how well products are sealed when presented for retail sale.

You will be able to quickly discern from e-mail replies (or lack thereof) or phone conversations whether the manufacturer of the supplements you consume, or are considering consuming, has its act together. Examine labels and choose supplements that are free of common fillers and additives, such as colorings, waxes, preservatives, and other chemicals. They'll be listed under "inactive" or "other" ingredients. You'll be surprised to discover just how prevalent these agents are in many of the leading vitamin brands and discount products available through big-box retailers and in supermarkets and drugstores. Understand that premium quality supplements are considerably more expensive than the giant bottles found on the shelves of warehouse stores. Many, but not all, products in the latter category offer minimal potency and bioavailability (ease of digestion and utilization by the body) and bring literal accuracy to the expression "pissing away your money."

Chapter Summary

1. Meat and Fowl: Choose local, pasture-raised animal products (or, next best, USDA-certified organic animal products) to avoid today's poor quality mass-produced feedlot animals fattened up with grains and laden with hormones, pesticides, and antibiotics.

2. Fish: Emphasize wild-caught fish from remote, pollution-free waters. Oily, cold water fish (anchovies, herring, mackerel, salmon, sardines) have the highest level of omega-3 fatty acids. Choose only approved farmed fish (coho salmon, shellfish, domestic trout, and certain other domestic species), and avoid other farmed fish (including the popular Atlantic salmon), fish at the top of the food chain (shark, sword), fish caught by environmentally objectionable commercial methods, or imports from Asia (both wild-caught and farmed).

3. Eggs: Local, pasture-raised chickens deliver more omega-3 and other nutrients than commercially raised chickens. Egg yolks are one of the planet's most nutritionally-dense foods—enjoy!

4. Vegetables: Vegetables should play a central role in your diet and comprise the largest section of your daily "plate." Brightly colored foods have high levels of antioxidants, phenols, fiber, vitamins, minerals, and other micronutrients. Consuming vegetables (and fruits) helps promote alkalinity in your body, boosting immune function and reducing disease risk. Dark leafy greens are an excellent choice to consume regularly as a base for any main course. Eating vegetables liberally (and seasonal fruits with some moderation and selectivity) will still result in a satisfactory average total carbohydrate intake of 150 grams or less per day.

It's essential to select locally grown or organic vegetables for maximum nutritional value and health safety. Be strict about going organic with vegetables (and fruits) that have a large surface area (leafy greens) or a soft open skin (bell peppers, carrots, winter squash, berries, peaches). You can be less strict with plants that have a tough, inedible skin (bananas, avocados, melons, oranges).

5. Macadamia Nuts: Macadamias earn special distinction due to their superior nutritional profile of mostly monounsaturated fats, as well as phytonutrients, fiber, antioxidants, and numerous vitamins and minerals. Macadamia nuts are deeply satisfying—an excellent snack choice for appetite control—and have been found to minimize disease risk. Other nuts, seeds, and their derivative butters are a healthy component of Primal eating, but some moderation is warranted due to their caloric density and a desire to regulate O6 intake.

(continued)

Chapter Summary (continued)

6. Coconut Products: Coconut's medium-chain fatty acids offer exceptional health benefits and are difficult to obtain, even in a healthy diet. Coconut oil, milk, flakes, and other derivatives can be great substitutes for offensive SAD ingredients. Coconut oil is excellent for cooking due to its high saturated fat composition.

7. Fruits: Fruits offer an outstanding source of fiber, vitamins, minerals, antioxidants, and other nutrients. Choose wisely by sticking to locally grown, in-season, pesticide-free fruits that are high in antioxidants. Fresh berries offer excellent antioxidant and nutrient levels. Some moderation is warranted with fruit due to year-round availability of highly cultivated modern fruits that are extra sweet. This is particularly true for those with fat reduction goals, since fruit is easily converted into fat in the liver.

8. Herbs and Spices: Herbs and spices offer tremendous macronutrient and antioxidant values and can enhance your enjoyment of meals. Strive for organic sources of herbs to avoid pesticide risk.

9. Moderation Foods: Certain modern foods are acceptable, provided they are not overemphasized: coffee; high-fat dairy (preference for raw, fermented products); approved fats and oils; other nuts, seeds, and their derivative butters; supplemental carbs (sweet potatoes, quinoa, wild rice); and water (obey your thirst).

10. Sensible Indulgences: Enjoy with full attention and awareness, and never feel guilty. Red wine and dark chocolate (75 percent cacao or greater) offer numerous health benefits, making them superior choices to enjoy in a responsible manner.

11. Supplements: Supplements can play a critical role in adapting Primal recommendations into the realities of hectic modern life. Supplements offer a convenient source of concentrated nutrition that helps account for nutrient deficiencies (e.g., depleted soil or objectionable conventional growing and production methods) in today's food supply. The following categories offer comprehensive protection and added support for even the healthiest of diets: multivitamin/mineral/antioxidant formula, omega-3 fish oil, probiotic formula, protein powder/meal replacement, and vitamin D.

CHAPTER 5

Primal Blueprint Law #2: Avoid Poisonous Things

"Drop Your Fork and Step Away from the Plate!"

In This Chapter

I detail the health risks of eating "poisonous things." In Grok's day, poisonous plants could drop him on the spot. Today our poisons are factory-produced items in bright packages that kill more insidiously over decades. We explore the cultural factors that default us to eating an unhealthy diet and consider strategies for resisting these manipulative influences.

I pay particular attention to dispelling the Conventional Wisdom tenet that grains (wheat, rice, bread, pasta, cereal, corn, etc.) and legumes (alfalfa, beans, lentils, peanuts, peas, and soy products) are healthy, countering these assumptions with extensive research and details indicating the problems grains and, to a slightly lesser extent, legumes cause due to their relatively recent introduction into the human diet.

Grain and legume consumption offers minimal nutritional value and generates a high insulin response. The phytates in these foods inhibit the absorption of minerals. Glutens disturb healthy immune function and promote inflammation. Lectins inhibit healthy gastrointestinal function. Ironically, the whole grains we've been taught to emphasize can have a worse impact on your health in many ways than refined grains, since they contain higher levels of these harmful anti-nutrients.

Trans and partially hydrogenated fats, and excessive consumption of polyunsaturated fatty acids (PUFAs) wreak havoc at the cellular level, promoting inflammation, aging, and cancer. Also important to avoid are all sugary foods and beverages, and assorted other processed foods.

When you see the golden arches, you are probably on your way to the pearly gates.
—William Castelli, M.D
Director of the Framingham Heart Study

I'd like us all to reflect for a moment on our priorities and our vision of a long, happy, healthy, fit life. When the topic of food comes up in conversation with family, friends, or casual acquaintances, it's fascinating to hear the litany of rationalizations, knee-jerk defense mechanisms, self-limiting belief statements, and general confusion or ignorance from otherwise intelligent folks when it comes to eating healthfully. But then again, Conventional Wisdom has often led even the best and brightest minds in nutritional science astray.

It's truly remarkable how successful Madison Avenue has been at indoctrinating lifestyles that produce huge profits for giant multinational corporations—and devastating health consequences for consumers—into generations of society. The marketing messages are so pervasive in modern culture that it's difficult, even stressful, to take control of your health and swim upstream against such cultural norms as fast food, the all-American high-carbohydrate breakfast, and the massive overconsumption of all manner of sweetened sodas, juices, energy drinks, teas, and coffees.

Even noble attempts to do the right thing miss the mark: mass-market "health foods" such as nutritionally challenged meal replacements, energy bars, and other heavily processed "fuel" marketed to athletes, or purification/detox diets with dubious ideas, such as eating nothing but brown rice for a week (talk about a long, hot insulin bath!). Finally, many of our eating habits are driven by cultural, social, emotional, or stress-related triggers other than hunger.

While savoring the occasional moderate serving of a rich treat can be an acceptable element of enjoying life, it's an entirely different story to ingest junk food habitually and mindlessly just because it's part of Americana (hot dogs at the ballgame, popcorn at the movies). If you notice yourself treading in these waters (or worse, repurposing the classic quote from Sir Edmund Hillary about why he climbed Mt. Everest—"because it's there"—into an excuse), please give this topic some sincere reflection and take decisive action. Remember, your ancestors worked unimaginably hard to survive, thrive, and create the amazing opportunities we have today for living healthy, happy, active, and long lives. As I say here often, your genes want you to be healthy, and you deserve nothing less than the very best your genes have to offer.

The most common retort I hear on this thread is, "hey, everything in moderation." Sage advice indeed, but Mark Twain best put this proverb in perspective when he said, "everything in moderation, including moderation." As the Korgs prove dramatically, we live in a world where extreme measures are necessary just to avoid serious disease (remember, some three-quarters of today's American population will eventually die of heart disease or cancer), let alone enjoy optimum health, fitness, energy levels, and body composition.

I support enjoying the occasional indulgence, but why not make it from the list of approved foods of the absolute highest quality? Take a glance at the label of a Milky Way® compared to the label of a delicious, high-antioxidant, organic dark chocolate with no additives, chemicals, chemically-altered fats, or fillers (and check the disparity in carb count). This sensible and deeply satisfying indulgence can hardly be described as a sacrifice or compromise. You can walk past the candy machine without skipping a beat.

> *'Everything in moderation' is sage advice indeed, but Mark Twain best put this proverb in perspective when he said,* **'Everything in moderation, including moderation'.**

Going Against the Grain

Perhaps the most widely accepted and damaging element of dietary Conventional Wisdom is that grains are healthy—the "staff of life" as we've been led to believe our entire lives. While grains have indeed enjoyed massive global popularity for the last 7,000 years, they are simply not very healthy for human consumption. From two million years ago, when the first Homo erectus arose and steadily evolved into the first modern Homo sapiens between 200,000 and 100,000 years ago, and continuing until about 10,000 years ago, humans existed entirely as hunter-gatherers. Early Homo sapiens derived their food from 100 to 200 different wild food sources, including animal meats, fruits, vegetables, and nuts and seeds. Grains were notably absent.

Around 10,000 years ago, forces conspired to create a dramatic shift in the human diet. The widespread extinction of large mammals on major continents coupled with increases in population forced humans to become more resourceful in obtaining food. Those living by water utilized boats, canoes, nets, and better fishing tools to enjoy more bounty. On land, humans refined their toolmaking and hunting strategies to include more birds and small mammals in the food supply.

Escalating competition for animal-sourced food led to agricultural innovations sprouting up independently in the most advanced societies around the world (Egyptians, Mayans, etc.). As wild grains (which were a very small part of some earlier diets but difficult to harvest for any significant yield) and, much later, legumes became domesticated, humans derived more and more calories from these readily available high-calorie sources, a trend that has continued to the present day—with dire consequences.

Loren Cordain, Ph.D., author of *The Paleo Diet*, explains:

> For better or for worse, we are no longer hunter-gatherers. However, our genetic makeup is still that of a paleolithic hunter-gatherer, a species whose nutritional requirements are optimally adapted to wild meats, fruits and vegetables, not to cereal grains. There is a significant body of evidence which suggests that the human genetic makeup and physiology may not be fully adapted to high levels of [cultivated] grain consumption. We have wandered down a path toward absolute dependence upon [cultivated] grains, a path for which there is no return.

Culturally, the cultivation of grains is the key variable that allowed modern civilization to develop and thrive. Large populations could now live permanently in proximity, and labor could specialize, leading to continued exponential advancements in knowledge and modernization. However, as Cordain elaborates, "[Grains] have allowed man's culture to grow and evolve so that man has become earth's dominant animal species, but this preeminence has not occurred without cost.... Agriculture is generally agreed to be responsible for many of humanity's societal ills, including whole-scale warfare, starvation, tyranny, epidemic diseases, and class divisions."

Dr. Jared Diamond, evolutionary biologist, physiologist, and Pulitzer Prize-winning professor of geography at UCLA, and author of *Guns, Germs and Steel*, goes so far as to say that agriculture was "the worst mistake in the history of the human race" and that "we're still struggling with the mess into which agriculture has tumbled us, and it's unclear whether we can solve it."

Costs to the individual were also significant. The flourishing of agriculture paralleled a reduction in average human life span as well as body and brain size, increases in infant mortality and infectious diseases, and the occurrence of previously unknown conditions such as osteoporosis, bone mineral disorders, and malnutrition. As cultural and medical advancements have eliminated most of the rudimentary health risks faced by early humans (infant mortality, predator danger, minor infections turning fatal, etc.), we can now live long enough to develop, suffer, and die from diet-related diseases, including atherosclerosis, hypertension, and type 2 diabetes (it used to be called *adult-onset diabetes* until millions of kids started developing it in recent years!).

> ❝ *The wise man sees in the misfortune*
> *of others what he should avoid.* ❞
> **—Marcus Aurelius**

The Base of the Disease Pyramid

Grains offer the great majority of their calories in the form of carbohydrate, so they cause blood glucose levels to elevate quickly. High-carbohydrate foods such as sugar and grains (and to a lesser extent, legumes) have been recently and suddenly introduced to the human food supply (that's right, even 10,000 years ago is "recent and sudden" in evolutionary terms) and yet are consumed in massive quantities. These sugars and grains shock our delicate hormonal systems, which are better adapted to what today would be considered a low-carbohydrate, high-fat diet.

Please realize that mismanaging your Homo sapiens genes by consuming a high-carbohydrate diet occurs even when you take care to emphasize whole grains over refined grains. Yes, brown rice and whole wheat toast burn slower than soda, but your body still has to produce a requisite amount of insulin to deal with the wildly excessive level of daily carbohydrate intake that is typical today.

A grain-heavy diet stresses the all-important insulin regulation mechanism in the body. After consuming that bagel, scone, muffin, French toast, or bowl of cereal (all derived from grains) and a glass of juice for breakfast, your pancreas releases insulin into the bloodstream to help regulate blood glucose levels. Even after the routine meal just described, many Americans technically become temporarily diabetic, with blood glucose levels soaring to clinically dangerous levels. You know the drill by now. After your meal, insulin is released into the bloodstream to promote the storage of glucose as muscle glycogen or direct its conversion to fat. Experience this often enough and you gain weight and develop insulin resistance and Metabolic Syndrome.

If, instead, you were to have a Primal Blueprint breakfast consisting of a delicious cheese-and-vegetable omelet with some bacon, you would enjoy a moderated insulin response, leading to balanced energy levels for the hours after your meal instead of a sugar high and insulin crash. Furthermore, with blood glucose levels balanced, you would be able to access and burn stored body fat for energy until your next insulin-balanced meal.

Phytates We Hate

There is sufficient evidence that this overreliance on grains—as well as on simple carb and sugar products in general—leads to numerous vitamin, mineral, and nutritional deficiencies. Most grains contain substances called phytates that easily bind to important minerals such as calcium, magnesium, and zinc in the digestive tract, making them more difficult to absorb. Ironically, the unprocessed—and, therefore, supposedly healthier—"whole" grains are typically the highest in phytates. Mineral deficiencies are common in underdeveloped nations that depend almost entirely on grain for their sustenance (humans across the globe obtain an average of 48 percent of their calories from grains, according to Worldwatch.org; the most impoverished nations get up to 80 percent of total calories from grains).

Grains also interfere with vitamin D metabolism and promote related deficiencies of vitamins A, C, and B12. These nutrients are not present in grains (again, ironically, unless they have been processed and then "fortified" by adding back the missing vitamins—albeit at a much reduced nutritional value). Deficiencies of these basic vitamins are prevalent mainly in third-world countries (see the recurring theme?). However, even Western eaters with more balanced diets, but who still rely too heavily on grains, miss out on eating more nutritious foods, such as meats, vegetables, fruits, nuts, and seeds. In the United States, 45 percent of citizens get zero daily servings of fruit or juice, and 22 percent get no daily vegetables.

Gluten, Lectin—Immune Affectin'

Certain grain (and also some legume and dairy) proteins mimic those found in viruses and bacteria, triggering an autoimmune (your immune system attacking healthy cells by mistake) response when ingested. Gluten—the large, water-soluble protein that creates the elasticity in dough (it's also the primary glue in wallpaper paste)—is found in most common grains, such as wheat, rye, and barley, and also in beans. Researchers now believe that as many as a third of us are probably gluten-intolerant or gluten-sensitive. That third of us (and I would suspect many more on a subclinical level) "react" to gluten with a perceptible inflammatory response. Over time, those who are known to be gluten-intolerant can develop a dismal array of medical conditions: dermatitis, joint pain, reproductive problems, acid reflux and other digestive conditions, autoimmune disorders, and celiac disease. And that doesn't mean that the rest of us aren't experiencing some milder negative effect that just doesn't manifest itself so obviously.

Grains, and legumes, also contain high levels of mild, natural plant toxins known as lectins. Researchers have found that lectins can inhibit healthy gastrointestinal function by damaging delicate brush borders that line your small intestine. Brush borders (named for their resemblance to paintbrush bristles; also known as *microvilli*) are where most of the nutrients from the food we eat are absorbed. They contain digestive enzymes that help break down carbohydrates as the final component of their digestive process, and allow appropriate forms of nutrients (glucose, amino acids, fats, vitamins, and minerals) to become absorbed into the bloodstream from the intestine.

Lectin damage to brush borders allows larger, undigested protein molecules to infiltrate the bloodstream. The ever-vigilant immune system sees these unfamiliar protein molecules (not necessarily lectins, but anything you ingest that was supposed to be fully processed in the digestive tract before entering the bloodstream) and sets up a typical immune response to deal with them. Unfortunately, these undigested protein molecules can resemble molecules that reside on the outside of healthy cells, leaving your immune system confused as to who the real enemy is. An autoimmune response ensues, something experts believe is the root cause of many common diseases such as rheumatoid arthritis, lupus, Hashimoto's thyroiditis, multiple sclerosis, and a host of other conditions.

The millions of folks who have been diagnosed with celiac disease or gluten intolerance will not do well switching to a diet heavy in legumes or even so-called "gluten-free grains." They are simply exposing themselves to other kinds of lectins, and of course too much insulin production.

The Holes in the Whole Grain Story

You are likely well aware of how unhealthy refined wheat flour, white rice, pasta, and other grains that have been stripped of their natural fiber and other nutrients during the manufacturing process are; and how whole grains have been lauded as the centerpiece of healthy eating by Conventional Wisdom for decades. Surprisingly, whole grain foods can be considered *less healthy* than their stripped-down cousins for many reasons.

When you ingest a refined product, such as Wonder Bread®, soda, or candy, you get empty calories and a big insulin hit—but that's all you get. Furthermore, the eventual total insulin production is the same for a slice of white bread as it is a slice of whole wheat bread. The only thing in whole grain's favor is a very minimal amount of protein and micronutrients. However, the nutritional advantages of eating whole grains are simply insignificant—especially in comparison to eating any vegetable, fruit, nut, seed, or organic animal food with far more nutritional value calorie for calorie (and, unlike whole grains, they also taste good!).

Whole grains present further problems precisely because they are whole; by definition having all three edible components intact: the endosperm (starchy), the bran (fibrous), and the germ (oily). Whole grains deliver higher levels of harmful phytates, glutens, and lectins that promote inflammation and offend your immune and digestive systems. While you get that highly touted dose of fiber from your whole grains, this, too, can be negative. Excessive fiber intake (practically automatic when you emphasize whole grains) can increase appetite and interfere with healthy digestion, mineral absorption, and elimination (more on this in the book's Q&A supplement at MarksDailyApple.com). You can obtain optimal amounts of fiber from Primal foods (veggies, fruits, nuts, and seeds), and also eliminate the risk of overdoing fiber intake.

For purposes of weight control and preventing disease, a gram of carb from a whole grain is no better than a gram from a refined grain, and could even be worse. I'm not suggesting that you choose refined grains over whole grains; I'm suggesting you ditch all grains in favor of Primal Blueprint foods!

Say Good-Bye to Fatigue, Illness, and Suffering

Understanding that the long-term effects of chronic hyperinsulinemia (high insulin levels in the bloodstream) are such conditions as general systemic inflammation, obesity, diabetes, heart disease, and cancer should be enough to convince you that it is critical to pursue a more natural way of eating. Eating low-carbohydrate, grain-free meals will not only result in immediate gratification in the form of regulated energy levels, but can also help you succeed with long-term weight management and quite possibly save your life.

> *High insulin levels promote fat storage and disease. Moderated insulin levels (typical of Primal Blueprint eating) stimulate fat burning and good health. It's that simple.*

The single most important requirement to improve your fat metabolism and succeed with long-term weight management is to reduce the total amount of insulin you produce. High insulin levels promote fat storage and disease. Moderated insulin levels (typical of Primal Blueprint eating) stimulate fat burning and good health. It's that simple.

At the risk of sounding overly dramatic or redundant, we must understand that the reasonable, "evolutionary" voice challenging Conventional Wisdom about grains is being battled by billions of dollars in corporate and government propaganda pushing us to conform to dietary habits that we are not suited for, that do not nourish us, and that are downright destructive to human health.

If you are one of the fortunate folks who are less sensitive to glutens, lectins, and phytates than most, you might take exception to my wholesale damning of foods that are a dietary centerpiece across the globe. Absent acute symptoms, I'll still argue that we are all genetically "allergic" in some way to foods that are not aligned with the Primal Blueprint. Perhaps you can try eliminating grains for 21 days, taking note of any general improvements in your condition. I'll bet your energy will be more regulated after meals, your digestion and elimination will improve, and the frequency of minor illnesses or inflammation conditions will subside, and you will be more successful controlling your weight. There simply are no good reasons to base your diet on grains—and a lot of reasons never to eat most grains again.

> *More die in the United States of too much food than of too little.*
> —**John Kenneth Galbraith**

Polyunsaturated Fatty Acids (PUFAs):

Conventional Wisdom has unwisely transitioned away from saturated fats to widespread consumption of PUFAs over the past several decades. PUFAs are easily oxidized and quickly go rancid (on the shelf and in your body!) particularly when heated during cooking. Oxidized PUFAs have a pro-inflammatory effect on your system, leading to assorted health problems and a disruption in healthy immune and hormone function.

The endocrine system is especially vulnerable to the effects of PUFA ingestion, leading to symptoms such as a slowed metabolism, low energy levels, and sluggish thyroid function. Heavy consumption of PUFAs in the modern diet is blamed as a leading contributor to insulin resistance, obesity, diabetes, heart disease, cancer, immune problems, arthritis, and other inflammatory conditions. Strictly avoid the following categories of PUFAs, replacing them with the approved fats and oils discussed in the previous chapter.

Canola Oil: Canola oil is touted as a great cooking and eating choice due to its high monounsaturated content. Unfortunately, canola oil is a heavily refined, genetically engineered product derived from the rapeseed plant. This plant is believed to be toxic to humans and animals—particularly harmful to respiratory function. Most canola oil is put through a deodorizing process that converts some of its natural omega-3s into harmful trans fats. The popularity of canola oil today is a classic example of Conventional Wisdom taking facts (canola has a high monounsaturated content; monounsaturated fats are healthy) out of context or otherwise distorting them at the expense of our health.

Margarine: Margarine is comprised of offensive ingredients and processed with chemical additives at high temperatures. While most all margarines today have the "trans fat-free" distinction proudly adorning the label, the PUFAs that some margarines contain still potentially raise LDL, lower HDL, and suppress immune function and insulin sensitivity. Research strongly suggests an increased risk of cancer and heart disease from margarine use. Foods that are now trans fat-free are instead being made with interesterified fats, which are no less dangerous. While long-term research has yet to be conducted on these chemically-altered interesterified fats, a 2007 study published in *Nutrition Metabolism* showed that interesterified fats had similar negative effects to trans fats.

Other Vegetable & Seed PUFA Oils: Includes corn, safflower, sunflower, soybean, cottonseed, and others. These oils, popular in packaged and frozen foods, as well as in bottles, are heavily refined in an offensive manner. They contain poor omega-6:omega-3 ratios and are believed to disturb endocrine function. They are a poor choice for cooking since they are highly vulnerable to oxidation when heated.

Vegetable Shortening: Similar to lard in appearance but chemically produced to create a trans fat. The brand name Crisco is an acronym for "crystallized cottonseed oil." Bad stuff—stay away!

Trans and Partially Hydrogenated Fats

Perhaps the most overtly offensive and dangerous element of the modern diet is the widespread consumption of toxic processed fats: partially hydrogenated, hydrogenated, and trans fats. The three are not quite the same but are very similar—and all evil. I'll use the term partially hydrogenated, because it is more widely used in food manufacturing and a more familiar term on food labels than plain hydrogenated. Partially hydrogenated fats are actually more objectionable than fully hydrogenated fats.

Trans and partially hydrogenated fats are found in almost every processed food product in the supermarket, including frozen dinners, breakfast foods, sweets, and desserts; packaged snacks (e.g., crackers, chips, and cookies); deep-fried foods; pastries and baked goods (e.g., donuts, croissants, and cupcakes); and, peanut butter, soups, and even grain products (e.g., bread, cereal, pasta, and rice mixes). A commonly cited estimate is that 40 percent of all products in a typical supermarket contain trans or partially hydrogenated fats.

Partially hydrogenated fats are easily oxidized to form free radical chain reactions that damage cell membranes and body tissue and that hamper immune function. Because your brain, nervous system, and vascular system consist primarily of fat-based membranes, any dysfunction in these critical areas can be devastating. Trans fats are not recognized as foreign by the body, so they are incorporated into cell membranes and asked to function as natural fats. Of course, they don't function normally; they just take up space usually reserved for healthy fats and wreak havoc on homeostasis.

Many scientists consider the cell membrane to be the brain of the cell (as opposed to the more common assumption that the nucleus runs the show), because the membrane receives feedback from the outside environment (e.g., ingested nutrients such as glucose entering the bloodstream, the presence of a virus attacking healthy cells, or increased blood flow due to exercise stimulus) and takes consequent action (e.g., triggers the expression of certain genes or the release of certain hormones).

When you have cell membranes comprising natural molecules and you replace them with synthetic dysfunctional molecules, such as partially hydrogenated fats, the intricate signaling system is compromised. Plain and simple, the routine and prolonged ingestion of these toxic agents is a major contributor to the alarming increase in diet-related cancers and many other diseases and adverse health conditions. Many experts believe there is a direct connection between consuming processed foods and obesity (beyond their direct contribution to caloric excess), theorizing that insulin resistance could be exacerbated by dysfunctional fat molecules accumulating in cell membranes.

Research suggests that consumption of trans and partially hydrogenated fats promotes inflammation, aging, and cancer. *The New England Journal of Medicine* reviewed numerous studies and reported a strong link between trans fat consumption and heart disease (including the strong tendency for trans fats to significantly raise LDL cholesterol levels and lower HDL levels). Harvard Medical School estimates that partially hydrogenated fats may be responsible for as many as 100,000 premature deaths each year in the United States. The United States Academy of Sciences says that there is "no safe level" of trans fatty acids in the American diet. The good news is that when you change your diet to eliminate these toxic agents, over time your cells will repair or replace these dysfunctional molecules with healthy ones.

Other Foods to Avoid

Grains...Oh, Did I Already Mention Them?

Wheat, corn, rice, oats, barley, millet, rye, breakfast cereals, pastas, breads, pancakes, rolls, crackers, and the like. Buoyed by Conventional Wisdom, I consumed grains with reckless abandon as a major percentage of my dietary calories for some 40 years. It wasn't until I completely eliminated grains from my diet that some epiphanies occurred. Those occasional stomach cramps that I always attributed to stress? They were more likely due to wheat allergies (their severity triggered by stress, of course). That sluggish feeling I had after pasta dinners that I attributed to fatigue from a hard day training or working? It was actually my brain experiencing glucose depletion from the postmeal insulin flash flood in my bloodstream. The bloating that caused me to loosen my belt buckle after big meals that I attributed to eating big meals? This represented a mild allergic reaction to gluten. The mild arthritis in my fingers that I first began to notice on the golf course in my 40s and chalked up to the aging process? Likely due to the pro-inflammatory nature of the lingering amounts of grains still remaining in my diet.

These routine tribulations that I had long considered a regrettable but inevitable part of life completely disappeared once my transition to a completely Primal Blueprint diet took hold. I've met very few people who eat a lot of grains yet who also claim to enjoy ideal weight, experience perfectly satisfactory and steady energy levels, and never feel digestive distress. At the very least, it's worth completing the aforementioned 21-day exclusion period to determine your sensitivity—and get a glimpse of your potential upside—from eliminating grains from your diet. Chances are, even if you are at a decent launching point now, you will experience a noticeable stabilization of daily energy levels, improved immune function, and a reduction in minor digestive distress.

Legumes

Alfalfa, beans, lentils, peanuts, peas, and soy products are classified as legumes. While legumes can serve as a decent source of protein, fiber, potassium, and antioxidants, they also provide significant levels of carbohydrate and those pesky antinutrient lectins. As *Paleo Diet* author Dr. Loren Cordain explains, "most legumes in their mature state are non-digestible and/or toxic to most mammals, when eaten in even moderate quantities." The fact that legumes need to be altered for human consumption through cooking, soaking, or fermenting should be our best clue to avoid or strictly minimize their consumption (all truly safe fruits and vegetables can be eaten either raw or cooked). To tiptoe into a sensitive subject, the beans that are consumed liberally by many world cultures (kidney, pinto, black beans, lentils) come with the annoying by-product of flatulence, caused by the fermentation of indigestible carbohydrates.

While soy has achieved great popularity as a healthy alternative to meat, unfermented soy products contain compounds that may interfere with thyroid hormone production and have demonstrated an estrogenic (feminizing) effect in certain tissue. Some soy products have decent nutritional value, and certain fermented products may be less objectionable (tempeh, natto, etc.).

That said, there is simply no good reason to ever consume legumes. Well, except as a source of supplemental carbs for that select group of mega calorie burners, without any excess body fat, who are not negatively affected by the lectins and who are looking for ways to replenish depleted muscle glycogen.

I understand that many people have a strong affinity for legumes and that legumes enjoy a reputation as a healthful food category, particularly among vegetarians, who otherwise have limited protein options. It will not be a disaster if you occasionally dip your vegetables in hummus at a dinner party, fry some tempeh with vegetables for a main course, or enjoy side dishes of peas, lentils, or steamed beans. However, emphasizing legumes in your diet is an inferior strategy to having vegetables, fruits, nuts and seeds, and animal foods as your primary meal and snack choices.

Processed Foods

Anything with chemical additives or that's been heavily altered from its natural state requires little discussion. Realize that you have been pummeled with marketing messages your entire life to consume branded, boxed "food" that has contributed directly and tragically to the obesity, illness, and death of those in your family and community. Knowing what our ancestors didn't eat is as important as knowing what they did: Grok never touched refined sugar, trans or partially hydrogenated fats, grains, legumes (well, maybe some occasional wild grains or legumes in small amounts), desserts, processed foods, or anything with hormones, pesticides, antibiotics, herbicides, fungicides, preservatives, or other chemicals.

Sugar

I recognize how addictive sweets are. After all, our genes were programmed to appreciate those rare sweet natural sugars our ancestors discovered on occasion. Unfortunately, today we are bombarded by sugar everywhere. Sugar products greatly stress your insulin sensitivity and reinforce an addiction to both sugar and all simple carbs.

No discussion of sugar would be complete without mention of high fructose corn syrup (HFCS). Fructose has long been considered a superior sweetener to table sugar (sucrose), since it is the primary sugar in fruit and generates a lower insulin response (fructose must be converted into glucose in the liver before it can be utilized in the bloodstream, thus muting both the glucose and insulin spikes). Unfortunately, the fructose that sweetens most processed foods and beverages today—HFCS—is derived from corn, not fruit. This inexpensive and extremely sweet chemically processed agent is found in the vast majority of sodas, energy drinks, teas, juices, baked goods, desserts, and snack foods in your grocery store.

It has been well-established that HFCS is even more lipogenic (fat-promoting) than glucose, since it is readily converted into either glucose or triglycerides in the liver. Diets high in HFCS have been shown to substantially increase triglyceride levels, increase risk of obesity (particularly in kids, since their soda consumption is so excessive in relation to their body weight), and contribute to the development of serious health problems such as type 2 diabetes, Metabolic Syndrome, and non-alcoholic fatty liver disease (NAFLD).

Many health-conscious consumers believe that honey or agave nectar are superior alternatives. Unfortunately, honey has a similar effect on blood sugar levels as table sugar, while agave has a higher fructose concentration than even HFCS (and thus prompts undesirable triglyceride production). There's no free ride here!

Artificial sweeteners are to be strictly avoided also, not only due to the health risks of ingesting chemically processed agents, but because they trick the brain into thinking you have just consumed a very sweet food or drink. As a result, your confused hormone response system stimulates an inappropriate insulin release and the "high-low, high-low" cycle begins. Some research suggests that your brain will seek even more "replacement" calories in reaction to being tricked with a sweet food that provides no caloric energy. Supporting this theory are the ever-increasing obesity rates despite widespread use of non-caloric artificial sweeteners in beverages and other foods (which, absent any other variables, should predict a collective decrease in caloric intake and obesity).

All forms of natural and processed sugars and sweeteners have a deleterious effect on your insulin system and general health. The less you eat sweeteners of any kind (yes, even the somewhat less objectionable stevia), the less you will crave them. Try cutting way back on sweets and sodas for even a couple of days and notice how your life improves immensely. See if you can maintain this sugar low for 21 days to begin to reprogram your genes to not need or want these agents. If you can do away with sweet desserts altogether, you'll be well on your way to eliminating the addiction.

Chapter Summary

Avoid the following:

1. Poisonous Things: Make a sincere effort to reject the powerful manipulative influence of corporate advertising pushing you in the direction of poor food choices and cultural traditions favoring unhealthy meal habits. Processed carbohydrates, including sugars, grains (wheat, rice, bread, pasta, cereal, corn, etc.), and even legumes should be eliminated or strictly moderated due to their effect on insulin levels and immune function and their inferior nutritional value to natural plants and animals.

2. Grains: While grains (and legumes) have been presented as healthy staple foods for thousands of years of civilization, our genes are maladapted to ingesting them because they elicit a high insulin response compared to the foods that have sustained human life for two million years: vegetables, fruits, nuts, seeds, and animal products. The regular pattern of stimulating high blood insulin levels from a diet of excessive grain and sugar products leads to difficulty burning stored body fat (hence, lifelong weight gain) and serious long-term health problems, including heart disease and diet-related cancers.

Grains offer minimal nutritional value in comparison to vegetables, fruits, nuts, seeds, and animal products, ironically making grains a leading cause of nutritional deficiencies across the globe. Objectionable agents in grains compromise health mildly to severely, depending on your sensitivity. The phytates in grains can inhibit the absorption of minerals. Glutens can disturb healthy immune function and promote inflammation. Other lectins can inhibit healthy gastrointestinal function. Whole grains are no healthier than refined grains, and can have a worse impact on health in many cases due to higher levels of these three agents.

3. Polyunsaturated Oils (PUFAs): In recent decades, we have unwisely transitioned from saturated animal fats to PUFA oils. PUFA oils oxidize easily, particularly when heated during cooking. They are pro-inflammatory, have unfavorable O6:O3 ratios, hamper healthy immune and hormone function, lower HDL and raise LDL cholesterol, and are associated with obesity, diabetes, cancer, and heart disease. Strict avoidance of canola, margarine, other vegetable and seed PUFAs, and vegetable shortening is critical to health.

(continued)

Chapter Summary

4. Trans and Partially Hydrogenated Fats: These chemically altered molecules found in heavily processed foods are highly toxic to the body and are a major contributor to inflammation, accelerated aging, and many cancers. Trans and partially hydrogenated fats promote rampant oxidation and free radical damage in the body and disturb the healthy composition and function of cell membranes.

5. Other Foods: Legumes are often incorrectly considered vegetables. While offering some nutrient value, they can stimulate a high insulin response, may also contain offensive lectins, and are best replaced with primal foods. Sugary foods and beverages (particularly high fructose corn syrup) are devoid of nutrition, stimulate excessive insulin, and are leading factors in the modern decline of human health.

PRIMAL
BLUEPRINT
SUCCESS STORIES

Some of the most rewarding elements of the Primal Blueprint movement are the astonishing Success Story submissions we receive at MarksDailyApple.com each week. We publish a story every Friday, but the submissions have become so frequent we can only share a portion of them. Nevertheless, I read every single one and they touch me profoundly. It's mind blowing to realize how big the movement has become and how much momentum has been created from word of mouth on Internet blogs, forums, and local community meetup groups.

While I hope this book is everything you were looking for, I would love for you to take things further by joining the MarksDailyApple.com community. These success stories are a mere sampling of the hundreds you'll find online. Who knows? Maybe someday you'll be compelled to send us a story and photos to join the ranks of people who have transformed their lives living Primally.

SUCCESS STORY:
MALIKA DUKE
Ft. Worth, TX

> **"** *I was starting to think I'd have to settle for the 'fluffy mommy look' forever.* **"**

Malika submitted a sequence of stunning photos chronicling her Primal transformation over time. Describing her starting point in May of 2010, Malika says, "After having three kids, I was starting to believe that I'd have to settle for the 'fluffy mommy look' forever. I'd completed a double round of an intense 90-day home workout program that glamorized "muscle confusion", but I was not happy with the way my body looked afterward. Since I'd worked incredibly hard, I suspected that the problem lay in my diet," Malika relates.

"Interestingly, I was at the same age (32) where my father (eating a traditional Caribbean diet high in rice and beans) was first diagnosed with diabetes. The disease has rendered him legally blind, compromising his independence, self worth, self esteem, and enjoyment of life. Diabetes also took the life of my grandmother in 2008, and affects my sister, mother (high cholesterol and blood pressure), aunt, uncle, two cousins and others in my family who refuse to seek change or entertain life after grains. My motivation to go Primal was to have diabetes and related conditions stop with me in the family bloodline!" asserts Malika.

Malika continues, "We had some family arguments over such a sudden dietary change, particularly when the food bills got higher from eating uncured bacon, sausage and farm-fresh eggs. After a short time however, there wasn't much for my husband to argue about. I mean, come on—what red-blooded American male would argue for whole wheat pasta instead of spinach, tomato and onion in bacon fat with a big honking piece of rib-eye?!"

Body composition results for Malika and her family were immediate and dramatic. "I didn't have a scale to weigh that old fluffy mommy, but I dropped all the way down to my current 151 pounds (69 kilos) and I'm seeing muscles that I thought were lost forever! My husband seems to have recovered from his totally undiagnosed Irritable Bowel Syndrome, and thanks me at least once a week for his newly uncovered eight-pack! My ten and eight year old's have leaned out from a pudgy 137 lbs (62 kg) and 110 lbs (50 kg), to 106 lbs (48 kg) and 84 lbs (38 kg), respectively. Things have gone so well that we've created a community to help women and families transition to a Primal Blueprint lifestyle!" concludes Malika. Check out her Website, featuring numerous helpful videos from Malika, FitRichWoman.com.

NICK LASZLO
South San Francisco, CA

> " *I'm actually looking forward to turning 50,*
> *and I've never felt or looked better!*
> *What a sharp contrast from when I turned 40...* "

Nick, 49, is a recovered alcoholic, "former fattie", and former elite long distance runner. After reaching his peak as an athlete in his 20s, Nick sustained a series of injuries, burnout and then "plunged into a 20-year exercise in self-pity", featuring substance abuse, pizza, fast food, high blood pressure, high cholesterol, and a long-term bout with Hepatitis C.

During his steady decline in health and fitness, Nick was cranking along in what he calls a "successful facade of a highly-paid software engineer." Losing his job in March of 2010 inspired Nick to take action and turn his life around. He quit drinking and took a long look in the mirror, noticing how well 36 percent body fat obscured the elite athlete trapped inside. Nick laced up his running shoes again, thinking that running, his "trusted best friend from the past", would make everything right. Alas, it wasn't so easy to return to single digit body fat. He tried starvation diets, diet pills and dangerous amounts of stimulants to no avail.

Good results started to happen as he dabbled in primal-style eating: He dropped 55 pounds (25 kilos) (going from 36 percent to *six percent* body fat, and gaining eight pounds of muscle) and his blood work normalized. However, he still had bouts of binge eating and a sense that things weren't ideal. After discovering *The Primal Blueprint* at a bookstore one day in 2010 and implementing its principles, Nick enjoyed breakthroughs in energy, metabolism, general health, and competitive success as a masters (age-group) long distance runner.

While Nick puts in more miles training for master's competition than might typically be recommended by the Primal Blueprint, he is careful to moderate his pace, avoid chronic patterns, and also integrate Primal-style strength and sprint workouts into his training regimen.

"Here I am today, looking forward to turning 50, and feeling tons better than when I was 40," commented Nick. "I currently earn my living as a personal trainer specializing in weight loss at a local health club. I give each new client a 'homework assignment' after our first appointment: Go out and buy Mark's book! *The Primal Blueprint* has changed my life and I know it will change theirs too," Nick concluded.

July 11, 2010   December 4, 2010

551   698

165 lbs   130 lbs

SUCCESS STORY:
MICHELLE MATANGI
New Plymouth, New Zealand

"I finally feel freed from my obsession with food, and can do the odd 24-hour fast with no problems."

Michelle, aka "Dollface" the prolific Primal blogger (primaljourney. blogspot.com), relates a compelling story of struggling for years to be healthy and fit. Her travails began a decade ago at age 21, with job stress, depression, weight gain, and of course the obligatory prescription meds from her physician. Michelle blames antidepressant medication for contributing to rapid weight gain, as she hit 87 kilograms (191 pounds) at 5'6". Upon adopting the Atkins Diet, she dropped many kilos in short order, but didn't feel healthy. "Lot's of diet coke and artificially sweetened chocolate, and continued anxiety and depression," remembers Michelle.

Michelle shifted gears, went back to grain-based eating, and endured several years of "constant hunger, and steady weight gain up to a morbidly obese 107 kilos (235 lbs). I was eating every 2-3 hours and constantly hungry!," Michelle relates. Realizing she had done better on a low-carb program, Michelle intensified her Internet research and discovered MarksDailyApple.com. "I was glued to the site for days!," remembers Michelle. "I eliminated grain foods, and added plenty of veggies, protein, and fat. No diet coke this time, just soda water and herbal teas. Furthermore, as I got deeper into the Primal Blueprint, I realized it's all about lifestyle, not just dieting. I now weigh 69 kilos (152 lbs) and finally have my anxiety under control."

Michelle continues, "The Primal way feels so natural—coming from a person who absolutely had to eat every 2-3 hours or I would get lightheaded and even dizzy! Now I can do the odd 24-hour fast with no problem. I finally feel freed from my obsession with food, and the handcuffs of my eating time-table. This is one of the best things about going Primal."

Michelle takes to care to not let her stunning before/after transformation photos and her incredible passion for Primal living get in the way of reality when communicating with others. Asked the secret to her succcess, she shoots straight: "Sometimes it feels impossible, stuck in a fat body, to imagine how you could ever be thinner. It can be a tough pill to swallow when you realize there is no magic pill, and you have to make some major changes if you want real results.

Sure, I still face daily challenges in a world driven by Conventional Wisdom and refined foods everywhere. But when I make conscious choices and focus on the satisfaction of eating Primal foods, it's easy to stay on track. That and I keep a pair of my old size 20 jeans around; they're a great reminder of where I've been and how far I've come!," concludes Michelle.

SUCCESS STORY:
DAVE PARSONS

Roosevelt, NJ

"I EAT MARK'S APPLE EVERY DAY. IT MAKES IT OKAY TO BE WHO I AM…AND BE A MEMBER OF THE PRIMAL LIFE CLAN!"

"Unconquerable Dave" as he is known at MarksDailyApple.com wows us with regular updates in his inimitable ALL CAPS writing style:

DEAR MARK, A PIC IS WORTH 1,000 WORDS…STARTED ~300 POUNDS…DOWN TO 200…NOW THERE AIN'T MUCH LEFT TO LOSE…..I REMEMBER THIS SIZE WHEN I WAS 18 YEARS OLD. GROK ON AND THANK YOU FOR THE ILLUMINATION! LATER BROTHER. STAY IN THE LIGHT. GROK RULES!

Dave, 54, first contacted me after losing 40 pounds (18 kilos) in six months. He related how his passion for cooking (SAD stuff, over past years) "just about slayed my entire family!" After four months of transitioning to Primal-style eating, he got into the groove with a simple approach, "If I can't kill it, find it, or gather it, I don't eat it. Makes it real easy to eat well! My body tells me what it wants and I listen. The wife and kids still around are impressed with my new attitude and look.

While most of Dave's early results came from Primal eating with only mild exercise, he relates that as weight came off and energy increased, he was able to resume some significant strength training. "I like the Primal approach way better than being a gym gorilla. I have my own outdoor Primal gym of trees and rocks and stuff," Dave relates. Averse to the gym or not, Dave's progress reports include some impressive gym numbers, such as a 404-pound (183 kilo) deadlift and 18-inch biceps. It's hard to top Dave's images to capture the essence of living Primally, but he makes a good attempt with words in closing a recent update:

"To steal words from Walt Whitman...
'I too am not a bit tamed, I too am untranslatable,
I sound my barbaric YAWP over the roofs of the world.'"

Everyone in the Primal community hears your YAWP Dave! May it echo to many more folks. Grok On brother!

SUCCESS STORY:
DEANNA EBERLIN
Corning, NY

"The biggest change in my life, beyond what I eat, how I exercise or how I sleep, is the simple freedom that the Primal Blueprint has afforded me."

Deanna is one of our longest duration success stories, still going strong over four years. Deanna relates that she started trending toward obesity in third grade, "the last time I felt normal". She reached 200 pounds (91 kilos) at age 18, feeling generally unhappy about life and her dead-end jobs. Fed up and tipping the scales at 250 pounds (114 kilos) ("I stopped weighing myself after that"), Deanna kicked off a new direction by ditching grains and engaging in Chronic Cardio. On a diet of six treadmill miles and 1,800 calories a day, Deanna dropped to 140 pounds (64 kilos), at which point she reached a frustrating plateau.

While Deanna's methods delivered substantial results on the scale, they were both short of her ultimate goal and seemed unsustainable over the long term. After some ruminating and Internet research, Deanna ultimately decided to "overcome my initial fat phobia" and begin transitioning to a Primal lifestyle. Not just diet, but optimal sleeping habits, more play, and ditching Chronic Cardio for a Primal-aligned program. In only three months of going Primal, Deanna lost that pesky final 15 pounds (7 kilos) to reach 125 pounds (57 kilos). "Half of my former bodyweight - how freaky is that?!", exclaimed Deanna. Beyond the body composition improvements, Deanna reports having more regulated daily energy levels, ("I only eat 2-3 times per day instead of 5-6"), high energy mornings in the office - to the dismay of dragging co-workers!, and enjoyable evenings - "I don't pass out on the couch after dinner anymore."

We checked back with Deanna in early 2012, two years after her initial submission and four years into her Primal journey. "I've added five pounds of muscle, and have experienced some peripheral health benefits such as increased hair thickness and an improved complexion," Deanna related.

Currently Deanna is taking college courses in Health and Wellness. Her final thoughts extend out to readers with a few tips: "Focus on lifestyle change that is sustainable and forget the extreme stuff. Choose freedom: eat what you want, when you want; and if you don't feel like exercising one day, skip it. Finally, set ambitious goals. When I started I couldn't so a single pushup. Now I can do 20—real ones, not girlie! Believe in the power of the body to transform, and be patient with the process."

SUCCESS STORY:
WADE BAKER
Portland, OR

"Within a month of eating Primally, my lifelong symptoms of asthma disappeared, my gastric reflux abated, I dropped 15 pounds, and ceased all prescription medication."

    Wade relates a disturbing litany of health conditions prior to going Primal. At 5'10" and 325 pounds, with a BMI of 47, Wade was taking three asthma medications, suffered from severe acid reflux (taking expensive prescription acid reducers), and strapped up to a CPAP machine each night to deal with his sleep apnea.

Having struggled his entire life with excess body fat, Wade embarked upon yet another weight loss program in January of 2010, guided by a professional physical therapist, trainer and nutritionist. "I committed myself feverishly to Conventional Wisdom: daily torturous battles with my body at the gym and a low-fat, high-fiber, high-carb diet. I experienced some modest initial results, but had a sense that all those refined carbs were not healthy. I battled about this with my nutritionist/trainer, who swore that my instincts were wrong and that I would be doomed to failure if I broke from Conventional Wisdom," Wade relates.

After a couple months of unease, Wade recalls, "I followed my gut and set out full-steam ahead down my Primal path. Within a month of ceasing my refined flour and sugar consumption and eating Primally, I began to see immediate and dramatic results. My lifelong symptoms of severe asthma immediately disappeared, my painful gastric reflux abated, I dropped 15 pounds that first month, and I was able to cease all prescription medication."

Concurrent to his dietary changes, Wade backed off of his Chronic Cardio patterns, taking his exercise heart rate down to 70 percent of max and establishing a rhythm of cardio and strength workouts balanced by sufficient recovery.

In eleven months, Wade dropped 105 pounds, humming along at a steady rate of 8-12 pounds of body fat lost per month. "No asthma, no gastric reflux, no painful sleep-deprivation headaches, no weakness from chronic workouts, no lethargy from insulin crashes, and no more annoying CPAP machine to sleep!," reports Wade.

Wade has checked in several times since his initial report nearly two years ago. "My life has dramatically changed. I almost never go hungry, and have no cravings—even when I skip a meal, which I often do. I have lost a total of 137 pounds following Primal Blueprint. I'm currently working with a personal trainer and getting into some heavy weights. My success has even convinced my trainer to start eating Primally, and he now recommends it to his clients!"

TOO GOOD
TO BE TRUE?

Hey, I thought the same thing upon receiving some of our more amazing photos (yep, they're real—we obtained signed affidavits from everyone!). "Sometimes being skinnier seems impossible to imagine when you're stuck in a fat body," as Dollface relates. However, with even a basic understanding of gene expression, these photos and stories begin to make perfect sense. How someone like Deanna, enduring obesity since adolescence, can shed half of her bodyweight in a couple years. Or how Nick can turn back the clock and rediscover athletic genes hidden for over two decades.

I know you love your morning granola and afternoon strawberry yogurt snack, but would you be open to tweaking some lifestyle staples for 21 days, to see if things could get even better? Granted, it's easier said than done for creatures of habit like us, but I hope these stories will get you dreaming big!

Remember, your hand is on the dial 24/7. You can offend your genes with all manner of modern challenges: Evening laptop sessions staring into a screen as bright to your eyes (and hormones) as the midday sun; or visits to a brightly-painted smoothie shop to obtain triple the amount of carbs Grok ate in a day—in just 20 minutes of slurping and scarfing.

Or, you can try as best you can to deliver the experience your genes expect to make you healthy (eating meat, fish, fowl and eggs; doing some occasional all-out sprints; hitting the sack soon after sunset), and reap the comprehensive benefits. The choice is yours!

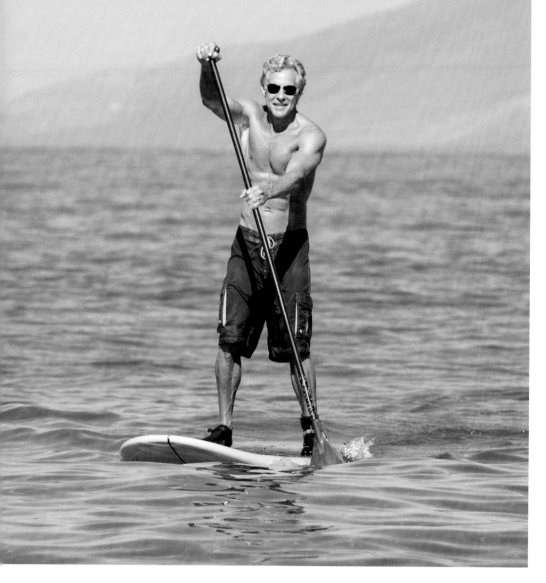

PRIMAL ESSENTIAL MOVEMENTS

Strength training can be simple, safe, and fun for everyone! Just focus on the **Primal Essential Movements**: pushups, pullups, squats and planks. These exercises work all the muscles in your body, and promote functional fitness for a broad application of athletic and daily life activities. Refer to the Bonus Material for details on the progression exercises for each movement to custom design an appropriate workout for your fitness level.

Pushups: Plank position, arms extended shoulder width apart, hands forward. Lower to ground, bending elbows at 45-degree angle backwards. Chest touches first! Keep body dead straight, core and glutes tight, head and neck neutral to torso. *PEM Mastery*: Male 50, Female 20.

Pull-ups: Elbows tight, chin tucked, shoulder blades retracted (protects spine). Raise body up, leading with chest, lower body quiet. Raise chin over the bar and gradually lower until arms are almost straight. *PEM Mastery*: Male 12, Female 5.

Squats: Feet shoulder-width or slightly wider, toes forward at comfortable angle. Lower by extending butt out/backward and keeping back straight – don't bend forward! Lower until thighs are parallel to ground. Stand back up completely, making sure your knees track in line with your feet. *PEM Mastery*: Male and Female 50.

Planks: Elbows on ground shoulder width apart. Raise onto toes with body horizontal, core and glutes tight. *PEM Mastery*: Male and Female 2 minutes.

CHAPTER 6

The Primal Blueprint
Exercise Laws

Move, Lift, and Sprint—Exciting
New Low-Tech Fitness Fads!

In This Chapter

I detail the rationale and benefits of the three Primal Blueprint exercise laws: Law #3, Move Frequently at a Slow Pace; Law #4, Lift Heavy Things; and Law #5, Sprint Once in a While. Following these laws will enable you to approximate the active lifestyle of Grok and develop what I call Primal Blueprint Fitness. Primal Blueprint Fitness represents a versatile and diverse set of abilities that allow you to tackle varied active lifestyle or athletic challenges safely and competently. In contrast, many pursue narrow, specialized forms of fitness that are minimally functional and often compromise general health (endurance athletes and bodybuilders fall in this category). Following the Primal Blueprint exercise laws will also help delay the aging process by preserving lean muscle mass, which correlates with enhanced organ function, a concept known as *organ reserve*.

I contrast the benefits of Primal Blueprint Fitness with the many drawbacks and health risks associated with Conventional Wisdom's fitness recommendations. Moving frequently at a slow pace is superior to an exhausting routine of Chronic Cardio. These workouts often lead to sugar cravings that compromise weight-loss efforts as well as hamper immune and endocrine function. Lifting heavy things involves brief, intense sessions (lasting 10 to 30 minutes) that promote optimal hormone secretion and prevent the catabolic effects of prolonged sessions that leave you exhausted and depleted.

Few things are more Primal than Law #5—run for your life once in a while! Brief, intense sprints (or other maximum efforts that are low or no impact) trigger optimal hormone balance, lean muscle development, accelerated fat metabolism, and incredible fitness breakthroughs. I discuss the best strategic approach for conducting workouts for each of the three Primal Blueprint laws, including form pointers for running and cycling and the benefits of going barefoot. Specific workout suggestions for strength training and sprinting are provided in the Bonus Material at the end of this book and online at MarksDailyApple.com, including a free downloadable ebook called *Primal Blueprint Fitness*.

Those who think they have not time for bodily exercise will sooner or later have to find time for illness.

—Lord Edward Stanley,
Three-time United Kingdom Prime Minister
(1799-1869)

The movements that dictated how our genes evolved were simple: squat, crawl, walk, run, jump, climb, hang, carry, throw, push, pull, and more actions we probably don't even have names for. This primal "training program" helped Grok survive the rigors of a hostile environment, explore new territories, track and exploit new types of food, build shelters, and basically become ripped.

Becoming super fit is as simple as blending lots of low-level movement with intermittent bouts of higher intensity efforts. There is little need for the incredible complexity of today's fitness scene—the outrageous gym equipment, obsessively detailed and regimented training programs, and fancy contraptions, such as cyclometers, GPS units, and calorie-burning meters. These gadgets, while possessing a high cool factor, can also lead you astray from the benefits of having a simple, varied, and intuitive approach to exercise. By the way, most young kids will employ many of Grok's movements without even thinking about it (squat, crawl, walk, etc.) when left outside to play in a suitable environment.

Unfortunately, commuting, work, digital entertainment, and modern comforts hinder our opportunities to enjoy spontaneous play and get fit naturally. Furthermore, Conventional Wisdom has brainwashed us to believe that a lean, fit body comes from either lucky genes or following a regimented, often overly stressful exercise routine. It's no wonder that many well-meaning enthusiasts have become either exhausted or totally turned off to getting fit. Millions more endure with flawed approaches that leave them disappointed and discouraged when they fall far short of their ultimate peak performance potential and ideal body composition.

At the bare minimum, you can get extremely healthy and fit on two hours a week of walking around, one abbreviated strength workout a week lasting 10-15 minutes, one full-length strength workout a week lasting around 30 minutes, and a sprint session every 7 to 10 days lasting 15-20 minutes (only a few minutes of that is hard effort). That's less than 3 hours out of the 168 at our disposal each week. You don't have to endure the fatigue and exhaustion that so many have suffered when following Conventional

Wisdom's recommendation to adopt a consistent and unnecessarily complex exercise program. You don't even have to be consistent; in fact, it's better if you are inconsistent with your workout routine. Heck, the old saying "All you need is a pair of shoes" doesn't even apply—you don't even need shoes! (See the sidebar "Happy Feet" later in the chapter.)

> *Pursue challenges that turn you on instead of worrying about what the magazines say is the "best" workout or the marketing hype that glorifies extreme events.*

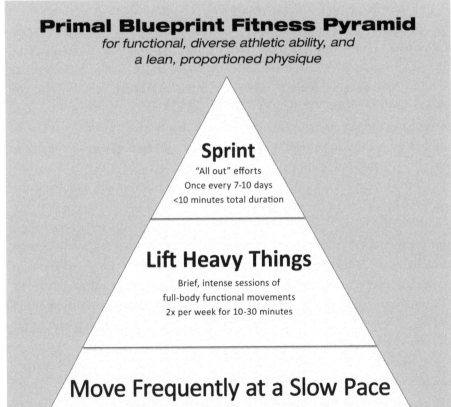

Primal Blueprint Fitness Pyramid
for functional, diverse athletic ability, and a lean, proportioned physique

Sprint
"All out" efforts
Once every 7-10 days
<10 minutes total duration

Lift Heavy Things
Brief, intense sessions of
full-body functional movements
2x per week for 10-30 minutes

Move Frequently at a Slow Pace
Walking, hiking, cycling, easy cardio
at 55-75% max heart rate for 2-5 hrs per week

While it's comforting to realize how well you can do with the bare minimum prescriptions, I'll also assert that you can take the Primal Blueprint exercise laws all the way to the top. If you are a devoted gym rat looking to get ripped, if you dream of auditioning for a swimsuit ad, or if you are competing at the elite level in team or individual sports (yep, including endurance sports), a comparatively minimal time commitment to the Primal Blueprint approach can produce vastly superior results (and decreased risk of injuries and burnout) compared to the traditional approach of frequent, prolonged strenuous workouts.

For example, an optimal exercise week for a very devoted exerciser could include a two-hour hike, another easy cardio session of one hour, two full-body strength-training sessions lasting no more than 30 minutes each, a sprint session with an accumulated five minutes of maximum effort, and a challenging "play" day (e.g., a pickup soccer, basketball, or Ultimate Frisbee game). This still only totals about seven hours of exercise.

If you are currently racking up a dozen or more hours of Chronic Cardio each week, or hitting the gym most every day for prolonged strength-training sessions isolating specific muscle groups, I encourage you to reframe your perspective from "more is better" to "intense is better." If you find yourself bouncing off the walls with extra energy because your new Primal schedule is too easy, *make your hard workouts even harder*—not longer or more frequent. Remember, the goal is to trigger optimal gene expression, not fill in all the blanks of your log book and teeter on the edge of injury and burnout.

For those interested in the effects of Primal exercise on weight loss, we must start with the critical assumption that 80 percent of your body composition success is determined by how you eat. Reprogramming your genes through dietary signals to derive most of your energy from stored fat will continuously push you towards your ideal body composition regardless of whether or not you work out hard. Also understand that low level cardio sessions alone do not raise your metabolic rate significantly enough to stimulate significant fat reduction. However, low level cardio workouts greatly enhance your ability to metabolize fat—both during exercise and at rest. Meanwhile, brief, intense strength and sprint sessions elevate body temperature and stimulate an increase in your metabolic rate, not only during the workout but also for many hours afterward.

Put everything together and you have a formula for successful long-term weight management: eating Primally and moving frequently at a slow pace (optimizing your fat-burning system) and lifting heavy things and running really fast occasionally (stimulating lean muscle development and increasing metabolic rate). This "round-the-clock" concept of reprogramming genes (through Primal Blueprint eating and exercise habits) is the true secret to natural, effortless, long-term weight loss and/or weight management. The story stands in sharp contrast to Conventional Wisdom's "calories in, calories out" model where you hope the 600 calories burned during your 50-minute step aerobics class will somehow lead to weight loss. Recall that Kelly Korg inhaled nearly double that on her quick visit to Jamba Juice!

Primal Blueprint Fitness

With a balanced regimen patterned after Grok and designed to promote optimal gene expression, you will develop what I call Primal Blueprint Fitness. This means you have a broad range of skills and attributes (strength, power, speed, endurance) that allow you to do pretty much whatever you want (or, in Grok's case, survive the various challenges of primal life) with a substantial degree of competence and minimal risk of injury.

By breaking free from the cycle of carbs fueling stressful, sugar-burning Chronic Cardio workouts, you can easily get into the ideal body fat percentage range of 8 to 15 percent for men and 12 to 20 percent for women. This is true no matter who you are or how plump your family tree is. For women, a Primal Blueprint Fitness program will tone your entire body—not just lower body fat levels but also give you some noticeable definition in your arms, legs, and core.

While many female exercisers are concerned exclusively with weight management and not inclined toward competitive athletic endeavors, you may surprise yourself—and gain some street cred with the neighborhood kids—when you display your aptitude on the soccer field or in a footrace. When you expand your horizons beyond "jogging at a strenuous pace for five songs on my iPod," your body will begin to show the effects all over, most notably by correcting the common trouble spots of excess butt, hip, thigh, and abdominal fat.

For the competitor, you can expect to branch out beyond your bread-and-butter skills to become a more complete athlete. Those who rely on bulk to hoist mucho plates or post up under the basket will become leaner and improve their power-to-weight ratio (how strong you are in relation to your body weight). This translates into more pull-ups, a higher vertical leap, and more quickness on your first step. Those who tend to be slight of frame and lacking in power will add a bit more muscle and improve pure strength and explosiveness, expanding their repertoire not only to outlast the competition but to out-power them.

Power-to-weight ratio is a critical Primal Blueprint Fitness benchmark because it has a strong functional component. A skinny dude like the late Bruce Lee was by reasonable definition more powerful than Hulk Hogan because of having a superior power-to-weight ratio. American Brian Clay, 2008 Olympic decathlon gold medalist, is the quintessential Primal athlete. At five feet eleven inches and 174 pounds, Clay is smaller than many of his competitors but is capable of a stunning versatility of athletic performances. While his physique is certainly impressive and looks great on the beach, it is not overly bulky nor overly defined like the vein-popping magazine cover models. However, Clay can sprint, run hurdles, high-jump, pole-vault, and throw such implements as shot, discus, and javelin at very respectable levels when his scores are considered against individual event specialists. In the SPARQ (speed, power, agility, reaction, and quickness) test commonly used to evaluate NFL prospects, Clay achieved a phenomenal score of 130. In comparison, Reggie Bush, a remarkable physical specimen who won the Heisman Trophy for USC and became a running back for the New Orleans Saints and Miami Dolphins, scored a 93.

> *Instead of following a strict schedule, align your workout decisions with your energy and motivation levels.*

Others point to the diverse athletic demands of boxing as fodder for the "greatest all-around athlete" distinction. Basketball stars, such as Kobe Bryant and LeBron James, blend an incredible array of skills—speed and endurance, strength and quickness—to perform seemingly superhuman feats. (Ever try a 360-degree slam dunk—even on a low basket? It ain't easy!). CrossFit.com, a popular exercise Web site, idealizes the ultimate athlete as a combination gymnast, power lifter, and sprinter. For the last word, I'll echo the Primal Blueprint philosophy about dietary habits. The ideal body that you build comes down to personal preference within the broad guidelines of the Primal Blueprint. Do the exercises that turn you on the most—in your mind, your heart, and your genes!

Regarding the specific workout plan to reach your Primal Blueprint Fitness goals, it is better to make sure your workout decisions align with your energy and motivation levels than to follow a strict schedule. Sprint once in a while when you are super motivated and energized. Take a walk around the block or hike up to the radio tower on Sunday morning if you feel the urge, or stay home and read the newspaper in bed if you're dragging and just don't feel like working out.

This unstructured approach might feel uncomfortable if you are under the influence of flawed Conventional Wisdom that values consistency, gadgetry, and judging your fitness progress by the obsessive tracking of quantifiable data such as miles covered, calories burned, reps completed, time in target heart rate zone, or placing in the race. Grok knew nothing of this superficial silliness. His motivation to exercise was completely pure: to acquire his basic needs of food and shelter or to satisfy the innate human desire for adventure, competition, and play and for exploring the boundaries of the human spirit, regardless of what measured results came of it. I urge you to determine the success of your fitness program by how much fun you are having and how much personal growth you experience from striving for your goals. Pursue challenges that turn you on instead of worrying about what the magazines say is the best workout or about the marketing hype that glorifies extreme events, such as the marathon or Ironman® triathlon, as ultimate athletic accomplishments.

Organ Reserve: The Key to Longevity

If you fall somewhere short of fitness freak on the continuum, keep in mind that the benefits of a sensible exercise program extend far beyond competitive success and looking good. The more lean muscle you maintain throughout life, the better your organs will function, up to an obvious point of diminishing returns; e.g., a bodybuilder has heaps of excess muscle that serve little or no functional purpose and require a lot of caloric energy to sustain. Optimal organ function correlates with maximum longevity and excellent health.

Organs, like muscles, adhere to the "use it or lose it" natural law. When you hit the deck for 50 push-ups, the conscious decision to engage these muscles in a work effort calls your heart, lungs, liver, adrenals, and other organs into action. Blood chemistry changes as you burn glycogen and fat, process oxygen, and produce metabolic by-products (e.g., lactic acid) at an accelerated rate. You are asking your organs to keep up with your active lifestyle, in the process strengthening them to better withstand the demands of daily life and the natural aging process.

In contrast, when your activity diminishes, as in the classic paradigm of aging, muscles and organs can atrophy. Their function decreases because they are given no reason to remain at 100 percent efficiency. An unfit person has lower bone density, less lung capacity (the quantity of air you can exchange on each breath) and stroke volume (the amount of blood your heart pumps with each beat) than a fit person. The aging process—at least in America—should really be called the "process of physical decline largely due to inactivity and lifestyle habits that result in mismanaged genes."

Because all of your organs and body systems work synergistically, you are vulnerable to the often fatal effects of your weakest link. For example, an unfit accident victim or a surgery patient who loses a lot of blood and has a heart operating at only 45 percent of potential capacity will often fare differently than a fit person with superior heart function suffering the same trauma. Bones break more easily among the unfit. Pneumonia is a common cause of death among the elderly often due to the inability of their weakened lungs to help clear the germ-laden mucus effectively through coughing.

> *Walking is the best possible exercise.*
> *Habituate yourself to walk very far.*
> —**Thomas Jefferson**

Primal Blueprint Law #3: Move Frequently at a Slow Pace

While you can benefit from low-intensity aerobic exercise almost indefinitely (e.g., hiking the Pacific Crest Trail or Appalachian Trail all summer is pretty darn good for your overall health), you can still obtain outstanding health and fitness benefits by engaging in a moderate amount of low-intensity aerobic movement (hike, walk briskly, cycle gently—or jog if you are really fit). You should shoot for a bare minimum of two hours and hopefully up to five hours of low-intensity aerobic movement per week, knowing that even five-minute work breaks or 15-minute strolls through the neighborhood with your dog contribute meaningfully to your genetic requirements for frequent movement.

If you can manage a single long hike on the weekend and a few short walks or cardio machine sessions during the week, you will dramatically reduce your risk of heart disease (in comparison to being sedentary), support optimal metabolism, better control your weight, and, in conjunction with the other two types of workouts, achieve broad athletic competency that characterizes Primal Blueprint Fitness.

Remember that these recommendations are averages. I will occasionally go for extended periods of time (thanks to injury or travel) doing no exercise whatsoever. I suffer no ill effects, experience no change in body composition (because I am eating Primally), and invariably pick up right where I left off when I resume normal training. At other times, when the stars align and I have the free time, I'll benefit greatly from doing vastly more than the recommended average (e.g., when going on a backpacking trip or another active vacation).

My definition of low-intensity movement is sustained exercise at a range of 55 to 75 percent of maximum heart rate (I will discuss in detail just what this means shortly). With this casual aerobic exercise, your heart and other energy systems work a little harder to handle the extra fuel and oxygen delivery demands, but not so much that you are overstressed. The specific biochemical signals created by this low-level aerobic activity produce numerous health and fitness benefits.

Improved Fat Metabolism: You train your body to efficiently utilize free fatty acids for fuel, a benefit that is realized 24 hours a day, with a higher metabolic rate and a preference for fat over glucose (provided you eat Primally). Low-level aerobic exercise also helps balance blood glucose levels and regulate appetite.

> " *I love running cross country.…*
> *On a track, I feel like a hamster.* "
> **—Robin Williams**

Zoning: "In" and "Out"

To determine your 55-75 percent exercise zone numbers, you must perform a strenuous maximum heart rate test (get medical clearance first), or use a formula to estimate your max. I recommend a new formula (from University of Colorado) as follows: 208 minus (0.7 times age) = Estimated Maximum Heart Rate. For example, Ken Korg at 40 has an estimated max heart rate of 180 beats per minute [208 - 28 (.7 x 40 = 28)]. Ken's low-level aerobic workouts should thus be conducted in a heart rate range of 99 beats per minute (180 max × 55 percent) to 135 beats per minute (180 max × 75 percent).

Fifty-five percent reflects the bare minimum exertion level to legitimately consider your effort "exercise." An unfit person can reach this walking to the mailbox. 75 percent feels surprisingly easy, particularly if you've been engaged in Chronic Cardio and regularly exceed that number. At 75 percent pace, you break a moderate sweat, can easily converse without getting short of breath, and finish feeling refreshed and energized instead of slightly fatigued and hungry, as you might after more strenuous workouts.

Monitor your heart rate during workouts with a wireless unit or a pulse check as follows: place your finger against the carotid artery on the side of your neck and count how many beats occur in exactly 10 seconds (on your watch or indoor clock). Multiply that number by six to determine your heart rate in beats per minute. You don't have to monitor every minute of every workout, but make it a regular practice to keep yourself honest. It's easy to drift too high when going by perceived exertion alone, since 75 percent is so comfortable. Exceeding 75 percent routinely can alter your workouts from healthy to chronic.

The best thing about heart rate training is that it individualizes your experience to ensure you get an optimal workout. This critical "individual" element—one that can make or break your entire exercise program—has long been ignored by group class instructors and social groups working out together. Generally speaking, asking a class or group of workout partners to keep pace together is a recipe for failure, for *all but the fittest members of the group*. As a final note, exceeding 75 percent occasionally, when you feel great and want to really go for it, is just fine—as long as adequate rest and recovery are observed.

Improved Cardiovascular Function: You increase your capillary network (blood vessels that supply the muscle cells with fuel and oxygen), muscle mitochondria, and stroke volume of your heart (more blood pumped with each beat) and also improve oxygen delivery by your lungs.

Improved Musculoskeletal System: You strengthen your bones, joints, and connective tissue so you can absorb increasing stress loads without breaking down. This is critical to your ability to perform and recover from your high-intensity Primal sessions.

Stronger Immune System: You enhance the function of your immune system by stimulating beneficial hormone flow and building a more efficient circulatory system.

Increased Energy: You finish workouts feeling energized and refreshed, rather than slightly fatigued and depleted from a schedule of moderate to difficult intensity workouts conducted too frequently.

> *Chronic Cardio—a program I followed for nearly 20 years as a marathoner and later as an ironman triathlete—is bad for your health, period.*

A Case Against Cardio

In contrast to the comprehensive benefits of frequent, comfortably paced exercise, getting more serious about working out can really mess you up if you have a flawed approach. Chronic Cardio at heart rates above 75 percent of maximum places excessive stress on your body, the kind of stress to which you are not genetically adapted. I'd estimate that the vast majority of folks you see working out on cardio machines, jogging through the neighborhood, or keeping pace in the group class are exceeding 75 percent (often by a wide margin) for the duration of nearly every session.

While an aerobic workout at 75 or even up to 85 percent of maximum heart rate might not feel terribly difficult at the time, a sustained pattern of Chronic Cardio can lead to numerous problems with metabolism, stress management, immune function, and general health. As exercise intensity increases, your preferred fuel choice shifts from primarily fat at intensities below 75 percent (fat burns well in the presence of oxygen, and fat stores are abundant—even in the skinniest marathoners!) to an ever-increasing percentage of glucose (quicker and easier to burn when oxygen is lacking due to your quickening pace). You'll recall that a major goal of Primal Blueprint eating and exercise is to reprogram your genes to burn more fat—not less.

A routine of Chronic Cardio requires large amounts of dietary carbohydrates each day to support it. While the risks of excess fat storage and hyperinsulinemia (overproduction of insulin) are moderated somewhat by a heavy exercise schedule, they are still significant because of your altered dietary habits throughout the day.

When muscles are depleted of glycogen (remember, stored glycogen is converted back into glucose for exercise fuel), your brain sends a powerful signal to replenish with quick-energy carbohydrate foods. Our brains have a tendency to tell us to overcompensate by eating a little too much. This is a genetically programmed survival adaptation against starvation risk, handed down to us from Grok. If you are looking to reduce body fat primarily through vigorous cardiovascular exercise (as Conventional Wisdom promises), you are quite likely to fail unless you slow down your pace and alter your diet to limit your carb intake.

Besides the weight-loss issues, Chronic Cardio increases the production of cortisol (in all but the most genetically gifted endurance athletes), which breaks down muscle tissue and suppresses production of key anabolic hormones, such as testosterone and human growth hormone. This hormonal imbalance caused by overexercising contributes to fatigue, burnout, immune suppression, loss of bone density, and undesirable changes in fat metabolism. Furthermore, the stress of Chronic Cardio increases systemic inflammation (a strong contributing factor to heart disease, cancer, and nearly all other health problems) and increases oxidative damage (via free radical production) by a factor of 10 to 20 times normal. This can lead to acceleration of the aging process. It's ironic that many in their 40s and 50s start engaging in marathon or triathlon training in hopes of improving health and delaying the aging process, when, quite often, it has the exact opposite effect.

Born to Walk—and Sprint

For those heavily indoctrinated into the Conventional Wisdom that Chronic Cardio is the path to health, fitness, and weight control, consider again the premise of the Primal Blueprint. Because Grok was a lean, strong, extremely active dude, he probably was capable of running long distances at a respectable pace, similar to today's gung-ho endurance athletes, but he most likely very rarely decided to do so. When the concept of organized hunting came along, it appears that Grok relied more on superior tracking ability (using his highly evolved brain) and walking or slow jogging (using his superior fat-burning system), rather than literally chasing down his prey. In fact, squandering valuable energy reserves (and increasing glucose metabolism by a factor of 10) by running hard for long periods of time would have hastened his demise. Imagine Grok chasing some game animal all-out for a few hours and—oops—not succeeding in killing it. He's spent an incredible amount of energy yet now has no food to replace that energy. He has suddenly become some other animal's prey because he is physically exhausted.

> ❝❝You have to stay in shape. My grandmother, she started walking five miles a day when she was 60. She's 97 today and we don't know where the hell she is. ❞❞
> **—Ellen DeGeneres**

A 2007 Taiwanese study published in the *British Journal of Sports Medicine* revealed that an intense sustained workout (working at 85 percent of maximum effort for at least 30 minutes) disrupted immune system function, destroyed some white blood cells, and triggered whole body inflammation for up to 72 hours. In contrast, there are literally hundreds of scientific studies confirming the benefits of conducting occasional short-duration, intense workouts (such as interval workouts—spacing work efforts between a particular rest interval). Intervals and sprints quickly and efficiently improve key performance factors including VO2 Max (how efficiently you process oxygen during peak exercise effort), competitive performance, and body composition.

I cannot emphasize strongly enough the importance of *slowing down* the pace of your cardio workouts to improve your health and fitness. Note that I'm speaking to the vast numbers of fitness enthusiasts in the gyms and on the roads who generally take their pace to "slightly uncomfortable" in the name of pursuing Conventional Wisdom's definition of "getting a workout." If you already like to take your time and smell the flowers on your walks, hikes, and bike rides, congratulations! Just get ready to add a few sprint workouts into the mix. That's where huge benefits will accrue for little investment. As I detail shortly, slowing down (and adding workouts from Laws #4 and #5) will not only improve health but will also lead to outstanding fitness breakthroughs.

I am fully aware of the many loud and passionate voices extolling the psychological and lifestyle virtues of devoted endurance training and agree that pushing and challenging your body with inspiring competitive goals supports mental, emotional, and also physical health (albeit with the significant caveats already discussed). An exercise physiologist friend of mine countered my "case against cardio" position recently by reminding me that Hawaii Ironman finishers are vastly healthier than the average population. While true, let us not forget, in the words of Jay Leno, the "average" we are dealing with: "Today there are more overweight people in America than average-weight people. So overweight people are now average. Which means you've met your New Year's resolution."

Furthermore, I'll assert that an old has-been like myself (goals: eat Primally, with no processed carbs; nail a couple brief, intense strength workouts each week—in the gym or outdoors; conduct one all-out sprint workout; and hang with the young guns for a two-hour Ultimate Frisbee match on weekends) possesses far superior health and comprehensive fitness to the lean, ripped (but often emaciated) physical specimens that strut in their Speedos down the main drag of Kailua-Kona, Hawaii, every October during Ironman week (seriously, they really do strut around shirtless and in Speedos).

> *If you start to feel good during a marathon, don't worry, that will pass.*
> **—Don Kardong,**
> **U.S. Olympic marathoner and author**

Yes, today's ironmen can all drop me like a shot in a long-distance swim, cycling, or running race (it would've been a different story back in the day, but I digress...), but their endurance superiority comes at great cost. Collectively, they tend to suffer from recurring fatigue and adrenal burnout, frequent overuse injuries, too-common minor illnesses from suppressed immune function (I get a cold maybe once every five years; a fair number of Ironman

Chronic Cardio Drawbacks—Pocket Reference

A consistent schedule of frequent medium-to-high-intensity (75 percent of maximum or higher) sustained workouts can overstress the body and lead to these negative consequences:

Hormone Imbalance: Chronic Cardio raises cortisol and lowers testosterone and growth hormone. This compromises optimal fat burning, muscle development, energy levels, and sex drive. Burnout is a common consequence of pursuing the "runner's high" too frequently.

Injuries: Recurring muscle fatigue, repetitive impact, restrictive footwear, and inflammation from excessive catabolic hormones released in response to Chronic Cardio traumatizes joints and connective tissue.

Metabolism: Burning more sugar (at above 75 percent of maximum heart rate) drives eating more sugar drives producing more insulin drives storing more fat.

Stress: Excessive oxidation and triggering of the fight-or-flight response compromise the immune system and accelerate aging and disease risk.

Use It or Lose It: Chronic Cardio compromises development of power, speed, strength, and lean mass and leads to muscle imbalances and inflexibility. Total fitness is sacrificed in favor of narrow, minimally functional aerobic endurance.

triathletes get five every year), and, last but certainly not least, high overall life stress scores—something often touted as the number one heart attack risk factor.

Having spent many years immersed in the type A community of driven fitness enthusiasts and competitive endurance athletes, I am aware that many heads will nod in agreement with my message—and then turn around and plug along with their familiar exhausting training regimens. If serious exercise is a centerpiece of your life, I don't wish to deprive you of your passion. That's right, go ahead and hammer that three-hour group ride or that 15-mile trail run with the big boys or big girls, but only do these things once in a while. This will produce far superior fitness benefits and eliminate the risk factors of repeating highly stressful workouts too frequently.

"But This Feels Too Easy!"

Granted, those with competitive endurance goals may not be satisfied to putter along exclusively at a slow pace and think they can take down the competition with that approach. The most direct performance benefits occur from the intense workouts that approximate the challenge of your competitive goals. However, whether you are a casual fitness enthusiast or a professional athlete, you must establish a strong base of low-level aerobic conditioning before you can introduce more stressful, higher intensity workouts.

With a strong aerobic conditioning base in place, you then have the ability to absorb and benefit from the occasional intense workouts that lead directly to competitive success—if you've chosen such goals. The tertiary benefits of low-level work (better balance, strong postural muscles, increased mitochondria development and capillary profusion, and strengthening of bones, tendons, and ligaments to prevent injury) might not be as readily apparent as the direct competitive application of beating your personal record at a time trial, but one cannot happen without the other.

This concept of base first, then intensity has been proven successful by the training regimens of the world's greatest endurance athletes of the last 50 years, beginning with the pioneering work of New Zealand running coach Arthur Lydiard. Lydiard's prize students, including 1960 and 1964 Olympic track gold medalist Peter Snell (today one of the world's leading exercise physiologists, in Dallas, Texas), showed that long-duration, low-intensity training, coupled with intense interval training and adequate rest (rest was another far-out concept for the '60s), could lead directly to Olympic gold medals and world records at races as short as 800 meters (which lasts less than two minutes).

When I completed my career as an elite marathoner and triathlete and transitioned into a career as a personal trainer, my training regimen shifted dramatically. I was still out there moving for several hours a day, but I went from banging my brains out with super fit training partners to dawdling along with a succession of clients on my daily calendar.

Unlike many of today's fitness trainers who stand there and count reps, I got outside with my unfit to moderately fit clients and did their workouts with them. Bike rides that I previously hammered at 20-plus mph for hours were now conducted at 13 mph (it seemed like any slower and we'd tip over!). The long, hard trail runs of my marathon days were replaced with easy jogs where my heart rate barely exceeded 100 beats per minute (only 50 percent of my max). With a young family and a career filling my days, I rarely had time to do my own specific workouts. I made the most of these opportunities by conducting extremely intense interval sessions once or twice a week—on cardio equipment or with a few quick laps around the track. Usually these sessions lasted around 20 minutes—until my next client came strolling in.

When I jumped into the occasional long or ultra-distance endurance race, the results were shocking to me. My "by chance" regimen of very, very slow workouts coupled with occasional very short, intense workouts was effective beyond my wildest dreams. I was able to place among the top competitors in the world in my age group and very close to the standards set by top professionals of that era. Indeed, the Primal Blueprint parameters literally took shape in my mind as I blew by my rivals (who were putting in big Chronic Cardio miles, just like I used to) at races despite what most experts and prevailing Conventional Wisdom would deem ridiculously inadequate preparation.

Primal Blueprint Law #4: Lift Heavy Things

The popular Conventional Wisdom concept of following a strength-training routine that calls for strenuous workouts several days a week is flawed. Your body thrives on intuitive, spontaneous, and fluctuating workout habits—not ego-driven regimentation organized around an arbitrary time period of seven days that has no special relevance to your fitness progress. It's the signals created when your muscles are challenged beyond what they are used to that prompt genes to make those muscles stronger. Get creative and integrate the "lift heavy things" law into daily life, aside from your formal sessions. For example, come fall, try raking your leaves vigorously—it's an unsurpassed shoulder, core, and abs session, and it will get your yard clean to boot!

Regarding the particulars of how to balance upper- and lower-body efforts, "push and pull" workout groupings, light weight with high reps or heavy weight with low reps: it doesn't matter that much! This is not rocket science. The idea is to challenge your body on a regular basis with brief, intense workouts involving full body, functional exercises. The specifics of your workout are based on personal preference. You can do just fine using a park bench and monkey bars, hitting a fancy gym with a high-priced personal trainer, or getting busy in your garage with a few basic weights, stretch cords, or creative "Primal" implements such as kettlebells, slosh tubes, and sandbags. Check out MarksDailyApple.com for hundreds of interesting and challenging resistance workout ideas.

> " *Challenge your body on a regular basis with brief, intense workouts involving full body, functional exercises. The specifics of your workout are based on personal preference.* "

Personally, I'm a devoted gym rat, but my faithful appearance at the local gym a few days a week has a heavy social element. Some days I'll be in there for an hour and 15 minutes, shooting the breeze, preening, and trash-talking with my pals—interspersed with some embarrassingly low-effort exercises where I barely sweat. Other days, when I'm feeling fired up, I'll push it hard for 25 minutes of maximum effort sets with short rest. After these workouts, I have trouble slipping my sweatshirt on and sticking my key in the ignition to drive home, but I am exhilarated and recovery is quick. These hard days are few and far between, but they make a big difference. Overall, once you get the Primal Blueprint eating strategy dialed in, you see that it does not require that much time to maintain excellent all-around functional muscle strength and an impressive physique. It's simply a matter of establishing a reasonable baseline commitment of regular workouts, with the occasional super effort that stimulates a fitness breakthrough.

A high-intensity, short-duration workout will stimulate the release of adaptive hormones—particularly testosterone and human growth hormone—

that get you lean, energetic, and youthful. Work hard and complete your session in less than an hour, even (or especially) if you are an experienced lifter. That's right—go against the Conventional Wisdom of long, drawn-out workouts of the same old sets with the same weight and repetitions. A 30-minute session is actually plenty for most people.

> *Always align the difficulty of your sessions with your energy level, and don't push yourself beyond what you are motivated and inspired to do. On the other hand, if you feel energized and ready to ramp it up a notch, go for it!*

As you improve your fitness, keep your focus on increasing intensity (more resistance, shorter rest periods, or tougher exercises) rather than extending the duration of your workouts. Repeated workouts that extend beyond an hour (I've seen some hard-core lifters routinely go for two hours or more!), where you lift moderate weights to failure again and again, can stimulate the release of cortisol that leads to fatigue, breakdown, and the metabolic problems already discussed at length. Again, think about Grok: he moved some big rocks, which gave his body a shock. But when the quick job was done, he could relax and have fun, basking in the sun.

Always align the difficulty of your sessions with your energy level, and don't push yourself beyond what you are motivated and inspired to do. On the other hand, if you feel energized and ready to ramp it up a notch, go for it! You will notice after your first couple of sets whether your reps to failure are worse or better than normal. If you are feeling—and performing—significantly worse than normal, consider skipping or sharply curtailing the workout. If you are feeling significantly better than normal, push yourself beyond your typical routine to achieve a fitness breakthrough.

I should point out that if you are new to strength training, you might get too tired to complete 30 minutes of high-intensity effort. Instead, you can work up to it by either compressing your workout time further or taking longer rest intervals between your hard efforts. Even a workout as short as seven minutes can produce outstanding benefits. I know of an ex-collegiate gymnast, still in competitive shape with an amazingly cut physique, who claims only to work out for seven minutes a few times a week, with no resistance equipment, in a tiny floor space in his living room.

Impossible? Get a load of his routine: three sets of 20 handstand push-ups, followed by three sets of 20-clap push-ups and 10 one-armed push-ups with each arm, followed by 10 Russian circles, transitioning immediately into 10 leg flairs, then five handstand push-ups, followed by....well, you get the picture! His many years of intense daily training have given him a fitness base to accomplish a phenomenal amount of work—and maintain exceptional fitness—with a minimal time commitment. Oh, and he eats right, too!

If you are spent after a 10-minute workout, congratulations! You've pushed yourself to the max and elicited a desirable fitness response in your body. By the way, those seemingly inconsequential hikes and walks will actually contribute substantially to your ability to hit it hard in the gym, thanks to the well-established connection between the cardiorespiratory and musculoskeletal benefits of comfortable aerobic exercise and your ability to perform at peak intensity.

I suggest you shoot for an average bare minimum of one comprehensive 30-minute session and an abbreviated session of 10-15 minutes per week. If you are a "more is better" gym rat, I'll argue in favor of increasing the intensity of these three sessions rather than adding additional workouts.

Feel free to experiment with the types of exercises that are most fun for you and with a routine that fits most conveniently and comfortably into your daily lifestyle. If you like altering your routine per the popular buzzword "muscle confusion," that's fine. If you are a creature of habit and prefer to do the same workout over and over, that's fine too—as long as it adheres to the "brief, intense, full-body functional movements" description. *The Primal Blueprint 21-Day Total Body Transformation* offers descriptions and photographs of what I call the Primal Essential Movements—four simple, safe, bodyweight resistance exercises (pushups, pull-ups, squats, and planks) that can get you super fit in less than an hour a week. We'll also cover these briefly in the Bonus Material at the end of this book.

Realize that this concept of sporadic, intuitive exercise means you have permission to take—and will, in fact, greatly benefit from—vacation time. The more extreme your goals and training regimen are, the more effort required to balance your overall stress levels on both a micro (daily or weekly) and macro (annual) scale. As I discovered for myself (the hard way), trusting the body's need for balance and intermittent stress can lead to results that are superior—in weight loss or peak competitive performance—compared to the die-hard trainaholics who never miss a workout and never get sufficient rest.

To make sure you are adhering to the Primal philosophy, I suggest paying close attention to your energy level and even your emotional state in the hours after a strength workout. After even my toughest sessions, I feel alert, energized, and positive—basically a natural buzz—for hours afterward. My muscles, while certainly not eager to repeat the workout in the immediate future, feel pleasantly relaxed, loose, and warm. In contrast, if your muscles feel stiff and sore after strength sessions, or you feel like taking a nap, raiding the fridge, or snapping at your loved ones, I recommend conducting shorter, more intense workouts, perhaps less frequently. If you can only maintain high-intensity effort for seven minutes, then end your workout there and work up to more sets in the future.

In regard to body composition, remember your strength-training efforts fall into the fine-tuning 20 percent category, while 80 percent of your success is determined by how you eat. This is a sobering stat if you are working hard at the gym, eating poorly, and praying in vain for that six-pack to show up on your midsection. In this scenario, all that hard work in the gym will contribute mostly to a higher grocery bill (okay, and more fleeting pleasure from unrestricted caloric intake), but you'll be wearing the same size clothing on your trips to the market.

Strength Workout Specifics

Emphasize exercises that engage a variety of muscles with sweeping, real-life movements (squats, pull-ups, pushups, etc.) instead of a series of isolated body part exercises (this includes those ever-popular, narrow-range-of-motion ab machines!). Remember that you are striving to achieve a high power-to-weight ratio and balanced, functional, total-body strength. Follow an intuitive and fluctuating approach focused on maintaining a proper balance of stress and rest.

This approach is a simpler and safer alternative to popular routines designed to pack on more muscle than your body is naturally suited for or to produce disproportionate muscles ("Develop huge guns in six weeks!") in the interest of vanity over functionality. For example, I like to run on an inclined treadmill for a few minutes in stocking feet, without letting my heels touch the ground. This offers a real-life functional test for my calves and works the small muscles, tendons, ligaments, and connective tissue in my lower extremities that are otherwise artificially protected and unchallenged in high-tech running shoes. I gradually incline the treadmill to reach from two to five degrees and then steadily increase the speed, making sure my heels don't bear weight or provide propulsion.

Keep in mind that I just made this up one day, and you may or may not like it. However, I think it offers an important counter to the time spent working out and walking around in overly cushioned and arch-supported running shoes. Contrast the broad benefits of this exercise with something like donkey calf-raises. This narrow-range-of-motion exercise (sit with a weighted bar across your knees and lift your toes off the ground repeatedly) has minimal functional benefit; besides, I'll stack my calves up against any bodybuilder's!

Grok probably never warmed up for his "workouts," and I'm just not a big fan of doing extensive cardio warm-up periods. That said, because you will usually be starting your workout "cold" (maybe you just left an office where you were sitting all day or you just got out of bed), it does make sense to get a little blood flowing into your muscles before hitting the intense stuff. Therefore, your strength sessions should generally start with a brief three- to five-minute warm-up using light weights or calisthenics specific to the muscle groups you'll be working that day. A few sets of easy push-ups and some jumping jacks might be sufficient.

Because Primal Blueprint Fitness workouts are intended to recruit as many muscle fibers as possible and to build functional strength rather than sheer bulk, I wouldn't worry about following some predetermined and deliberate effort-recovery cycle. Instead, try to be slightly explosive with most of your movements. By that I mean you should apply a controlled dynamic force to each repetition such that you complete it at a speed that allows you to maintain form and a reasonable pace for the number of reps you intend to complete. Do that and, believe me, you'll slow down naturally on that final rep or two! This method will fully load the muscle and trigger the biochemical signal to grow stronger by recruiting new fibers.

While there are disparate schools of thought on the best strength-training techniques, I make this general suggestion here to align with the concept of optimal gene expression and prevention of the all-too-common burnout from chronic workout patterns. If you have specialized fitness goals or expert personal training support suggesting a different technique, I wouldn't be overly concerned. I'll default here to the big picture and assert that brief, intense workouts are the key to Primal Fitness success.

Much has been written about breathing while lifting weights, some of it relevant (to protect your back from damage) and some of it conjecture.

When you apply force, you should generally be either exhaling or holding your breath. This will form a sealed air space in the transverse abdominal muscles of your lower core that protect your lumbar spine. While some camps caution against holding your breath, there is no scientific support to affirm this is harmful. In fact, I find I can bang out two or three reps in a row more effectively when holding my breath and then can catch my breath during a recovery phase.

There are many excellent resources—from certified personal trainers, magazine articles, books, video Web sites like CrossFit.com, articles on MarksDailyApple.com, and even your imagination (observing certain obvious safety rules, such as spine stability)—to help you create an ideal total-body routine for your needs. The possibilities are nearly limitless if you observe the strategic rules of Primal Blueprint-style training.

If You Don't Know Squat, Try Hangin' with Grok

"What would Grok do?" It's hard to imagine Grok stretching much beyond a yawning feline-style spine elongation upon awakening, hanging lazily off a branch, or engaging in the timeless, all-purpose stretch of squatting down to the ground. Furthermore, recent research suggests that your central nervous system may be disturbed by a traditional static stretching routine before exercising due to something scientists call a *neuromuscular inhibitory response*. In plain-speak, your muscles might actually get weaker (by up to 30 percent) for up to 30 minutes after an inappropriate stretching session (poor technique and/or bad timing— like stretching "cold" muscles before exercise), and stretching might contribute to more injuries than it prevents.

If you are engaged in a chronic training pattern overworking tired muscles, the ensuing soreness and tightness might make you feel like stretching frequently. I have a better idea: *mellow out* and let your muscles recover! Muscle tissue repair is best accomplished through inactivity, extra rest and sleep, good nutrition, and brief, repeated exposure to cold water; this counters dated Conventional Wisdom that you should stretch and exercise moderately to speed recovery.

If you are exercising Primally, your muscles should feel supple and strong nearly all of the time. Sure, you'll occasionally get sore and stiff from challenging workouts (yep, this is a good thing). This is nature's way of telling you to get some rest.

Stretching certainly has a place in your routine when done correctly. For one, we must acknowledge the sedentary influences of modern life (such as the loss of hip flexor mobility that comes with sitting in a chair all day) and take corrective action through exercise and some specific dynamic stretches, which I will discuss shortly.

The best benefits of stretching may be obtained after workouts, or to otherwise go from active-to-inactive or inactive-to-active states. My two favorite stretches are the **Grok Hang** and the **Grok Squat**. The Grok Hang offers a safe, full-body stretch that leaves you feeling exhilarated every time. It's also an effective strengthening exercise—as Primal as they come. It's as simple as grabbing hold of a bar or tree branch (with overhand grip) and hanging for as long as you can support yourself.

The Grok Squat involves squatting down to the ground, lowering your torso between your bent knees (back straight ideally, or slightly curved) until your butt is nearly touching the ground and arms are extended in front of you. This natural movement provides a safe, gentle, efficient post-workout stretch for your feet, calves, Achilles, hamstrings, quadriceps, buttocks, lower and upper back, and shoulders. For thousands of years people have squatted as a natural "sitting" position in the absence of chairs (to say nothing of Barcaloungers!). For Grok—and millions of people today in the undeveloped world—squatting is the default position for resting, socializing, eating meals, and even eliminating.

Try a Grok Squat for 20 seconds and notice what a comprehensive effect you get from such a basic movement. If it's first thing in the morning or you're a little stiff from some intense activity or other stressor (e.g., jet or car travel), simply lowering into the position provides a good stretch. When I'm feeling warm and loose, I'll gently rock back and forth and/or extend my arms out farther to obtain a deeper stretch. One caution: if you haven't done this for a while, are overweight, or have joint issues, you can begin to ease into this stretch (and keep yourself from going too low or falling over) by holding on to a post or another stationary object.

Beyond the Grok Hang and the Grok Squat, there are certain other dynamic stretches (moving your body to achieve a stretch, as opposed to static stretches that place stress on a still muscle) that are very effective, particularly if you have any injuries or joint issues. In *The Primal Blueprint 21-Day Total Body Transformation*, I present a sequence of photos and descriptions of my pre-sprinting routine of dynamic stretches and technique drills.

Enthusiasts of yoga, Pilates, and other well-designed workouts that emphasize a balance of strengthening and stretching can discover effective routines that help improve flexibility, protect against injury, and overcome weaknesses and imbalances. What I want you to take away from this discussion is that static stretching may not provide much benefit and could even be counterproductive—especially prior to workouts when your muscles are cold. Even with stretches as simple as the aforementioned, be wary of any discomfort, skip or adapt the movements accordingly, and ease into and out of stretching positions.

> *My own prescription for health is less paperwork and more running barefoot through the grass.*
> **—Leslie Grimutter**

Primal Blueprint Law #5: Sprint Once in a While

Obviously, Grok's life featured the occasional brief all-out sprint, not for sport but rather to kill or avoid being killed. These bursts of speed were enhanced by the immediate flooding of the bloodstream with fight-or-flight adrenaline-like chemicals. When Grok survived a run to safety from a charging bear, the resulting biochemical signals prompted a cascade of positive neuroendocrine, hormonal, and gene expression events, the net effect of which was to build stronger, more powerful muscles and an ability to go a little faster the next time.

Modern research confirms the Primal Blueprint premise: the occasional series of short, intense bursts can have a more profound impact on overall fitness—and especially weight loss—than can a medium-paced jog lasting several times as long. This is because of increases in metabolic rate and appetite suppression (both due to elevated body temperature in the hours after workouts), development of more calorie-burning lean muscle tissue, and improved insulin sensitivity (working muscles learn not only to burn glucose efficiently for fuel but also to absorb glucose—transported by insulin—after workouts).

The profound benefits of sprint workouts really hit home for me back in the early 1990s, when I'd take my personal training clients to the Santa Monica College running track. We'd often share this beautiful facility with some of the world's greatest Olympic sprinters. These physical specimens were a sight to behold. Obviously, they were blessed with remarkable genetic gifts, but it was also clear they were training and living in a manner that brought out the best of their genetic potential. In getting to know some of these athletes and their coaches, it became apparent how remarkably different their training methods were from the prevailing templates of the fitness and nutrition industry.

These Olympians were not out there all day circling the track to exhaustion: their workouts consisted of minimal amounts of very slow jogging, casual stretching (between competition-specific drills), unhurried efforts to fuss with their equipment (e.g., starting blocks or resistance tools), and, finally, a brief series of explosive efforts—lasting seconds, not hours. Their banter during these sessions was light; they were always smiling, laughing, joking, and clowning around in between the intense focus of their main sprint sets. They also spent some serious time in the gym working very hard with weights, but these track and gym sessions were interspersed with frequent easy or rest days, including occasionally sleeping in until double figures and taking daily naps. Their training diets were not laden with tofu, frozen yogurt, and energy bars; they were more likely to feast on chicken and ribs after a workout. Carl Lewis, considered by many to be the greatest Olympic athlete of all time, with nine sprint and long jump gold medals to his credit, reportedly trained only an hour per day at his peak. And yet sprinters are among the leanest, most well-muscled people on the planet.

Introducing sprinting into your exercise routine is not as easy as lacing up a pair of shoes and heading out the door to go jogging. Sprinting is a physically stressful activity that requires a significant fitness base, muscle strength, and flexibility. To reduce injury risk, beginners are advised to choose exercises that are low or no impact. Sprinting up a steep hill (and walking down to commence repeat efforts) offers a lower impact option than flat running, while stationary cycling presents a no-impact option. I don't recommend outdoor cycle sprints (except for expert riders) due to the danger factor. You can also choose cardio machines (VersaClimber, elliptical, StairMaster, etc.), but I prefer running because the weight-bearing nature (and thus the increased degree of difficulty) of the activity offers maximum benefits, such as improved bone density and greater stimulation for muscle gain (or toning for females) and fat loss. If you are significantly overweight as you start this program and/or your knees aren't strong enough, cycling or using an elliptical machine might be the best way to start.

For running sprints in particular, you'll want to start the first few sessions gently, gradually increasing the speed and intensity of your sprints over time. You also need significant recovery time after sprint workouts. I recommend conducting a sprint workout approximately once every seven to ten days, and only when you have high energy and motivation levels. That's right, even as little as two to three sprint sessions per month can produce outstanding fitness benefits and break you out of Chronic Cardio ruts that may have lasted years. I'm talking about frequency of maximum intensity workouts here. I also recommend supplementing your all-out efforts with "wind sprint" sessions, consisting of brief repetitions (8-20 seconds) at 75-85 percent of maximum effort. These efforts are only moderately strenuous and will condition your muscles, tendons, and joints to perform better during the occasional all-out sessions, as well as improve your technique.

Running is the best but comes with a higher risk of injury if you are out of practice (i.e., you haven't chased down any animals or scored any touchdowns in the last few decades).

Novices can start with three to four sprints, short of full speed, with long rest periods in between efforts. You will likely experience some muscle soreness in the days after these efforts, but your body will quickly adapt to your new workout routine. You can then build up to a workout that includes six to eight all-out sprints. You should never push your body through an intense workout if you have any symptoms of fatigue, soreness, compromised immune system, or another malaise. As discussed with strength training, your sprint sessions should be intuitive, intermittent, and spontaneous—just as they were in primal life for Grok. The occasional sprint workout will elicit the most desirable gene expression effects—much more so than workouts performed come heck or high water just because it's Tuesday.

One final note: this isn't about speed—it's about effort. It doesn't matter if you aren't covering ground quickly, as long as you exert yourself to the point of going all-out for that brief interval. Age is not an issue here. Whether you are 20 or 75, you can find a form of sprint workout that fits your style. For some people, it's simply walking fast up a steeply inclined treadmill for 30 seconds.

Clouseau-Robics and Doberman Intervals

While I've discussed the fight-or-flight response in the negative context of excessive aerobic exercise or hectic modern life, you should realize that eliciting a stress response is desirable with your sprint workouts. The difference here is that the brief, intense stress is exactly what your genes crave to build fitness and strength and to optimize metabolic function.

Imagine if every so often someone rudely interrupted your jog around the track by turning a vicious Doberman loose! I guess now you'd run as fast as possible, right? Or, like Inspector Clouseau, say you hired a martial arts master as a personal assistant to launch surprise attacks when you least expect it. Preposterous as it sounds, this type of sporadic intense "life-or-death" stimulation just might produce far superior fitness benefits than filling in all the blanks in your training log.

Sprint Workout Specifics

Your sprint efforts should last between 8 and 20 seconds, with duration, recovery, and number of repetitions determined by your ability level. Sprints of 8 seconds or less are fueled by pure ATP in the muscle cell, sprints of 8 to 20 seconds are fueled by lactic acid, and maximum efforts lasting longer than 20 seconds are fueled by glucose. While the scientific particulars may only be relevant to athletes trying to hone sport-specific skills and mimic competitive circumstances (track-and-field events of varied distance, football, soccer, etc.), you might like to vary your routine over time to include short, medium, and longer sprints.

Longer sprints with short rest develop your anaerobic lactic acid buffering system (a desirable ability for a half-mile or mile race), while the shorter sprints with long rest periods develop your pure speed and explosiveness (such as for a 100-meter race). All types of sprint training will stimulate your fat-burning systems, lean muscle development, and beneficial hormone flow, particularly the release of testosterone and human growth hormone (HGH). In this case, even though you will not be burning fat during the actual sprints, your body will become more efficient at burning fats to recover over the long term.

Because the weight-bearing aspect of running makes it significantly more difficult than cycling, running sprints should be shorter than cycling sprints. I prefer going all-out for about 15 seconds (after gradually ramping up my speed) and then taking a full rest period of one minute between efforts. I'll complete six to eight of these efforts, typically on grass, at the beach on hard sand or even in soft sand. Sometimes I'll get lucky and discover a clean path of freshly upturned deeper, soft sand from the beach tractor—begging to be blemished by my footprints! These options stimulate a variety of muscle groups, helping me enjoy a cross-training effect as I have to lift my knees higher to generate maximum turnover.

Ideally, you should sprint on a natural surface, such as a grass athletic field or the beach; use a running track or cement road if you can't find a suitable natural surface. While I like uneven surfaces to develop balance and foot strength for walks and hikes, don't risk it for sprinting. Use a smooth, straight, safe course with excellent footing. I strongly recommend making an effort to minimize your dependency on bulky running shoes and strengthening your feet by going barefoot, if possible, or using specially designed shoes that encourage a fuller range of motion.

On other days, my cycling sprints might consist of six to eight one-minute all-out sprints with two-minute recoveries. Regardless of your specific workout choice, the entire sprint session—including brief warm-up and cool-down periods—will require less than 20 minutes. The Sprint Workout Suggestions in the Bonus Material section offer several options for novice, intermediate, and advanced workouts, including an exciting plyometric workout, a stadium steps workout, and a couple of low- or no-impact sprint options, such as sprinting up steep hills or on a stationary bike.

Proper Running and Cycling Form

While form concerns are relatively minimal in running and cycling compared to other sports, you must respect these important basics:

Running: Torso faces forward at all times, shoulders and pelvis square to your forward direction. Refrain from side-to-side swiveling of the hips or the shoulder girdle. Arms and hands are relaxed as pumping is initiated from the shoulders. Elbows are bent at 90-degree angles. Don't let arms or hands cross the center line of your body. Focus on fast turnover by striding in a motion similar to pedaling a bicycle. Lift foot quickly off the ground in a dorsiflexed position, drive knees high, and then initiate the next stride quickly. Your heel should nearly kick your butt during the recovery phase of the stride. Envision your foot clearing the height of your opposite knee on each stride.

When you experience the inevitable tightening up midway through your sprint, focus on keeping your face, arms, and hands loose and relaxed. Notice in videos or photographs of Olympic sprinters how their jaws are slack and their hands are soft and open. Be aware of your breathing rhythm and resist the temptation to hold your breath or pant shallowly. Take deep, powerful breaths by focusing on a forceful exhale.

Cycling: Strive for a rhythmic cadence in a range of 80 to 100 revolutions per minute. Most recreational cyclists pedal at far too low a cadence, putting excessive strain on the muscles instead of balancing the cardiovascular and muscular load with an efficient cadence. Focus on applying circular force to the pedals rather than just stomping down. I highly recommend a clip-in pedaling system to achieve a proper circular stroke. Maintain a level pelvis at all times. Do not rock your pelvis from side to side in an effort to impart more force. Keep your upper body virtually still, with arms, chest, neck, and head relaxed and supple.

Be sure that your seat height is appropriate. A quick test is to place your heel (unclip it from the pedal) on the pedal axle when it's at the very bottom of the pedal stroke. You should be able to extend your leg fully (with pelvis level) and barely touch (or barely miss) the pedal axle. A seat that is too high or too low will stress the knees and also lead to rocking. Resist the temptation to tense your muscles when the effort becomes difficult. Breathe deeply by inflating your diaphragm fully on the inhale. Because you are bent over, you should feel your diaphragm pressing against your rib cage when you inhale; then relax and allow a natural exhale.

Happy Feet

One of the most annoying non-Primal elements of today's fitness movement is shoes. You heard me, shoes are lame. Sure, typical athletic shoes provide substantial support, cushioning, and general protection, but they also immobilize your feet inside the shoe—much like being in a cast. Hence, the complex network of 52 bones (a quarter of the total in your entire body) and dozens of tendons, ligaments, and small muscles cannot work their magic to provide balance, stability, impact absorption, weight transfer, and propulsion.

Constantly wearing shoes during exercise and daily life leads to weakened feet, fallen arches, shortened Achilles tendons and calf muscles, imbalances between the hamstrings and quadriceps, an inefficient gait, and, of course, recurring pain and injury. The 43 million Americans who experience foot problems daily (we will spend an estimated $900 million annually on foot care products) offer another disturbing example of living in conflict with our ancestral heritage.

Granted, shoes are essential for contact sports or activities involving hard surfaces, such as football, soccer, basketball, volleyball, running on the road, and the like. However, for your purposes of conducting basic Primal Blueprint Fitness activities, going shoeless on occasion (and gradually increasing frequency over time) is possible and beneficial. Keep in mind that a lifetime spent in "casts"—desensitizing and weakening your feet for their primary functional purpose—will require that you proceed with extreme caution with your barefoot endeavors. Here again I'll make a concession for modern life (I don't think Grok had any broken glass to worry about on his hikes) by recommending the use of a unique and excellent product called the Vibram FiveFingers shoe.

The Vibram FiveFingers "shoe" consists of a lightweight, form-fitting rubber sole attached to a nylon-like sock and a hook-and-loop closure system. Vibrams slip onto your bare feet like fingers into a glove (with a hole for each toe) and offer excellent protection from sharp objects and

(continued)

Happy Feet (continued)

debris. Duly protected, you can simulate a barefoot experience by giving your feet a complete range of motion during activity. Search MarksDailyApple.com or VibramFiveFingers.com for details.

Make an effort to gradually introduce barefoot time into your workouts and everyday life, providing ample time for your feet to adjust and get stronger without undue shock. For example, on my first few long hikes in FiveFingers, I kept my "normal" shoes in a small pack just in case I needed them. Some mild next-day soreness in your arches is to be expected after your initial barefoot endeavors and is a natural part of the strengthening process (just as with muscle work). However, make sure you don't experience any pain during your efforts to get your feet more Primal. Be particularly careful if you are minimally active or overweight or if you have a history of foot problems or other medical issues. As with most other Primal activities, it is better to ease into a new form of exercise than to overdo it.

You can get some low-risk barefoot time by adopting the Eastern tradition of removing your shoes when you enter your house and otherwise using minimal footwear (flip-flop sandals or the like) whenever you don't need the protection or decorum of more substantial footwear. Try a short stint in stocking feet on the treadmill at your gym and see what you think! Consider complementing your shelf of "big" shoes with a pair of Vibrams or other choices from the rapidly expanding category of minimalist athletic footwear, using them first for walking around, then for short workouts, and gradually increasing your use as you remain pain-free. Hopefully, one day you'll work up to running some sprints barefoot—it doesn't get any more Primal than that!

> " *The only exercise some people get is jumping to conclusions, running down their friends, side-stepping responsibility, and pushing their luck!* "
> —**Author Unknown**

Chapter Summary

1. Primal Blueprint Exercise Laws: Mirroring the active lifestyle of Grok is not a complex endeavor requiring the extensive time, money, or specific equipment that Conventional Wisdom suggests. You can get extremely fit in as little as a few hours a week, provided you exercise strategically with a balance of extensive low-intensity movement, periodic high-intensity, short-duration strength-training sessions, and occasional all-out sprints.

Best results will come when your exercise routine is unstructured and intuitive, and workout choices are aligned with your energy and motivation levels. Always allow for sufficient recovery and pursue goals that are fun and inspiring. Weight loss goals can succeed by combining Primal eating and frequent low-level exercise (fine-tuning your fat-burning system) with occasional brief, intense strength and sprint sessions (to stimulate an increase in lean muscle and metabolic rate).

2. Primal Blueprint Fitness: Primal Blueprint Fitness means you have a broad range of skills and attributes (strength, power, speed, endurance—with power-to-weight ratio as a critical benchmark) that allow you to do pretty much whatever you want with a substantial degree of competence and minimal risk of injury. In contrast, narrow, specialized fitness goals are popular today (e.g., for endurance athletes and bodybuilders). These goals often compromise functional fitness and general health. By exercising—and eating—Primal Blueprint style, you will develop the unmistakable physique of a well-balanced athlete and eliminate the drawbacks of narrowly focused, overly stressful exercise programs.

3. Organ Reserve: Leading an active lifestyle and maintaining ample lean muscle mass correlates with optimal organ function and longevity, because your organs must keep up with the physical demands you place upon your body. In contrast, inactivity will accelerate the aging process to the extent that it becomes a greater risk factor than simply getting older.

4. Move Frequently at a Slow Pace: Two to five hours per week of low-intensity aerobic exercise (heart rate zone of 55 to 75 percent of max heart rate), such as walking, hiking, easy cycling, cardio machines or (if you are fit) jogging, offer excellent health benefits, including improved cardiovascular, musculoskeletal, and immune function and fat metabolism. In contrast, Chronic Cardio (75 percent of max heart rate and up) workouts can place excessive stress on your system, deplete the body of energy (leading to increased appetite for quick-energy carbohydrates), inhibit fat metabolism, promote overuse injuries, and generally result in a burnout condition. Slowing down workout pace and moving around more in daily life lead to improved fitness and health.

(continued)

5. Lift Heavy Things: Best results in strength training come from a sporadic routine of brief, intense workouts. These workouts will stimulate the release of adaptive hormones, such as testosterone and human growth hormone, helping improve body composition and delaying the aging process. Exercises should focus on real human movements (lunges, squats, plyometrics, push-ups, pull-ups, planks, and other body weight resistance exercises) instead of isolations on narrow-range-of-motion gym machines. Session difficulty should be aligned with energy and motivation levels: push hard when you feel like it and take it easy or skip workouts when you are tired. With this approach, you will avoid the risk of injury, exhaustion, and burnout that comes from trying to follow a consistent schedule of long-duration workouts several times a week. Complete sessions should last around 30 minutes, even for experienced strength trainers. A mini-session of as little as 10 minutes can be extremely beneficial.

6. Sprint Once in a While: No workout is more Primal than an all-out sprint. Efforts like these fueled human evolution through survival-of-the-fittest! Today you can enjoy excellent fitness, body composition, and health benefits from intense sprinting, modeling the "use it or lose it" principle. All-out sprint sessions should be conducted sporadically when energy and motivation levels are high. Intensity is the key—efforts should last between 8 and 20 seconds, with complete rest between efforts to ensure maximum performance. Novices can do low-impact options, such as uphill sprints or stationary bicycle sprints. All-out sessions can be supported by less strenuous wind sprint sessions that improve technique and resiliency of muscles, tendons, and joints.

7. Form and Feet: Proper form in running and cycling is imperative. For running, the body should always face forward, the center of gravity should be stable, and wasted motion (i.e., side-to-side movement) should be eliminated. Focus on striding in a circular motion (a la cycling) with center of gravity always balanced over feet. For cycling, ensure proper seat height and apply circular force while pedaling at a rapid, efficient cadence of 80 to 100 rpm. Make an effort to minimize bulky shoes that restrict natural foot motion and weaken stabilizing and propulsion muscles.

CHAPTER 7

The Primal Blueprint
Lifestyle Laws

If You Don't Snooze, You Lose

In This Chapter

I detail the five lifestyle laws of the Primal Blueprint: Law #6—Get Adequate Sleep; Law #7—Play; Law #8—Get Adequate Sunlight; Law #9—Avoid Stupid Mistakes; and Law #10—Use Your Brain. While Grok's diet and exercise patterns were clearly major influences in shaping how his (and our) genes evolved, there were other environmental and behavioral forces that were no less important in perfecting the DNA recipe for a healthy, vibrant human being.

Law #6, Get Adequate Sleep, delivers obvious benefits but is widely compromised today. Good sleep entails a basic understanding of the physiology of sleep cycles, establishing consistent habits, taking advantage of the benefits of napping (when you need one), and applying effective time-prioritization skills. Law #7, Play, is a widely neglected lifestyle law that can deliver widespread benefits and make you quantifiably more productive when balanced effectively with work. Law #8, Get Adequate Sunlight, is an area where Conventional Wisdom has let us down, scaring us into avoiding the outdoors due to the misinterpreted risks of skin cancer. Obtaining optimal levels of vitamin D, synthesized from sun exposure on your skin, is critical to cellular health and cancer prevention.

Law #9, Avoid Stupid Mistakes, explains how our obsessive desire to control or eliminate all sources of potential danger has made us lazy and inattentive. Cultivating the skills of hypervigilance and risk management is essential to avoid self-inflicted trauma and unnecessary suffering. Law #10, Use Your Brain, is about pursuing creative intellectual outlets unrelated to your core daily responsibilities and economic contribution. Finding more stuff to do with your brain may seem counterintuitive to many of us who feel our brain function is maxed out each day. However, the unrelenting pace of modern life and intense pressure to achieve and consume strongly conflict with our genetic makeup and can lead to feelings of restlessness and discontent. Making time for hobbies and personal growth challenges will keep you refreshed and excited about life.

I am two with nature.

—Woody Allen

Primal Blueprint Law #6: Get Adequate Sleep

For billions of years, the evolution of nearly all life forms on earth has been driven by the consistent rising and setting of the sun. This circadian rhythm (from Latin: circa, meaning "around"; and dia, meaning "day") governs our sleeping and eating patterns, as well as the precise timing of important hormone secretions, brain wave patterns, and cellular repair and regeneration based on a 24-hour cycle. When we interfere with our circadian rhythm via excessive artificial light and digital stimulation after sunset, irregular bed and wake times, jet lag, graveyard shift work, and alarm clocks, we disrupt some of the very processes we depend upon to stay healthy, happy, productive, and focused.

Admittedly, aligning your sleep habits with the rising and setting of the sun is a challenge in today's world. Depending on where you live and the time of year, your sleep time might increase to the tune of two to six hours a day. Can you say, "Ain't gonna happen anytime soon?" This is not to say you have to turn in at sunset in order to be healthy. For one thing, modernization has substantially lowered our activity level and the overall degree of difficulty of daily life (I know commuting is tiring, but imagine walking home from the office every day!).

Conventional Wisdom usually recommends seven to eight hours per night, while those in the evolutionary health movement call for more. *In Sleep, Sugar, and Survival*, authors T.S. Wiley (anthropologist and medical theorist), and Bent Formby, Ph.D. (biochemist, biophysicist, molecular biologist), urgently call for nine-and-a-half hours per night for seven months per year, with less sleep acceptable during the long daylight hours of summer. In addition to obtaining the requisite number of hours, your sleep must be of high quality—not harmed by a disruptive environment, objectionable meds or foods, or behaviors that elevate stress hormone production (vigorous exercise, screen time, or other high stimulation) in the hours before bed. Calm, quiet, dark evenings, and consistent bed and wake times are critical factors for high quality sleep.

Sleep was long thought to be a passive state, but we now understand sleep to be a dynamic process. The brain is active during sleep (but responding to internal stimuli, not external), and it drifts in and out of various sleep stages, or cycles. Our natural sleep pattern is to progress from light sleep (rapid eye movement (REM), when you dream and can be woken easily) into escalating stages of deeper sleep cycles (non-REM sleep, when you are out like a light and experiencing maximum restorative hormone flow, balancing of brain chemicals, and cellular repair in muscles and organs). This cycling of REM into non-REM sleep is repeated throughout the night, with each complete cycle believed to last about 90 minutes.

If you divide your night's sleep into three equal time periods, your first third is characterized by the highest percentage of non-REM sleep, while the final third of your sleep time is characterized by a lengthening of the REM cycles and a shortening of the deep sleep cycles (the middle cycle is a balance between the first and the last). Waking up naturally involves letting the cycles play out until finally, after a period of exclusive REM sleep, you wake up effortlessly (REM sleep is characterized by increases in heart rate, respiration, and muscle and brain wave activity, making it easy to rise from this more alert state).

The sleep hormone melatonin presides over you falling asleep and going through the various sleep cycles. Melatonin is manufactured in the pineal gland near the center of the brain. As light diminishes, the pineal starts to convert the feel-good hormone serotonin, which has kept your mood elevated all day (and which is why so many of us take SSRI meds—to avoid depleting serotonin), to increasing amounts of melatonin, so that your mind and body slow down and you become sleepy.

With the morning light stimulating your central nervous system, melatonin production is then suppressed and serotonin begins to increase. With melatonin predominating at night, the areas of the brain involved in emotional and social function get the rest they need, helping you face the next day mentally refreshed. A study from Dr. Sophie Schwartz and colleagues presented at the 2008 Forum of European Neuroscience suggested that getting a good night's sleep can help the brain "harden up weak memories which otherwise might fade in time." Other hormones released during sleep, such as human growth hormone, help your body burn fat and repair muscle tissue.

We hold these truths about quality z-time to be self-evident. However, we are not walking our talk in modern life. A recent study cited by the Harvard School of Public Health found that an increasing percentage of Americans are seriously deficient in sleep (40 percent of Americans get less than five hours of sleep per night), and an incredible 75 percent of us suffer from some form of sleep difficulty each night. Chronic sleep deficit may lead to weight gain by affecting how your body processes and stores carbohydrates and by altering hormones that affect your appetite and metabolism. It can negatively affect your mood, concentration, and memory retention during the day, making you less productive and more irritable, impatient, and moody. Insufficient sleep can also lead to hypertension, elevated stress hormone levels, irregular heartbeat, compromised immune function, and drastically increased risk for obesity and heart disease.

Our natural (or actually I should say, "learned") inclination to be constantly entertained is difficult to balance with our need for adequate restoration. It's not until we are truly exhausted that sleep moves up the hierarchy of wants and needs. It shouldn't have to be that way. Sure, you can get away with some occasional departures from your routine with no ill effects. Just as with your dietary choices, if you can observe a consistent bedtime 80 percent of the time, the 20 percent of the time when you stay up late, wake up super early, or otherwise skimp on perfect rest will probably be handled by your body more easily. On the other hand, if you have a habit of disrespecting consistent sleep time habits, you create momentum in the wrong direction and will struggle to achieve basic health and fitness goals, especially losing excess body fat.

How to Get an "A" in "Zs"

Here are some important measures you can take to get optimum amounts of high-quality sleep. Visit MarksDailyApple.com for more discussion on this topic, including some helpful tips to beat jet lag.

Create an Ideal Sleeping Environment: It's critical to make your bedroom an area of minimal stimulation and maximum relaxation. Your bedroom should be used only for sleeping (well, okay, that other stuff, too)—with absolutely no computer, television, work desk, or clutter present. You should have a clear physical and psychological separation between your bedroom and other areas of the house where you do work or enjoy entertainment. Browse the Internet or page through design magazines to get a feeling for the beauty of contemporary minimalist bedroom styles.

Follow Consistent Bed and Wake Times: Establish a consistent, circadian-friendly routine to optimize hormone flows and ensure that you enjoy complete sleep cycles. Remember that melatonin floods your bloodstream on circadian cues triggered by darkness. For two million years, that meant sunset; today, it means *the time that you make it dark*. You experience the highest percentage of deep sleep at the outset of your night. Sorry, but if you miss bedtime, sleeping in to reach your typical hourly total will not completely catch you up.

If you are a night owl, you can probably develop some level of tolerance and effectiveness for a consistent, artificial light-induced late-night bedtime and an artificially darkened late-morning awakening. If circumstances require that your sleep habits depart from the earth's natural light and dark cycles, make a strong effort to sleep with an eye mask (check mindfold.com for a total darkness sleep mask) in a completely darkened room, since all of your skin cells (not just your eyes) are sensitive and responsive to light.

Wind Down the Night and Ease into the Day: Because everything you do after sundown is technically non-Primal, it's important to wind down calmly in the hours preceding your bedtime. Minimize your central nervous system stimulation before going to bed, so you can have a smooth, relaxing transition from your busy day to downtime. Reading is a time-tested popular method to wind down, but choose fiction or something light to promote maximum relaxation.

It may also be helpful to decompress your busy brain by writing down your thoughts before bed. Take 5 or 10 minutes to write out everything from your day: accomplishments, to-do tasks, stresses, and worries. It's easier to arrive at solutions if you don't try consciously to force them. Get them down on paper, and then let your sleeping mind do the work for you. You'll wake up feeling clearer and more positive.

" *No day is so bad it can't be fixed with a nap.* "
—Carrie Snow,
stand-up comedian

In the morning, awaken gradually and naturally coming off a complete REM-dominant sleep cycle. Staying in bed for a few minutes to read or talk ("Again, your name was…?") or starting your day with some light breathing and stretching exercises is preferable to springing up after the fourth snooze alarm and rushing into action. A brief warm shower can help stimulate your central nervous system naturally and get blood circulating—a particularly good idea if you are going to exercise soon after awakening. Hard-core Grok disciples can even try a cold-water plunge upon awakening in the summer months—beats a high-carb breakfast any day as a morning energizer!

Eat and Drink the Right Stuff: Eat your last meal a couple hours or more before bed, so digestion does not interfere with your sleep process. If you are a wine drinker, one fine glass with dinner may help you relax and unwind in the evening hours. The same goes for herbal teas. Chamomile in particular is touted for its mild sedative effect. By all means pass on the carbs—all day long and especially before bed. Insulin will interfere with melatonin production.

Napping: It's Not Just for Cats Anymore

If you are able to obtain all of your requisite sleep at night, there is probably no reason to routinely take naps during the day. On the other hand, if you do have obstacles (job requirements, young children, noisy surroundings, etc.) that prevent you from getting adequate nighttime sleep, napping can help you sustain the focus, energy, and productivity you need for an active life.

> *A nap of 20 to 30 minutes will recalibrate your brain's sodium/potassium ratio, a critical factor to recover from nervous system fatigue and wake up feeling refreshed.*

Many cultures across the world have appreciated nap time throughout their history, especially warm weather countries in Latin America, Asia, the Mediterranean, North Africa, and the Middle East. Furthermore, more than 85 percent of mammals have *polyphasic* sleep habits, meaning multiple sleep-wake incidents. Anthropologists believe that Grok likely experienced disruptions to nighttime sleep (primal dangers, caring for young), and took advantage of afternoon downtime for napping. Unfortunately, it seems the fast pace of modern life (combined, perhaps, with some weird puritanical guilt factors) prevents napping from being a culturally acceptable lifestyle habit.

Because the rhythm of sleep cycles is so critical to brain and body restoration, napping can produce remarkable benefits in a relatively short time by helping you catch up on non-REM sleep cycle deficiencies, shortcutting you into the deep sleep cycles characterized by theta brain waves. Many experts recommend a nap period of 20 to 30 minutes. This time frame is believed to be sufficient to recalibrate your brain's sodium/potassium ratio, a critical factor to recover from nervous system fatigue and wake up feeling refreshed. A nap of this length will not result in the unpleasant grogginess you might experience from a prolonged siesta, nor will it interfere with falling asleep that evening. Notable nappers throughout history include Winston Churchill, John F. Kennedy, Napoleon, Albert Einstein, Thomas Edison, Leonardo da Vinci, and Lindsay Lohan.

> *Art is older than production [making things for practical use] for us, and play older than work. Man was shaped less by what he had to do than by what he did in playful moments. It is the child in man that is the source of his uniqueness and creativeness.*
> **—Eric Hoffer, American social writer and philosopher (1902-1983)**

Primal Blueprint Law #7: Play

Few would argue the importance of play, yet compliance among many health-minded people is low in this area. We have been so heavily socialized into regimented, technological, industrialized life that scheduling time for play (now there's an oxymoron!) is a big challenge. I don't know about you, but I don't think the word *playdate* existed when I was a kid. Oh, we had play-dates in my neighborhood, all right—365 of them, to be exact. They lasted from the final school bell till the dinner bell, not deterred by mud, rain, sleet, or snow (no kidding, I'm from Maine!). We didn't need our moms making transportation arrangements via e-mail or cell phone. We just needed air in our lungs, bike tires, and basketballs.

As the challenges and responsibilities of making a living or managing a family accumulate in our adult years, we collectively adopt the belief that play is for youth. The truth is that play is for everyone, particularly those absorbed in the incredible complexity and breakneck pace of modern life. Regular play—time away from work, home duties, school, and other scheduled and unscheduled responsibilities to express the childlike elements of your basic nature—helps quench your thirst for adventure and challenge (physical and mental), improves health, relieves stress, strengthens your connection with friends and community, and simply enhances your enjoyment of life.

Learning disability specialist Dr. Lorraine Peniston enumerates many research-proven psychological benefits of play, including:

- Perceived sense of freedom, independence, and autonomy
- Enhanced self-competence through improved sense of self-worth, self-reliance, and self-confidence
- Better ability to socialize with others, including greater tolerance and understanding
- Enriched capabilities for team membership
- Heightened creative ability
- Improved expressions of and reflection on personal spiritual ideals
- Greater adaptability and resiliency
- Better sense of humor
- Enhanced perceived quality of life
- More balanced competitiveness and a more positive outlook on life

There is plenty of evidence attesting to the fact that we can be more productive when we carve time for play into our busy schedules. A New Zealand study reported that people were 82 percent more productive following a vacation and enjoyed enhanced quality of sleep—but that 43 percent of Americans had no vacation plans in 2007 due to work pressures (and it's probably worse now). A 2006 study published in the *Sunday Times* (England) noted that the percentage of married couples citing lack of quality time due to overwork as the basis for divorce has more than tripled in recent years, even while the traditional leading reasons, such as violence and infidelity, have dropped sharply. Australian research suggests that frequent breaks from a sedentary workday produce numerous health benefits, including weight control and favorable blood levels of triglycerides and glucose. A study published in the *New York Times* suggests that enjoyable leisure activities boost immune function even more powerfully than stressful events suppress it.

For the majority of us who move far less than we are genetically programmed to, busting loose outdoors, in fresh air and sunlight, for some relatively unstructured physical fun will produce the best physical and psychological benefits. If you are one of the few who have a physically demanding job or daily routine, mellower pursuits (drawing trees in the park, skipping rocks in the pond) might indeed be the ticket.

> ❝❝*We don't stop playing because we grow old;*
> *we grow old because we stop playing.* ❞❞
> **—George Bernard Shaw, Irish playwright**
> **and political activist (1856-1950)**

My favorite activity of the week is a regular Sunday afternoon pickup Ultimate Frisbee game with my son and several other families at the park. It is a great sport, requiring diverse athletic and strategic skills, and is fun for players of all ages and ability levels. I'd say it's a safe sport, too, except for my freak accident that resulted in a serious knee injury in 2007—possibly attributed to a still-17-year-old brain directing a 54-year-old body to get some big air for a circus catch! Most important, my enjoyment of play time has prompted me to reframe my main reason for exercising: I train Primally so I can play hard at whatever I want whenever I choose, whether it's at Ultimate, snowboarding, soccer, stand-up paddling, or golf.

If you can take the spirit of this message to heart, you can make something happen that will change your life. Let's be clear that I'm not advocating selling the shop and becoming a surf rat. All work and no play makes for a dull boy, but all play and no work makes for a foreclosure. Balance is important in all areas of life, and it's up to you to define your level of work-play balance. It might help to keep this popular sentiment in mind: "No one ever said, 'I wish I'd spent more time at work' on their deathbed."

Primal Blueprint Law #8: Get Adequate Sunlight

While the dangers of excessive sun exposure are well recognized and heavily promoted by today's medical community, it's important to challenge Conventional Wisdom's blanket statement to shun the sun—or lather up with tons of sunscreen as do English Channel swimmers with their lanolin.

Adequate exposure to sunlight helps our bodies manufacture vitamin D, which helps regulate growth in virtually every cell of our bodies and prevent a variety of diseases. Vitamin D is essential for healthy teeth, bones, and nails; eyesight; the absorption of other key nutrients, such as calcium and vitamins A and C; and immune function. Vitamin D has also been shown to play a role in the prevention of breast, prostate, and colorectal cancer; cardiovascular disease; diabetes; autoimmune diseases; and inflammatory conditions, such as arthritis.

Perhaps the most exciting revelation about vitamin D has to do with its critical action on Gene P53—the "proofreader" gene. P53 acts as a spell-checker during each of the hundreds of millions of cell replications that occur each day, informing the cell when something has gone awry and instructing it to make necessary changes. Many scientists believe P53 is an important first line of defense against the kinds of mutations that can develop into cancers. The bottom line is that generously exposing much of your body to direct sunlight on a regular basis is essential for health and the prevention of skin cancer.

Early humans spent hundreds of thousands of years absorbing power-ful equatorial rays over their entire bodies every day. As we migrated farther away from the equator, genetic adaptations occurred (the lightening of skin pigment and hair over many generations) to help us continue to absorb sun optimally even when it was less plentiful. Just as we've suffered devastating health consequences from the relatively recent shift in the human diet away from hunter-gatherer to grain-based, the same dynamic holds for our sun exposure—except this lifestyle alteration has been even more abrupt. Only in the last couple of centuries of industrialization have millions of people in the civilized world gone for long periods of time with little to no direct sun expo-sure. Consequently, there has been an alarming increase in health problems related to vitamin D deficiency.

The symptoms of vitamin D deficiency are not as overt as the disturbing image of scurvy-stricken sailors staggering around lacking vitamin C (which was, interestingly, partly a result of their high grain consumption), but the health consequences are devastating nonetheless. The risk increases for those with confined lifestyles (spent in the home, office, or auto—witness Ken Korg), those with dark skin living distant from the equator, children with vi-tamin D-deficient mothers, the elderly, or people who are house- or hospital-bound. Recent research suggests that vitamin D levels are also low in those with obesity and Metabolic Syndrome.

Dr. Joseph Mercola, Internet health advisor (mercola.com) and author of *The No-Grain Diet*, states:

> The dangers of sun exposure have been greatly exaggerated and the benefits highly underestimated. Excess sun exposure is not the major reason people develop skin cancer (many believe poor diet, exposure to other environmental toxins such as swimming pool chlorine, and insufficient sun are more significant risk factors). [A study from the Moores Cancer Center at UC San Diego suggested that] 600,000 cases of cancer could be prevented every year by just increasing your levels of vitamin D.

Granted, the "fell asleep slathered in baby oil at the beach" burn-and-peel ordeals are indeed bad news. Medical experts suggest that even a few severe sunburn episodes in your early years (who hasn't fallen asleep on the beach or chaise lounge as a teenager?!) can generate sufficient ultraviolet radiation damage to potentially lead to the development of carcinoma (less serious growths that are easily removed from skin surface) or melanoma (a more serious form of cancer) in later decades. But there is a happy medium between too much sun and too little.

> *Regular exposure of large skin surface areas to sunlight during the months of peak solar intensity at your latitude (enough for a slight tan) remains the primary way to obtain an ample amount of vitamin D.*

Regular exposure of large skin surface areas to sunlight during the months of peak solar intensity at your latitude remains the primary way to obtain an ample amount of vitamin D. For most people, maintaining a slight tan indicates that you are obtaining adequate vitamin D exposure, while a burn is, of course, unhealthy.

Contrary to Conventional Wisdom, dietary efforts to obtain vitamin D are almost inconsequential compared to sun exposure. Vitamin D experts recommend you obtain around 4,000 International Units (I.U.) per day, but the SAD provides only around 300 I.U. per day, and the vaunted glass of milk provides only around 100 I.U. By contrast, 20-40 minutes of direct sunlight can produce around 10,000 I.U. of vitamin D, which can easily be stored in your cells for future use. In the winter months when the sun's rays are of inadequate intensity to promote vitamin D production, supplements can be useful. For the extremely sun challenged, supplements, along with carefully chosen artificial tanning lights, can boost vitamin D production. Blood tests are available to determine how your vitamin D levels compare to recommended levels. Search MarksDailyApple.com for "sun exposure" and "vitamin D" for numerous detailed posts.

The variables of season, climate, and skin tone are substantial and should be carefully considered on a daily basis to ensure you obtain adequate sunlight while avoiding risk factors of excessive exposure. Generally, the goal is to expose the large surface areas of your skin (arms, legs, torso, back) to direct sunlight *for about half the amount of time it takes to sustain a slight burn.* This is a pretty low-risk endeavor that allows for plenty of individual flexibility.

Exposing your large skin surface areas is the key. If you are worried about wrinkling and cancer risk on the skin areas that are at most risk of overexposure and are most visible and sensitive—face, neck, and hands—go ahead and cover them with clothing or sunscreen routinely. They represent an extremely minimal amount of your vitamin D potential anyway. Just be sure to bag enough rays during the summer months to manufacture plenty of vitamin D, because in latitudes outside the tropics, there are four to eight months during the year when vitamin D production is impossible. Check the Lifestyle Laws Hacks in the Bonus Material for sun exposure strategy details.

How to Screen Your Opponent

If you find yourself spending enough time in the sun to encounter a burning risk, you should have a protection plan. Unfortunately, Conventional Wisdom lets us down again by touting sunscreen as a fail-safe method. Credible research has shown that most sunscreens have historically not blocked the UVA rays that can cause melanoma, instead blocking the UVB rays that cause burning. So, without burning as a deterrent, you spend more time in the sun bagging UVA rays and increasing cancer risk. Bad news!

Furthermore, many of the popular agents used in sunblock products may have toxic properties, especially when you consider the standard recommendation to reapply these synthetic chemicals frequently to your porous skin. Octyl methoxycinnamate (OMC), a chemical contained in 90 percent of sunscreen products, could damage living tissue if it penetrates your outer layer of dead skin. Titanium dioxide, another popular

(continued)

sunscreen compound, has been named a "potential occupational carcinogen" by the U.S. government due to unclear toxic danger.

Nevertheless, worries about skin cancer are valid, particularly for those with fair skin, red or blond hair, and light eyes, or those with numerous moles; these folks are six times more likely to develop melanoma than those with darker features.

If you must be out in the sun for extended periods of time, it is far preferable to use clothing, especially technical fabrics touted as providing extra sun protection, to minimize your exposure to harmful UVA rays—and to prevent burning. There are numerous apparel brands touting enhanced SPF (sun protection factor) effectiveness; search the Internet or visit a high quality specialty sports store to find some. If you are partial to good ol' cotton, realize that it, too, will offer significant SPF effectiveness. Examining your skin after a day in the sun to make sure it's not burned will reveal just how well your clothing protects you. As a backup to clothing protection, use a premium sunscreen that protects against UVA, UVB, and the newly described UVC rays. Check out the EWG's Sunscreen Guide, which ranks safe and effective sunscreens, and opt for an opaque zinc-based cream that entirely blocks all rays.

Beyond exposing yourself sensibly and being careful to always use protection (can you believe I slipped that line past my editors?!), a diet high in antioxidants and with a moderated O6:O3 ratio can go a long, long way toward reducing or eliminating any damage caused by sun exposure. In fact, one of the more common testimonials from people who have adopted a Primal Blueprint eating strategy is, "I can stay out in the sun longer without burning." On the flip side, a bad diet could be an even more profound risk factor than sun exposure for skin cancer. Research published by the National Academy of Sciences indicates that dietary O6:O3 ratio is critical to skin cancer prevention. Furthermore, excess consumption of PUFA and chemically-altered fats has been known to exacerbate the growth of tumors and other inflammation-related health conditions.

In a future book, I'll address the topic of sun exposure in great detail and help you formulate a customized sun exposure plan. For now, I want you to second guess Conventional Wisdom's knee-jerk, fear-based reaction to skin cancer dangers and the view that the sun is evil.

Primal Blueprint Law #9: Avoid Stupid Mistakes

Despite common Fred Flintstone-like depictions, early man was far from a numbskull. Grok was most certainly attuned to his surroundings and was skillful at avoiding mistakes or getting into situations likely to endanger health. It is a common faulty assumption that our hunter-gatherer ancestors lived "solitary, poor, nasty, brutish, and short" lives. This was the description advanced by 17th-century English philosopher Thomas Hobbes, when he argued for the need to have government structure in civilization instead of living off the land hunter-gatherer style.

Research suggests that Grok and his family were actually generally healthy (robust is the apropos term), productive, and so appreciative of their lives that they felt the need to express themselves through art. There may even have been a selective benefit within tribal units for grandparents—meaning that getting older may have actually had an evolutionary advantage, such as babysitting or the transfer of important knowledge and history.

So, if they were so robust and if our genes truly evolved to allow us to live long lives, then why was the average life span relatively short? I had always assumed that it was due to events like death from childbirth, infections, accidental poisoning, or even tribal warfare. But then I got a real-life experience of what might have affected life span more than anything else. Far from nasty and brutish, it was the mundane lapses in judgment, even minor ones, that likely spelled doom for many primal humans.

My unusually bad dive during an Ultimate Frisbee match in September 2007 resulted in a torn quadriceps muscle, displaced kneecap, ruptured prepatellar bursa, and smashed nerve. An X-ray revealed no other tendon or ligament damage, and my orthopedist said the soft-tissue injury would heal in 8 to 12 weeks. He advised me to use pain as my guide and come back slowly. Because I had no pain at all (smashed nerve, remember?), I felt like I was recovering fairly quickly—to the point of even resuming my beach sprints in early December, followed by a snowboarding trip over Christmas break. But despite wrapping the knee every day and taking it fairly easy (wink, wink—and again no pain), I came home with a very swollen, black-and-blue knee. By the end of the week, I was unable to bend it more than a few degrees.

An MRI revealed a large organized hematoma over the quad and knee-cap; it needed to be removed surgically, otherwise I would carry it with me forever. During surgery, it was discovered that the original torn quad muscle had never repaired itself and was leaking blood into the space, causing the hematoma. So my surgeon removed the hematoma and stitched the quad back to the patellar tendon.

Here I was, 54 years old, looking forward to living well past 100, but I was effectively incapacitated for more than four months by an injury caused by a random fall. (Truth be told, I had second thoughts as soon as I jumped.) Of course, I had the luxury of modern surgical procedures to repair the damage and eventually recovered fully. Had this happened 10,000 years ago, my inability to run away from a predator might well have spelled the end for me—all because of a momentary lapse of judgment. Even today, a small accident that active younger folks barely sneeze at (e.g., a fall from a ladder while hanging the holiday lights or turning an ankle on a staircase) can mean something entirely different for someone elderly and sedentary.

" I drive way too fast to worry about cholesterol. "
—Stephen Wright, American Comedian

The Darwin Awards—Long Live Natural Selection

As society continues to modernize exponentially, we are arguably exhibiting less and less common sense in avoiding stupid mistakes. I believe part of the reason is that deep down, we know we can afford to make them. Our intricate system of safety nets in modern society has compromised our capacity to take responsibility for our role in the "accidents" that occur and are chronicled by the news media daily.

Look no further than YouTube or the Jackass movies and television shows to confirm that we are actively inviting unnecessary struggle and suffering into our lives. It's all in the name of expressing the youthful sense of adventure that has been stifled by the constraints and predictability of the modern world. The "Darwin Awards" satirical book and Web site annually bestow special distinction on those who "improve the gene pool by removing themselves from it" with particular brilliance. Here are some of my favorite winners from recent years:

Hot Rod: A Texas motorist spilled a gas can in the back of his car. While searching for the can at night, he flicked on a cigarette lighter to get a better view, igniting the vehicle.

Nacho Libre: A Pennsylvania man was critically injured when, distracted by a plate of nachos on his lap, he crashed his motorcycle into a telephone pole.

CSI—Alternate Ending: A police officer in Illinois was trying to show another patrolman how their fellow officer had accidentally killed himself. While reenacting the shooting incident from the previous week, he forgot to unload his gun and shot himself in the stomach. While driving himself to the hospital to seek treatment, he was killed in an auto accident.

Up, Up, and Away: A Catholic priest in Brazil attached a lawn chair to dozens of helium balloons and launched his homemade craft. Winds picked up and he drifted out to sea. Well prepared for this potential adversity, he fired up his satellite phone to call for help but could not figure out how to operate his GPS unit to provide an accurate location for rescuers. Rescuers were unable to locate him—ever…although bits of balloon were found later on mountains and beaches.

Off the Falls: A man attempted to pilot a rocket-boosted jet ski off the side of Niagara Falls. The idea was for the rocket to launch the jet ski beyond the danger of the falls and then deploy a parachute and float to safety. The damp air caused both the rocket and parachute to fail as he rode off the edge of the falls. Miraculously, he survived the 160-foot drop but drowned because he didn't know how to swim and was not wearing a life jacket.

Each of us must admit that we have brought various levels of misfortune and trauma into our lives from lapses in concentration or critical thinking. As we attempt to reflect on these stupid mistakes, often we default to blaming bad luck instead of reenacting the chain of events with a deep, honest assessment of our accountability. In fact, the concept of taking responsibility seems to have all but disappeared from modern life. If we truly deconstruct those times when we have been the victim of circumstances, it's quite likely we can discover that exact moment when we were distracted, made a poor choice, or ignored the clear warning signal that might have helped us to avoid the entire incident.

Hypervigilance and Risk Management

Each of us possesses the genetically hard-wired skills of hypervigilance and risk management. Like any other skill—or muscle—we have to use and develop them or they will atrophy. Unfortunately, the obsessive effort society makes to diffuse all forms of risk and danger suppresses the use of these natural instincts: endless warning signs on roads and in public venues, safety hazard labels on every consumer product, and sensationalized news reports about the dangers of toxic playground bark or pajamas catching fire. Furthermore, continued technological innovations in the name of comfort and convenience collectively push us toward running on autopilot, often to our detriment, through various mundane elements of daily life.

Drive through Europe and you'll notice very few warnings or safety precautions on the roadways—even high in the Alps they don't bother with guardrails. Take a spin through the canyons near my home and you will see miles upon miles of safety barriers, guardrails, runaway truck ramps, and diamond-shaped yellow signs with admonitions and icons warning you of assorted dangers that lurk around every corner. Nevertheless, every year tragedy strikes our local community with fatal accidents (typically induced by alcohol and/or speeding) on these obsessively protected roads.

Meanwhile, the historic traffic fatality rates in France, Germany, Great Britain, Switzerland, and Scandinavia—per capita and per vehicle miles driven—are significantly lower than those of the United States. Interestingly, some progressive traffic engineers, in the US and abroad, are popularizing the concept of *shared space* as a tool to reduce accident rates. The concept relies on human instincts, such as eye contact, in favor of traditional traffic signals and signs. For example, the removal of bike lane striping on a roadway may actually make cycling safer by increasing driver vigilance. This seemingly counterintuitive concept speaks to the power of nurturing our natural instincts to navigate potentially hazardous situations effectively when we are not pacified by excessive safety measures.

As we strive to succeed in modern life, we must be willing to take personal responsibility for our actions instead of defaulting to speed-dialing a personal injury attorney whenever we come to misfortune. If you get hit by a motorist running a red light, it most certainly is his fault, but you may fare better if you remember to fasten your seat belt and look for oncoming traffic despite the color of the traffic light. I can't remember if an errant throw or overly aggressive defensive play was involved in my Ultimate accident, as I prefer to focus on the fact that I hurled myself through the air irresponsibly and then tried to come back into action too quickly afterward. When I take responsibility for my actions, my misfortune becomes a growth experience—an appealing alternative to feeling like a victim or placing any importance on the notion of bad luck.

Similarly, every time I encounter a dicey driving situation, I realize something upon further reflection when things calm down: whenever I mumble "asshole" to someone who has just cut me off, I should really be saying it to myself, too—for being in a rush, being too aggressive or impatient, or diverting my focus from the road momentarily. Maybe the motorists who incur my wrath truly deserve a little choice feedback, but I can find something I brought to the table most every time.

This theme also works in a discussion about dietary habits. You can blame lousy food options in airports, your distressing family medical history, or the limitations of your budget, but in each case you may be better served to accept some personal accountability. Take the extra time to pack healthy snacks for your travel. View your family history as a catalyst to cultivate hypervigilance and risk-management skills instead of as a curse. Take a deeper look at your lifestyle priorities, make some compromises, and stretch your food budget a bit to choose the very best of everything. In this way you can turn negatives into positives and create excellent leverage to be the best you can be, regardless of "bad luck" or other figments of your imagination that are vying for your attention.

> " *Everybody gets so much information all day long that they lose their common sense.* "
> —**Gertrude Stein,** American author and French art patron (1874-1946)

Primal Blueprint Law #10: Use Your Brain

While the modern world features plenty of complex thought and a constant and rapid progression in human innovation—technological and otherwise—our overstimulated lifestyles compromise our ability to use our brains with maximum effectiveness. In the workplace, the mismanagement of information overload from personal digital assistants (BlackBerry®, Droid®, iPhone®, iPad®, etc.), instant chat, and the like can stifle creativity and innovation, not to mention our levels of energy, motivation, and health. Consequently, many of us operate in a reactive mode, constantly and often futilely trying to keep pace with the information with which we are bombarded.

In Mark Bauerlein's book *The Dumbest Generation*, he blames digital technology for compromising the intellectual development of young people.

"When we were 17 years old, social life stopped at the front door. Now [via Facebook, texting, Skype, etc.] peer-to-peer contact…has no limitation in space or time," observes Bauerlein. Hence, time to read, daydream, free-associate, or gain an adequate understanding of current events, history, and other mainstays of cultural sophistication goes by the wayside.

If we back up and examine the true definition of stress as "stimulus," it's clear that we require a certain amount of daily stress to thrive, prosper, and be happy. Art De Vany, Ph.D., author of the *New Evolution Diet*, draws a compelling link between exercising our minds and our genetic nature as free, independent, adventurous human beings. "Modern life leaves our minds restless and under-utilized because we are confined, inactive, and comfortable," De Vany argues. "We cannot be satisfied with more and more, because we are evolved for another lifeway in which material goods do not matter. The result is that we are deeply unsatisfied with modern life and don't know why." Our genes simply don't know what to make of all our "stuff."

> *Modern life leaves our minds restless and under-utilized because we are confined, inactive, and comfortable.*
> **—Art De Vany, Ph.D.,**
> author of *The New Evolution Diet*

At first glance, few might agree that our minds are restless and under-utilized. Many of us end our days running on fumes, feeling like our minds will explode if we send or receive any more e-mail. Our minds are indeed overstressed, yet technically under-utilized, because we lack the balance that creative intellectual outlets, play, healthy diet, exercise, sleep, and other winning behaviors promote. Eight hours of brain power is probably a sensible limit to devote to your daily work efforts. However, engaging your mind with things that stimulate your creativity in other ways and that you have a passion for is critical to mental health and overall well-being. Here are few suggestions to model Primal Blueprint Law #10—Use Your Brain:

Pursue New Endeavors: Learn a foreign language or musical instrument, take dancing lessons, tackle a jigsaw or crossword puzzle, write a fiction short story—or anything else you can imagine outside of your comfort zone that sounds interesting and challenging.

Discipline Your Brain Use: Pay close attention to balancing your daily intellectual stimulation with rest. Make an effort to avoid (or power down) distracting influences and focus on a single peak performance task at a time.

Exercise the Muscle: Instead of outsourcing as much brain function as possible to technology, make a habit of challenging your brain during your routine daily endeavors. Replay your favorite song on your iPod and try to memorize the lyrics, bust out your school year book and try to recall the names of your long-lost fellow students, or use your head to add up numbers instead of always relying on a calculator or notepad. Do a Google search for Sheppard Software's "Place the States Game" and see how closely you can come to dropping individual states into their correct spot on a blank USA map. There are endless opportunities to keep the brain fresh throughout your day.

Chapter Summary

1. Get Adequate Sleep: Despite being a critical component of good health and stress management, sleep is regularly compromised in modern life due to the pull of technology and hectic schedules. Insufficient sleep can lead to numerous health problems and declines in cognitive function. Try to align your sleep habits as closely as possible with the rising and setting of the sun, with special attention to minimizing artificial light and digital stimulation after dark. Create a calm, dark, relaxing sleeping environment, observe gradual transitions into and out of sleep, and observe consistent bed and wake times. Occasional brief naps can produce many health benefits, including reduced risk of disease plus improvements to mood, concentration, and physical performance.

2. Play: The regimented nature of modern life leaves many adults—and even kids—deficient in play. The profound psychological benefits of play are integral to healthy cultures, communities, and individuals, including a direct relationship to work productivity. Engage in some unstructured outdoor physical exertion each day to counter the negative effects of a sedentary, technological existence.

3. Get Adequate Sunlight: A reasonable amount of daily sun exposure (defined according to many personal variables, including skin pigment and climate) can produce numerous health benefits and alleviate many health risks, because it enables your body to synthesize optimal levels of vitamin D. The dangers of sun exposure are overdramatized and many suffer from sun deficiency today. Risks of skin cancer are greatly minimized if you avoid sunburn and cover or screen the most vulnerable areas of face, neck, and hands.

Pursue a strategy of exposing the large surface areas of your skin (arms, legs, torso, back) to direct sunlight for about *half the amount of time it takes to sustain a slight burn*. Dietary sources of vitamin D are vastly inferior to sun exposure. Vitamin D supplements can be useful in the winter months when sunlight is of insufficient intensity to allow for vitamin D production. When you've had enough sun, clothing is the best protection, as sunscreens have some health objections and may be less effective than advertised.

4. Avoid Stupid Mistakes: Avoiding stupid mistakes was a critical survival factor for Grok, because margin for error was much lower. Today, modern life attempts to shield us from all manner of danger, yet—possibly desensitized by all these protection mechanisms—we still seem to find a way to invite trauma and tragedy into our lives by making stupid mistakes. You must practice your hardwired, evolution-perfected skills of hypervigilance and risk management to navigate successfully through even the mundane elements of daily life. This will prevent unnecessary suffering and ensure longevity.

5. Use Your Brain: Human innovation and overstimulation have compromised our ability to use our brains to maximum effectiveness. You must exert great discipline to leverage technology to your advantage instead of falling victim to it by spacing out, burning out, or otherwise misusing your greatest weapon as human beings: complex thought. Pursue new challenges, such as music, language, hobbies, or adventures that stimulate your brain and allow you to depart from your daily routine. This will keep you refreshed and energized for your core daily responsibilities and economic contribution.

CHAPTER 8

A Primal Approach to Weight Loss

Meet Ya at the Sweet Spot!

In This Chapter

I provide a step-by-step process for losing an average of one to two pounds (one-half to one kilogram) of body fat per week. You'll learn how to target protein, carb, and fat intake in order to ramp up fat metabolism, maintain high dietary satisfaction levels, and avoid the risk of depleting muscle tissue and suffering from the usual rebound-rebellion effect of severe caloric restriction. I discuss how deregulating food intake and fasting intermittently can be effective calorie-restriction tools and how exercise can accelerate progress toward your body composition goals.

I review two weight-loss case studies (Ken and Kelly Korg, naturally!), calculating their average daily caloric expenditure and optimal daily intake of each macronutrient—Primal Blueprint style—to produce targeted and effective fat loss. We'll examine a daily food diary of delicious, nutritious meals that contains a detailed caloric analysis and macronutrient breakdown for each meal plus a daily total. The case studies result in a loss of around eight pounds for Ken and Kelly (3.6 kg) in a single month. Finally, I provide troubleshooting tips for possible setbacks and plateaus that arise when trying to lose weight in the real world.

Desserts is just *stressed* spelled backwards.
—Anonymous

These are the critical elements of the *Primal Blueprint* weight-loss approach:

- **Minimize carb intake** to moderate insulin production and enable stored body fat to be burned for energy.
- **Optimize protein intake** to maintain or increase muscle mass.
- **Optimize fat intake** to achieve satiety, provide energy, and eliminate hunger.
- **Deregulate meal habits and engage in occasional Intermittent Fasting (I.F.)** to produce accelerated caloric deficits that lead to greater fat loss.
- **Exercise Primally** to fine-tune fat metabolism and build or tone lean muscle without the drawbacks of Chronic Cardio.
- **Avoid excessive regimentation or obsessing on results** in favor of appreciating the process and viewing body composition goals with a long-term perspective.
- **Remember** that optimal health is the underlying goal of living Primally. LGN (*looking good naked*) is just a pleasant side effect.

By now you've caught my drift that the Primal Blueprint is a way of life as opposed to a regimented, gimmicky crash course diet. I thought carefully about whether to put the presumptuous claim of, "effortless weight loss" on the cover. However, I believe deeply that if you honor the Primal Blueprint principles at least 80 percent of the time, long-term weight management will happen as a natural by-product of your enjoyable, stress-balanced lifestyle.

Easier said than done right? While we have literally thousands of success stories compiled at MarksDailyApple.com, we also communicate occasionally with folks whose progress is not always smooth and steady. I'd like to shift gears in this chapter and get a little more precise about macronutrient intake. Following the steps covered in this chapter will enable you to immediately reduce excess body fat without the struggling and suffering inherent in any fat loss program that's attempted with a carbohydrate-based low-calorie diet.

The idea is to hit the sweet spot where carbs have been reduced just enough so that your body prefers to burn fats and a moderate amount of ketones instead of relying so much on glucose. This carbohydrate sweet spot is between 50 and 100 grams per day for most people. Where you land in this range depends on your size, age, sex, and metabolism. Consume more carbs than that (up to 150 grams a day) and you'll maintain body composition quite easily without adding fat, but you'll have to work a little harder to burn it off. On the other hand, it's certainly healthy to take in less than 50 grams per day of carbs once in a while (as we said, you could actually live on zero carbs for quite a long time), but the idea is to stay just on the fringe of ketosis.

In the sweet spot, you will maintain high energy levels (no more insulin crashes), you can exercise (including regular intense sessions) without getting exhausted, and you won't exhibit any of the unpleasant by-products of sudden, severely carb-restrictive diets that put you into ketosis without having prepared you to effectively use those ketones as fuel. These include the annoying "ketone breath," insufficient vitamin/mineral intake (due to the severe restriction of vegetables and fruits), and poor compliance due to the deprivation and inconvenience involved in trying to bottom out on carb intake.

As you continue to eat in the sweet spot (or dip into the maintenance zone on certain days, no biggie), your eating habits will send signals to your genes to up-regulate fat burning processes and down-regulate fat storage processes. You'll become both fat-adapted and keto-adapted, able to derive energy minute-to-minute from your stored body fat. By eating in the sweet spot, you can expect to drop one to two pounds (one-half to one kilogram) of excess body fat per week. This may not seem like much in comparison to the headline on the flyer tacked to the telephone pole or the flashing Internet banner ad. However, unless you plan to lose water and muscle tissue (and I know you don't), losing one to two pounds of fat per week (your personal maximum rate within this range depends on your existing body weight, metabolic rate, and activity level) means an average daily deficit of 500 to 1,000 calories. You cannot realistically (or safely) lose any more than a pound or two a week of body fat without depleting muscle mass or becoming fatigued.

How to Lose like a Winner

The sensible limits on the rate of losing body fat is evident when you consider that one pound of fat contains 3,500 calories and adults only burn between 1,500 and 3,000 total calories per day. What about the "Biggest Losers" glorified on the television program, or in before-and-after magazine contests, who alter their body composition dramatically in a short time? These results are achieved with a combination of incredibly intense exercise coupled with severe caloric restriction, an approach that is simply inhumane and impossible to follow long term. Generally, these crash efforts result in a significant reduction in water retention and lean muscle mass, and just a bit of fat.

A crash weight-loss program (or any other form of extreme stress, such as a family crisis) prompts a fight-or-flight response in your body. Buzzed on adrenalin, you can triumphantly complete your six-, eight-, or twelve-week program (particularly when the bright lights of television and monetary incentives are there to motivate you). Afterward, you are likely to collapse in exhaustion when the fight-or-flight response wears off and your body's energy reserves are depleted. In this "post-traumatic stress" state, many become sedentary (or much less active, in any case) and tend to overeat—a genetically programmed reaction to an ordeal perceived as a starvation threat. Lo and behold, the "before and after" success story typically becomes a "before and after and back to before…and then some" reality! There is absolutely no reason to have to struggle or suffer to achieve your body composition and health goals. In fact, if you are, I can guarantee that your approach is flawed.

Before the disappointment of hearing "only a pound or two a week" gets etched onto your face, understand that when you embrace the Primal Blueprint as a lifelong transition out of flawed Conventional Wisdom's grain-based diet into something aligned with your genetic requirements for health, you'll realize there is no hurry here—you have complete control over your physique for the rest of your life. Fine tune eating habits or workout patterns for a few weeks and you can drop fat or add/tone muscle as simple as turning a number on a dial. Stay with the Primal Blueprint and you will always trend towards your ideal body composition.

Weight-Loss Macronutrient Plan

The plan is as follows: obtain a calculable level of protein sufficient to preserve lean muscle mass, strictly limit carbs to an average of 50 to 100 per day, and use fat as the main variable to obtain the satisfaction you need from your diet each day so that you aren't stressed or anxious about your weight-loss journey. To ensure your success and comfort during the fat-reduction period, please make an extra effort to have appropriate snacks available at all times. These include vegetables and certain fruits, and foods high in protein and/or fat (hard-boiled eggs, jerky, macadamia nuts, olives, sardines). If you're feeling deprived during your Primal journey, or have cravings for some of your old grain-based standbys, have a few celery sticks smothered in macadamia nut butter, a hard-boiled egg, a handful of beef jerky, then call me!

> " *Your appetite will guide you effectively to meet your protein requirements, just as your thirst does for hydration requirements* "

Protein

As you learned already, you need an average of 0.7 to 1 gram of protein per pound (1.5 to 2.2 grams per kilo) of lean body weight per day to repair, build, and/or maintain lean muscle mass effectively and to adequately support numerous other metabolic functions dependent upon dietary protein. For an active female with 100 pounds (45 kg) of lean body mass, this is only 400 protein calories per day. For an active male with 150 pounds (67.5 kg) of lean body mass, this amounts to only 600 protein calories per day.

I'm not asking you to undergo an expensive underwater body composition test to pinpoint your lean body mass and then carry around a calculator to nail your exact protein requirements every day. Your appetite will guide you effectively to meet your protein requirements, just as your thirst does for hydration requirements. That said, if you experience low energy or a perceived reduction in muscle mass, you may want to delve further into just what you are eating to be sure the levels are in proper range. Jot down everything you eat for a few days, and then use an online food calculator such as PaleoTrack.com or Fitday.com to determine how many grams of the various macronutrients you are consuming. I've provided some suggested meals with detailed nutrient breakdowns in this chapter to give you a feel for how healthy and satisfying the Primal Blueprint weight-loss plan can be.

Carbohydrate

Limiting your average carb intake to 50 to 100 grams per day will effectively moderate your insulin production and optimize your fat-burning process. At this level of carbohydrate intake, your body will be stimulated to burn more stored fats and manufacture a little extra glucose in the liver through gluconeogenesis. In this case, however, dietary protein will provide the substrate for gluconeogenesis instead of your precious muscle tissue. I've discussed the gluconeogenesis process as a bad thing in the context of the fight-or-flight response triggered by Chronic Cardio or a protein-deficient extreme diet, but it can just as easily be a wonderful energy-balancing mechanism when you eat Primally.

> *You can enjoy abundant servings of vegetables and some well-chosen fruit and still lose excess body fat—provided you ditch sugars, grains, and legumes.*

As an added benefit of this process, your liver will generate a moderate amount of ketones that will help spare muscle tissue and provide added fuel for cells that might otherwise require glucose. Hence, limiting your carbs to well under 100 grams per day will put you in a very mild (and desirable, because you'll be burning fat like crazy) state of ketosis. You probably won't even notice it, but for the appreciable increase in steady-state energy now available. If your batting average drifts above 100, your increasing blood glucose levels will start to redirect energy pathways more toward glucose burning.

I'm not asking you to split your carrot sticks down the middle or to skimp on salad portions to stay under 100 grams. As you can see from this chapter's examples, you can still enjoy abundant servings of vegetables and ample servings of well-chosen fruit (nutrient-dense foods that are particularly important to consume when you are restricting calories and exercising diligently) and land in the optimum range for insulin control and weight loss. The key to meeting this seemingly strict guideline effortlessly is to virtually eliminate processed carbs from your diet—then it's truly a breeze. If all you do is get rid of sugars, desserts, soft drinks, pasta, bread, cereals, and beans, (and starchy tubers such as potatoes—especially if you eat them and their derivatives frequently—for the time being) you won't even have to track the remaining carbs.

Really, It's All About the Carbohydrate Curve

Your body composition *success* is overwhelmingly dependent on controlling your carbohydrate intake and, consequently, your insulin output. Exercising correctly, managing your stress levels, and accounting for genetics are minor factors in the equation. Your *failure* to maintain desirable body composition may have assorted contributing factors—unlucky genetics, overly stressful exercise, insufficient sleep, emotional eating issues, and more—but an excess body fat condition *almost always includes excessive carbohydrate intake.*

Eat in the 100-150 gram Maintenance Zone and you won't gain fat (unless you have an extremely severe overeating problem...but even then it will be hard!). Eat in the 50-100 gram Sweet Spot and you will lose body fat, no matter who you are and how hard it's been to drop weight in the past. Really, it's all about the Carbohydrate Curve!

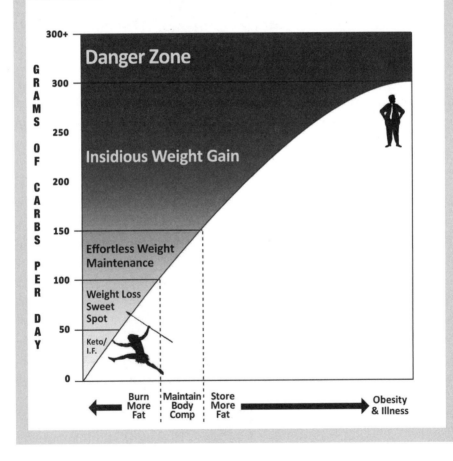

Fat

Coupling your protein requirements with your strict limitations on carbohydrates (at 50 to 100 grams per day during the fat-loss phase), it's easy to see how you can reduce body fat at an accelerated rate. Even an active male will be under 1,000 calories per day before considering fat intake. Hence, the variable for your energy needs and total calorie consumption ends up being fat. If you are committed to success, you will make a concerted effort to eat only what you need (in fat and in total calories) to feel satisfied and energized. Because fat has such a high satiety factor, a little will go a long way. Even something like a small handful of nuts can sustain you for hours when you skip meals or need a quick snack to keep you going. With the right meal choices and healthy snacks around, your intensive weight-loss experience will not involve the typical struggling and suffering of a "diet." After you reduce the amount of body fat you desire, you can consume even more liberal amounts of fat without worrying about gaining weight.

While the "eating fat is okay for weight loss" idea might seem contradictory at first glance, it is valid; without insulin, eating fat will not make you fat! If you don't produce insulin, your body has no way to store the excess calories as body fat. Note, however, that if I give you an inch and you take a mile—pounding high-fat foods all day "as directed by Mark Sisson"—you will not succeed in losing fat either. As you build up momentum with more and more weeks of eating low insulin-producing meals, notice how your genes become reprogrammed to not require regular high-carbohydrate feeding sessions to stay awake and functional. Your appetite will "self-regulate" to a point at which you eat when you are hungry and become comfortable eating only as much as you need to feel satisfied. As your old, ravenous "eat-every-three-hours" sugar-burner hunger gives way to the new "energy-all-the-time" fat-burning furnace you have created, capitalize on your progress now and then by skipping meals—noticing that you can actually crank away all morning without eating an All-American breakfast. In fact, your new breakfast might now be the 500 calories of fat you are currently sitting on or that's hanging over your belt (no offense) ready to be burned off as energy. Proceed with your dietary transition at a pace most comfortable to you and realize that this is the essence of Primal living: rejecting a dependence on dietary carbs as facilitated by the Standard American Diet and reclaiming your Homo sapiens genetic factory setting as a fat-burning beast!

Ken Korg: Suggested Eating for Primal Weight Loss

Let's look at a case study of our old friend Ken Korg, a 40-year-old, five-foot-eleven (177.5 cm), 197-pound (89 kg), moderately active male with 25 percent body fat (metric equivalent: 25 percent; sorry, still too much!) who wants to lose weight aggressively (near the maximum suggested rate of two pounds per week) following the Primal Blueprint. We'll calculate Ken's estimated daily caloric expenditure and suggested macronutrient intake based on Primal Blueprint guidelines. Then, I'll present a list of suggested meals and snacks with accompanying macronutrient analysis. The day's example will show how Ken can enjoy sensible, satisfying meals and snacks and still achieve a dramatic improvement in body composition by meeting the average macronutrient guidelines for a single month.

Throughout these examples, remember to focus on the concept of averages. While it's instructive to examine a detailed daily example of both expenditure and intake to understand how we can properly achieve caloric deficits, in reality you will have days when you exceed your carb limit, fall short of your protein limit, and exercise more or less than the averages in our calculations. Ultimately, this isn't about counting and tracking, but about developing an intuitive sense of what works best for you.

Caloric Expenditure

The basal metabolic rate (BMR) estimates were derived using a BMR calculator (bmi-calculator.net is one of many Internet resources). BMR factors your age and weight to estimate the number of calories your body burns if you simply stay in bed all day. An Activity Factor adding additional calories to the daily estimate is derived using the Harris Benedict Formula (also available at bmi-calculator.net), which takes into account typical levels of activity. You can input your personal variables and generate similar estimates for total daily caloric expenditure.

1. Basal Metabolic Rate: Number of daily calories Ken burns to support basal metabolic functions (at his age and body composition) = 1,923.

2. Activity Factor: Harris Benedict Formula for additional calories burned when "moderately active": BMR × 0.55 = 1,057.

3. Total Average Daily Calorie Expenditure: BMR (1,923) + Activity Factor (1,057) = 2,980

Macronutrient Calculations

- 197 pounds at 25 percent body fat = 148 pounds of lean body mass (67 kg)
- Moderately active = 0.7 grams per pound (1.5 grams per kg) factor for protein intake per pound of lean body mass
- 148 pounds × 0.7 = 104 grams of average daily protein intake
- Goal of losing 8 pounds (3.6 kg) per month = 932 calories per day average caloric deficit
- Desired average caloric intake per day = 2,048 (2,980 average caloric expenditure less 932 deficit)
- Desired protein grams = 104 (416 calories) – per previous calculations
- Desired carb grams = 75 (300 calories) – to get into the Sweet Spot on the Carb Curve
- Desired fat grams = 148 (1,332 calories) – to get back into the 2,048 daily total

You can see right away that the suggestions will not be difficult for Ken to follow. That amount of fat calories will provide ample energy and satiety at each meal, while the number of protein grams will ensure that his body recovers from exercise stress and continues to burn at his average daily rate of 2,980 calories—or higher. In his past dieting efforts, Ken tried to cut back on calories in general, slightly reducing normal intake of fat, protein, and carbs. More likely, he probably made a little extra effort to cut back on fatty foods but was not nearly diligent enough with carbs and possibly compromised some lean body mass (depending on how devoted his efforts were) by falling short of protein requirements.

Each time he tried to lose this way in the past, Ken's energy and exercise level declined slightly but insulin was still prevalent to drive consumed calories into fat cells. Hence, his body fat percentage has stayed pegged at 25 percent for years despite repeated efforts to reduce. Let's see how the results can differ when eating Primal Blueprint style.

Ken Korg Food Journal

Breakfast

Primal Omelet
Eggs (three medium) with cream (1 ounce) and shredded cheddar cheese (1 tablespoon)
Chopped mushrooms, red onions, and red peppers (3/4 cup total)
Topped with sliced avocado (2 ounces) and fresh salsa (2 tablespoons)
Fresh blueberries (1/4 cup)
Cup of black coffee

FitDay.com Analysis
Total Calories: 463
Protein: 23 grams, 89 calories (19 percent)
Carbs: 22 grams, 82 calories (18 percent)
Fat: 33 grams, 292 calories (63 percent)

Lunch

Primal Salad
Mixed salad greens (2 cups)
Chopped onions, carrots, jicama, red peppers, and cherry tomatoes (2 ounces each)
Chopped or shredded chicken (3 ounces)
Sesame seeds (1/3 ounce)
Chopped walnuts (1/2 ounce or 7 halves)
Oil-based dressing (2 tablespoons)

FitDay.com Analysis
Total Calories: 585
Protein: 31 grams, 124 calories (21 percent)
Carbs: 30 grams, 120 calories (21 percent)
Fat: 38 grams, 341 calories (56 percent)

Dinner

Salmon and Vegetables
Broiled wild salmon (6 ounces)
Steamed asparagus and zucchini (6 ounces each) with butter (1 tablespoon)
Red wine (5-ounce glass)

FitDay.com Analysis
Total Calories: 560
Protein: 39 grams, 157 calories (28 percent)
Carbs: 16 grams, 63 calories (11 percent)
Fat: 26 grams, 232 calories (41 percent)
Alcohol: 16 grams, 108 calories (21 percent)

Ken Korg Food Journal

Snacks

Hard-boiled egg
Macadamia nuts (1-1/2 ounces
or 17 nuts)
Venison jerky (one 4-inch strip)

FitDay.com Analysis
Total Calories: 437
Protein: 14 grams, 58 calories
(16 percent)
Carbs: 8 grams, 32 calories
(7 percent)
Fat: 41 grams, 347 calories
(79 percent)

Daily Totals

Calories: 2,045
Protein: 107 grams, 428 calories
(21 percent)
Carbs: 78 grams, 297 calories
(15 percent)
Fat: 139 grams, 1,212 calories
(59 percent)
Alcohol: 16 grams, 108 calories
(5 percent)

Ken Korg
Caloric deficit from average
daily expenditure (2,980) = 935
Projected net fat loss over
30-day period: **8 pounds**

To make up for the caloric intake deficit, Ken will derive his additional 935 daily calories from stored body fat—what is now his primary energy mechanism to fuel a busy day. Quite an improvement from his previous roller coaster of carbs, caffeine, insulin, fatigue, and insufficient exercise.

You Won't Believe What's Primal!

The diary entries for Ken and Kelly illustrate the concept that Primal Blueprint weight loss does not have to be a Spartan exercise of weighing and measuring bland food, choking down powdered "replacements" for real food, or otherwise engaging in repetitive, restrictive eating habits. While the rules of Primal Blueprint macronutrient intake are clear-cut, there is tremendous opportunity for flexibility within these guidelines.

At MarksDailyApple.com, we have hundreds of recipes, shopping tips, and detailed meal-planning strategies that will help you actually enjoy the process of eating healthy, perhaps to an even greater extent than you did your pre-Primal dietary habits. You may also enjoy *The Primal Blueprint Cookbook* and *The Primal Blueprint Quick and Easy Meals*. Take a glance at this list of recipes that are posted on the Web site—yep, they're all Primal-approved!

> *Primal Blueprint eating offers tremendous flexibility for personal preference, allowing you to actually enjoy the process of transitioning to Primal eating.*

- Arugula Endive Salad with White Wine Vinaigrette
- Spicy Thai Coconut Soup
- Broiled Halibut with Garlic Aioli and Steamed Broccoli
- Crustless Quiche with Spinach and Scallions
- Baked Mahimahi with Pesto and Tomatoes
- Grilled Flank Steak with Sauteed Beet Greens and Creamy Horseradish Beets
- Smoked Salmon with Asparagus and Poached Egg
- Spicy Korean Seaweed Salad with Shrimp
- Sauteed Broccoli Rabe with Sundried Tomatoes and Pine Nuts

Kelly Korg: Suggested Eating for Primal Weight Loss

Now let's evaluate Kelly Korg, our 40-year-old, five-foot-four (162 cm), 148-pound (67 kg), very active female with 27 percent body fat. While her goal of losing nearly eight pounds of body fat (3.6 kg) in a single month is ambitious for a female, she is fit enough to tolerate intense exercise and create substantial caloric deficits with sensible Primal Blueprint meals. She will actually reduce her total weekly exercise hours and corresponding calories burned in favor of a more sensible program with slower paced cardio, more rest, and shorter, more intense workouts.

Caloric Expenditure

1. Basal Metabolic Rate: 1,411

2. Activity Factor: Harris Benedict Formula for additional calories burned when "very active": BMR × 0.725 = 1,023.

3. Total Average Daily Calorie Expenditure: BMR (1,411) + Activity Factor (1,023) = 2,433

Macronutrient Calculations

- 148 pounds at 27 percent body fat = 102 pounds of lean body mass (46 kg)
- 1.0 grams per pound (2.2 grams per kg) factor for protein intake per pound lean body mass (due to high stress levels and history of heavy exercise requiring more protein than a moderately active person like her husband)
- 102 pounds lean mass = 102 grams of average daily protein intake
- Goal of losing 7.66 pounds of body fat per month = 894 per day average caloric deficit
- Desired average caloric intake per day = 1,539 (2,433 average caloric expenditure less 894 deficit)
- Desired protein grams = 110 (408 calories) – per previous calculations
- Desired carb grams = 79 (316 calories) – to get into the Sweet Spot on the Carb Curve
- Desired fat grams = 91 (816 calories) – to get back into the 1,539 daily total

You can see right away that the diet will be much more pleasant for Kelly to follow than her previous efforts to severely restrict calories interspersed with inevitable carb binges. The fat calories will provide satiety at each meal (missing from her last diet, which featured heavily processed high-carb liquid shakes). The protein calories will ensure that her body recovers from exercise stress and also maintains and even builds some attractive lean muscle tissue and that her metabolic rate stabilizes at 2,433 calories daily.

Kelly Korg Food Journal

Breakfast

Breakfast: Steak and Fruit
Flank steak (4 ounces)
Blueberries (1/2 cup)
Peach (1/2 of whole)
Green tea (1 cup)

FitDay.com Analysis
Total Calories: 238
Protein: 25.0 grams, 106 calories
 (44 percent)
Carbs: 15.7 grams, 56 calories
 (24 percent)
Fat: 8.5 grams, 76 calories
 (32 percent)

Lunch

Chicken Club Lettuce Wrap
Lettuce (3 large leaves)
Diced cooked chicken (4 ounces)
Sliced red pepper (1/2 cup)
Plum tomato (1 medium)
Avocado (1/2 of whole)
Mayonnaise (1 teaspoon)

FitDay.com Analysis
Total Calories: 397
Protein: 38.5 grams, 159 calories
 (40 percent)
Carbs: 17.2 grams, 62 calories
 (14 percent)
Fat: 20.5 grams, 176 calories
 (44 percent)

Dinner

Beef Stir-Fry
Sliced beef steak (4 ounces)
Olive oil (2 tablespoons)
Sliced zucchini (1 medium)
Sliced mushrooms (1 cup)
Spinach (1 cup)
Sliced bamboo shoots (1/2 cup)
Sesame seeds (1/4 ounce)

FitDay.com Analysis
Total Calories: 611
Protein: 37.6 grams, 150 calories
 (25 percent)
Carbs: 9.5 grams, 35 calories
 (6 percent)
Fat: 48.1 grams, 426 calories
 (70 percent)

Snacks

Hard-boiled egg (1 large)
Apple (1 large)
Almond butter (1 tablespoon;
   spread on apple)

FitDay.com Analysis
Total Calories: 283
Protein: 9.3, 35 calories
   (13 percent)
Carbs: 33.1 grams, 121 calories,
   (43 percent)
Fat: 14.8 grams, 127 calories
   (45 percent)

Daily Totals

Calories: 1,529
Protein: 110.4 grams, 450 calories
   (29 percent)
Carbs: 75.5 grams, 274 calories
   (18 percent)
Fat: 91.9 grams, 805 calories
   (53 percent)

Kelly Korg
Caloric deficit from average daily
expenditure (2,433) = 904
Projected net fat loss over 30-day
period: **7.75 pounds**

Weight-Loss Exercise Plan

While my view that 80 percent of your body composition success is determined by how you eat is difficult to prove scientifically, the anecdotal evidence is overwhelming. Go to the starting line of a major marathon or ironman triathlon and take note of the surprising level of excess body fat sported by many of these highly trained athletes. The same goes for the droves of gym rats and aerobics queens with flawed diets and physiques that belie their tremendous devotion to fitness.

There's no better proof that regardless of how many calories you burn, consuming excessive processed carbohydrates ultimately inhibits your ability to access and burn stored body fat efficiently around the clock. Instead, all that arduous training results in an increased appetite, again thanks to insulin-driven sugar cravings from poor food choices combined with, or as a consequence of, overly stressful workouts. Unless you are a genetically gifted, extremely devoted endurance athlete (i.e., racing at the front of a pack with a motorcycle escort), it's a vicious cycle that you cannot escape no matter how hard you exercise.

While it's true that exercise moderates the insulin response (i.e., a sugary energy gel consumed during a tough workout will be burned quickly and not prompt an insulin release like it would if you sucked it down at your desk), burning lots of calories (particularly with Chronic Cardio) and eating lots of carbs throughout the day will simply make you carb-dependent for energy. Invariably, left to its own devices, your body will want to overcompensate by tempting you to eat slightly more than you need to refill the tank, as if it's actually thinking, "what if this clown decides to do this again tomorrow? I'd better be ready!" This is how so many people have programmed their genes over the years, protecting them against depletion by stimulating an appetite increase in response to hard exercise.

Beyond the appetite increase, chronic exercise patterns have been scientifically shown to make you lazier throughout the day. Seriously—it's known as the *compensation theory*. Perhaps some of this compensatory behavior is conscious ("Sure, why not take the elevator? I already ran five miles this morning"), but there is also a subconscious component. The compensation theory asserts that you generally move less energetically throughout the day and are more liberal with your appetite and caloric intake. Buoyed by a deep down sense of accomplishment from your chronic workouts, you essentially grant yourself free license to chill out and pig out!

> ❝ *The bottom line is that you will not lose fat effectively with exercise-driven weight-loss efforts unless you moderate insulin production.* ❞

The bottom line is that you will not lose fat effectively with exercise-driven weight-loss efforts unless you moderate insulin production. Of course, a sensible exercise program will improve your health, sense of well-being, and muscle tone and somewhat minimize the negative effects of the high-carb diet by making you more insulin-sensitive, but it won't get rid of that spare tire. On the flip side, I have been able to maintain my ideal body composition effortlessly, even working out only one-tenth as much as I used to, since I evolved to eating very low-carb Primal Blueprint foods (getting increasingly observant over the past 10 years and eventually reaching what you might call very strict Primal in 2002). During my recovery from knee surgery in 2007, I was able to maintain my exact weight and eight percent body fat on zero exercise for a month and very limited exercise for a few more months after that.

Of course, we all have genetic differences that create the reality of "results may vary." Regardless, you must focus on the concept of triggering the ideal expression of your own genetic potential through the combination of Primal Blueprint diet and exercise behaviors. Consider an age when you were pleased with your fitness level and physique. It *is* possible to approximate your appearance and energy levels at age 18 or 21, reversing years or even decades of suboptimal diet and exercise practices, in a relatively short time.

Be content with uninterrupted gradual improvement in your body composition and a wholehearted enjoyment of the process. This improvement may not be a linear "pound or two a week" experience. Instead, you may have some months, or seasons, when you will really lean out and will face the inevitable plateaus (I'll discuss how to handle these shortly) over other periods of time. With this mind-set—that you are taking care of your health and constantly progressing toward your goals (at a speed you determine, mainly by dialing in your carb intake)—your motivation and compliance levels will be strong even years down the line.

By the way, you are welcome to pursue the program with more enthusiasm and discipline to produce accelerated results, but you must align your efforts with your fitness level. A serious athlete who has added a few pounds in the off-season can ramp up training easily and return to ideal weight relatively quickly. An old-time pro triathlete I coached was once asked how long it took to drop the typical seven pounds he'd gain during the off-season after he resumed his training program: "Couple long rides," he deadpanned. On the other hand, a novice unaccustomed to regular exercise must follow a more patient approach to avoid burning out. Following are some Primal exercise recommendations to turbocharge your weight-loss efforts.

> *Be not afraid of growing slowly,*
> *be afraid only of standing still.*
> **—Chinese Proverb**

Ramp Up Low-Level Activity

As discussed previously, when you exercise at moderate heart rates, you run little risk of fatigue or burnout. Increase your daily activity level in every possible way—walking or cycling instead of driving for nearby errands, taking the stairs, parking at the edge of the lot, strolling the neighborhood after dinner, and enjoying leisurely hikes on the weekends. One friend of mine makes business calls while walking briskly on a treadmill (a great icebreaker, by the way: "Hey, what's that hum in the background?"). Considering the average American watches 28 hours a week of television, we could possibly cure obesity if we all casually pedaled stationary bikes during our viewing time (and of course regulated our insulin production by eating Primally)!

Make Your Hard Workouts Harder

Focus on intense strength training and sprint sessions, ensuring that you are well rested and fully recovered between efforts. Remember, it's not frequency of your intense workouts that matters as much as quality. When you exercise a muscle to short-term exhaustion at 12 reps or deliver a max effort for 10 pull-ups, you'd be surprised what your body can do two minutes later if you repeat the effort. If you think you've pushed it to the limit at your typical 25-minute intense workout, take a 5-minute water break and then go back out there for another 8 minutes of high intensity. If you pat yourself on the back after your typical eight sprints, rest five minutes and go back and do a couple more!

Chill Out and Break Through

I cannot emphasize strongly enough how important it is for you to reject the Conventional Wisdom mind-set toward weight loss that obsesses on daily calories burned, strictly controlled portion sizes, and other anal-retentive nonsense. If you are hungry, eat (the right stuff). If you are motivated, exercise (the right way). And if you are tired, rest! When you are dragging, your energy is going toward rebuilding broken-down muscles and energy systems. Pushing a fatigued body through exercise will only lead to depletion, burnout, and undesirable sugar cravings.

> *If you are hungry, eat (the right stuff).*
> *If you are motivated, exercise (the right way).*
> *And if you are tired, rest!*

The key to the exercise component of weight loss is in expertly balancing stress and rest to allow for peak efforts to be reached in conjunction with adequate recovery and rebuilding. With athletes I advise, I call these peak efforts *Breakthrough Workouts*—sessions that are difficult and challenging enough to help you "break through" to a higher fitness level (or, in our context here, stimulate a reduction in body fat).

Whether you want to reduce your 10k time or drop 10 pounds, it comes down to directing optimal gene expression, primarily through diet, and secondarily through an effective workout plan with occasional Breakthrough sessions. From our understanding of the selection pressures of evolution, it's clear that taking fat off is more difficult than packing it on. Only by harnessing your energy with careful attention to stress management and the occasional bouts of brief, very intense, good old-fashioned hard work can you expect something different than the "same ol' same ol'": scale numbers, clothing sizes, race times, and so forth.

Shhh! Sisson's Six-Pack Secrets

"How to have washboard abs on a high-fat diet, no cardio, and no ab exercises" was the title of one of my most popular MarksDailyApple.com posts. In the weeks after the post, my shirtless photo accompanying the article was "tagged" and spread all over Facebook, necessitating a crash course on the amazing technology of social networking in order to protect my name and likeness!

While a "six-pack" is the universal hallmark of a lean, fit, well-toned man or woman, getting there following Conventional Wisdom protocol (grueling crunches and sit-ups to the point of nausea, burning endless calories on a treadmill, and then obsessively limiting what you take in) is too daunting to be a realistic goal for all but the most devoted (and least employed) gym rats. The truth is, we all have washboard abs…underneath whatever fat might currently be obscuring them.

I'm willing to bet many times the price of this book that you can bring to the surface impressive ripples you never knew existed (or at least haven't seen since your college intramural days) by hitting the sweet spot with your carb intake and naturally engaging your abs throughout daily life. In fact, washboard abs can be considered an effortless side effect of living Primally.

Grok had to have a great set of abs in order to be an effective thrower, climber, runner, jumper, crawler, and lifter. Not that abs themselves lift, throw, catch, or push—but the whole complex of abdominals (rectus and transverse abdominis, internal and external obliques, and pyrimidalis) provides the foundation for nearly every athletic and everyday movement you do. Thus, they are part of today's popular "core" training—the ultimate functional muscle group. Consequently, the best way to work your abs is to involve them in almost every other movement you do—every time you do it.

When you do push-ups, tighten your abs (pressing the navel toward the spine); the same is recommended during pull-ups, squats, lunges, curls, and other complete body exercises. Raking leaves, carrying your toddler, reloading the bottom drawer of the copy machine, lugging groceries out of the trunk and onto the kitchen counter, and infinite other daily activities—including simply sitting at your desk or in your car—can all be considered opportunities for a mini ab workout. I bet I did more than a thousand of these efforts sitting at my desk writing this book!

When you are engaged in basic movement, sitting or walking, you should tighten your belly as if you are going to be punched in the gut while blowing out the candles on your birthday cake. Hold it for 10, 20, or more seconds a few times every hour. Now do it while slightly tilted to one side. Repeat for the other side. For even better results and a stronger core, you can also simultaneously contract your buttock muscles. After a while, it will become second nature to squeeze your abs spontaneously. Engage your abs, eat right, and in no time you'll be sporting that six-pack!

Suggested Exercise Week Schedule

Walk, walk, walk. Hike, hike, hike. Move, move, move. This might seem like strange advice to help you get lean and ripped like our primal friend Grok. However, by now you should have a clear understanding of why ill-advised frequent moderate- to high-intensity workouts simply burn glucose and increase appetite and that your exercise program on the whole is only dealing with the 20-percent slice of the weight-loss pie. After all, walking around the block or hiking up to the water tower doesn't burn enough calories to contribute notably to weight loss. However, increasing your daily movement will build you from the inside out—toning muscles, joints, and connective tissue to enable you to thrive on the high-intensity workouts that strongly influence body composition.

Coupled with Primal Blueprint eating habits, your active lifestyle will refine your fat-burning skills so that you become an efficient fat-burning machine around the clock and easily reach your ideal weight in a matter of weeks or months, as seen with the Korgs' case studies. Best of all, as you scan the suggested daily meal plan (earlier in this chapter) and the weekly exercise plan (next), you'll see that it's easy to eat and exercise in a Primal manner for the rest of your life. Here's a sample of what Kelly and Ken did to "go Primal" with their workouts:

Sunday: Two-hour hike at low intensity. (The Korgs can do this together and get quality time as well.)

Monday: Easy 45-minute spin on stationary bike and 15-minute walk after dinner.

Tuesday: Thirty-minute intense strength-training session. Go for an 8 to 10 effort on a 10 scale. Try the, simple, functional, bodyweight resistance exercises I call the Primal Essential Movements (pull-ups, pushups, squats, and planks). These are described in the Bonus Material section at the end of this book. Further details are available at MarksDailyApple.com in the free download eBook, *Primal Blueprint Fitness*, as well as *The Primal Blueprint 21-Day Total Body Transformation*. Fifteen-minute walk after dinner.

Wednesday: Rest.

Thursday: Easy 45-minute stationary bike ride or hike.

Friday: Sprint session at grass field, school track, or even the beach. You can also sprint indoors on a treadmill, elliptical, or stationary bicycle. Duration, including warm-up and cool-down, is about 30 minutes. Choose from the recommended sessions based on ability level in the Bonus Material.

Saturday: Ten-minute intense strength-training session. Go for a 6 to 7 effort on a 10 scale.

Exercise Week Analysis

Total Duration: Around five hours—most of it comfortable cardio.
Total Calories Burned: Who cares! Enough to accelerate fat reduction and get in shape without suffering.
Muscle Groups Exercised: Arms, legs, core, and everything in between or attached.
Total Scenery Enjoyed: A ton more than someone on a treadmill or an elliptical or in a Spinning class.
Total Fun Had: Lots!

What a far cry from Kelly Korg's exhausting regimen of predawn high-intensity workouts, mundane malnutrition shakes replacing real meals, and the resulting fatigue, energy-level swings, and sugar cravings! Kelly, on the Primal Blueprint plan, could wake up leisurely with the rest of the family and enjoy herself with comfortable exercise sessions (possibly including some of her less than optimally active family members?). Instead of suffering several mornings a week, she could pick a few key opportunities with high-intensity Breakthrough Workouts that leave her exhilarated and accelerate her fat reduction. In six months' time, she'll have shed some 24 pounds of body fat and likely have added a few pounds of well-placed, lean, toned muscle tissue. She'll be happier and more energetic and she'll look better than she has in decades, with less effort and less struggle than before.

Meanwhile, Kelly's neighbor Wendy (remember her, the peppy network marketing enthusiast who dropped eight pounds in two weeks?) will almost assuredly weigh the same or more than she did when she started her cleansing diet six months prior. Furthermore, because 99 percent of network marketing participants lose money (from a survey of the largest and most reputed network marketing operations—after considering all expenses and inventory purchased from the company for resale), she'll probably have a lot of cleansing diet kits gathering dust on the garage shelves.

I.F. You Want to Lose *Even More Fat,* Try It!

As we reflect on the tidy examples of Ken and Kelly Korg nailing their daily caloric deficits with delicious, fulfilling meals, I must stress once again the concept of averages and expanding your timeline for measured progress out from a day or week to at least a month-by-month view. The meal diaries for Ken and Kelly obviously represent a good—make that perfect—day. In real life, your ability to optimize your meal choices and caloric intake will be more difficult than the examples (based on some of my own favorite meals) printed here. I realize there will be days, and even longer periods, when you slip away from ideal.

However, you can get back on track and even make up ground easily because of the metabolic leverage you create with Primal Blueprint eating habits. When your insulin production is moderated and your fat metabolism is optimized, you have a greatly reduced need to snack or even eat regular meals. As you'll see from my 72-hour personal journal sidebar in the next chapter, my own day-to-day caloric intake frequently varies by 250 percent or more! I didn't even realize this until I completed the journals and evaluations for this book.

When your body has reprogrammed gene expression to be able to get energy from fat whenever it wants, hunger tends to subside and blood sugar and energy levels stabilize. Why not tap into this new "skill" and take full advantage? You can not only easily make up lost ground when you slip a little, but you also accelerate the process of fat reduction to virtually whatever speed you want (up to the maximum mentioned previously) by engaging in a classic Primal strategy called Intermittent Fasting (I.F.).

Your choices of just when and how to practice I.F. should fit with your personality, lifestyle schedule, and unique habits and preferences. Both meticulous planners and spontaneous types can succeed with these varying styles. I suggest trying a mixture of unplanned meal skipping combined with structured fasts of 12 to 24 hours, or even longer for devoted and experienced fasters. There are few rules or strict guidelines to follow with I.F. Most readers will be well-served to simply break free of their habituation (does that sound nicer than "addiction"?) to regimented mealtimes and other cultural traditions, such as always having dessert after dinner, eating until you are stuffed, or freaking out if you skip a meal.

Numerous studies show that I.F. offers a multitude of benefits, including lowered blood pressure, improved insulin sensitivity and glucose uptake, loss of body fat (obviously), a decrease in oxidative damage, and even a kick-start for tissue repair. I fast when I feel a disturbance in immune function, such as a sore throat or stuffy head, and feel that my recovery is quicker. These benefits are achieved when certain genes are "turned on" to repair specific tissues that would not otherwise be repaired in times of surplus. One could surmise that this genetic adaptation allows certain cells to live longer (as repaired cells) during famine because it's energetically less expensive to repair a cell than to divide and create a new one. That might help explain some of the phenomenal longevity results produced by studies on animals eating restricted-calorie diets. With mice, longevity continues to improve as calories are restricted by 10 percent, 20 percent, and even 50 percent of normal.

Animal studies have shown that I.F. reduces spontaneous cancers, which could be due to a decrease in oxidative damage or an increase in immune response. Pockets of research around the globe strongly suggest that deregulated meal timing and generally moderated caloric intake produce many health benefits (particularly for those who are overweight) and promote longevity with virtually no negative side effects. How about that for an alternative to the zillion-dollar pharmaceutical and agricultural industries?

Whatever method of caloric restriction you engage in, the net effect is to send signals to your genes to up-regulate fat burning and down-regulate glucose burning, as well as to turbocharge your body's calorie processing system. It's a similar dynamic to that invigorating feeling you get from a splash in cold water, an afternoon nap, or an intense workout. Your body likes to be stimulated and challenged with these natural, positive stressors that fine-tune gene expression and numerous other functions and evolutionary skills. In contrast, your body rebels and weakens from *artificial* stressors such as jet travel, working long hours indoors, pushing through a long, uncomfortable cardio workout, or eating till you are full three times a day for your entire life. Here is a quick overview of some ways you can achieve I.F.:

Skipping Meals: Listen carefully and you may discover that you're not always hungry when your regular mealtimes come around. On these occasions, delay or skip meals until you experience actual hunger sensations. You will learn to appreciate food even more when you use it to truly nourish and energize yourself, instead of habitually shoving stuff down the pipe just because it's six o'clock or because everyone else is partaking at the alumni mixer.

Condensed Eating Window: Eat all of your meals within a set period of four to seven hours. This allows for a sustained fasting period (when you factor in sleep time) until the next day.

Early and Late: Enjoy an early morning meal and a late afternoon/early evening meal. This is a good option for people who have stressful jobs or otherwise have difficulty carving out a relaxed time period for lunch in the middle of the day.

Planned Fast: Enjoy dinner and then fast until the following evening (24 hours), or continue to fast until the next morning (about 36 hours). Many have success doing this once weekly. You may want to start by trying it once a month and work up to more frequently. Regardless of what approach you use, be sure that you don't overeat when you do sit down to meals. After a skipped meal or fasting period, you will be especially attuned to your body's hunger signals and satisfaction levels when you resume eating. Overeating is a largely psychological response to the anxiety of altering a familiar routine. Expert fasters typically ease out of their fast with several sparse meals to gently reengage the digestive system.

By seamlessly integrating Intermittent Fasting into your Primal Blueprint eating routine, you will prove to your conscious brain that you can survive quite nicely without constantly needing food. This is easy to handle when you control insulin production with Primal Blueprint foods and really, really hard when you are entrenched in a typical American diet with lots of carbs and insulin highs and lows.

If you have tried fasting or skipping meals in the past but (as with Kelly Korg) concurrently ate a diet moderate to high in carbs, you can likely relate to becoming irritable and exhausted when you miss even a single meal. In my days as an endurance athlete, I burned so many calories and relied so heavily on carbohydrate to refill the glycogen stores I drained daily, I'd feel like I was on the verge of a hypoglycemic coma if I did so much as skip breakfast or otherwise failed to stuff my face several times a day. Now I marvel at how often I forget to eat—and the fact that doing so has no impact on my energy levels. That's the true power of shifting from being a sugar burner to becoming an efficient fat burner.

I cannot emphasize the magic of this transformation enough. Freeing yourself from an addiction to regular doses of energy from ingested calories is the essence of "going Primal." Experiencing these Primal "symptoms" yourself ("hey, I'm actually not hungry!") will recalibrate your entire belief system about food and meals. Or as one friend of mine commented about his dropping excess body fat by eating Primally and being more sporadic with his meals, "hey, regular meals are overrated!"

If you take a moment to reflect on the principles of evolution and homeostasis, it's clear how messed up our modern eating culture is. It should not be hard for humans to sustain daily energy levels and optimal body composition—we just make it hard by constantly pumping our bodies with foods that we are not adapted to eat. Eat Primally for 21 days to allow your genes to up-regulate fat-burning mechanisms and get used to moderated insulin levels, then start playing around with Intermittent Fasting. I promise that you will experience this epiphany: that you are eating the way evolution designed you to (perhaps for the first time since you were an infant) and that it is easy and fun and leads to incredible breakthroughs in the frustrating challenge of fat loss and long-term weight management.

Weight-Loss Troubleshooting

If you are making a sincere effort to drop body fat with the Primal Blueprint and are not satisfied with your results, here are some suggestions to alter your routine and issues to investigate further that might be tripping you up.

Get into the Sweet Spot and Stay There!

When you limit your carbs to 100 to 150 grams per day, you can pretty much maintain your weight and body composition indefinitely. You will probably even experience a gradual and sustained reduction of body fat if you come from eating a typical Western diet of double or triple that many carbs and carry a bit, or a lot, of excess fat.

However, if the fat is not coming off quickly enough after a month or two of Primal Blueprint efforts, the best remedy is to tighten up the reins even further with your carbohydrate intake and stay in the sweet spot for several weeks.

While you may experience difficulty adjusting to the severe reduction of dietary "staples" (e.g., grains and pleasure foods including sweetened beverages and snacks), your body will quickly adapt to an eating style that is aligned with your genes. Yes, I know, getting your carbs down to 50 to 100 grams a day is easier said than done. It is on this issue that many people get stuck in the mode of "trying" to cut back instead of making a firm commitment to modify their habitual intake of certain foods and replace them with ample servings of foods that are more nutritious and technically more satisfying to your body than your favorite carb treats. For what it's worth, some investigators believe Grok's average daily intake of carbs was as low as 80 grams per day for months on end—and he thrived on that!

Keep in mind that there are days when you will go well above 100 or even 150 grams, thanks to the reality of prevalent carb choices and cultural traditions that can entice you away from a strict Primal Blueprint eating style. It will require great discipline to maintain an average of 50 to 100 grams (remember, most of us are accustomed to throwing down 300 grams per day or even more), but you only have to do it for a short time—say a month or two—depending on your starting point and how ambitious your goals are. By "great discipline" I'm not talking about suffering with a cloud of anguish and guilt hanging over your head; it's more like "eat reasonably generous amounts of eggs, meat, chicken, fish, nuts, and seeds, plus all the vegetables you want and fruits (with a little bit of restraint and selectivity), and stay away from all grains and processed foods."

If you find yourself struggling to meet your weight-loss goals, I strongly recommend using an online food calculator to know exactly where you stand instead of guessing. I find the mere act of having to write down everything I eat for one or two days increases my awareness of dietary habits and provides an effective check and balance against idle grazing or overeating when awareness is low. Chart everything you eat for a few days and then enter the results at PaleoTrack.com or FitDay.com to get a truly accurate indication of where your carb intake is. Even today, with what I consider a pretty decent knowledge of the macronutrient content of many foods, I continue to be surprised at some of the results that the online calculators spit out.

Moderate Stress Levels

Body fat reduction simply doesn't work well when you are skimping on sleep, working too hard, or experiencing high levels of emotional and psychological stress. Scientific research is validating the connection between lack of sleep and hormone levels that hamper fat metabolism or increase appetite. To succeed long term with changing your body composition, you must have the time, energy, and patience to devote great attention and care to the topic. Rushing through meals or reaching for sweet foods when you are stressed is not aligned with the simple lifestyle of the Primal Blueprint.

While the insulin control and intense sprint sessions might be the sexier elements of the Primal Blueprint weight-loss plan, you should not discount the importance of the supporting lifestyle elements that can make or break your success. Getting enough sleep (including naps, which trigger positive hormone flow, balanced appetite, more energy for and faster recovery from exercise), sunshine (vitamin D enhances all cellular function, including fat metabolism), and play, and relaxing and using your brain will assist your weight-loss goals on many levels. It's time to start walking your talk, stop burning the candle at both ends, and make the right choices to allow your genes to express themselves optimally.

Adopt a Positive Mind-Set

I believe there is a bigger picture to observe that involves optimism, positive thoughts, and enjoyment of the process when you pursue body composition changes. The subject of body composition is laden with failure, deprivation, restriction, self-limiting beliefs ("I have the fat gene"), and superficial judgment from society. Here's a sampling of Shape magazine article teasers: "Top 10 Moves For a Tighter Tush," "Firm Your Trouble Spots," "Get Flat Abs By August 1st." It's critical to approach the subject with a positive attitude and an appreciation for the process. Your primary motivation must be to enjoy a higher quality of life and better health. The by-product of a change in body composition is not something to obsess about, measure, and judge as success or failure each day or each week, but instead to experience effortlessly as a consequence of lifestyle change driven by ideals higher than wanting to look good in a bikini for your summer vacation in Hawaii (although there is nothing wrong with that goal if it's within a healthy big picture context).

Accept Your Plateaus, Then Carry On—Primally

After a few months of progress, you often arrive at a frustrating point where the weight stops coming off, or you stop building muscle. That makes sense from an evolutionary perspective, because the body is so well-tuned to adapt to any situation. Even with carefully restricted carb intake, your body may react to a sustained period of fat loss by taking subtle actions to drift closer toward homeostasis. For example, genes could "down-regulate" insulin receptors and other metabolic systems in the interest of preserving fat—a crucial survival mechanism for millions of years. In many cases, this plateau is just an example of the body saying, "I like this new weight. It's easy to maintain, I have more energy all the time and I never get sick."

Accept that your genetically ideal weight might include a bit higher percentage of body fat than that of a magazine cover model, and that there is nothing wrong with that. You might decide that it's not really worth the additional effort and focus to go beyond your "healthy, energetic, comfortable weight" to your ultimate ripped weight. Accept that plateaus are going to happen and exercise a little patience. Weight loss does not happen in a linear manner—there are simply too many variables and homeostatic forces at work. When I say you can "average a pound or two a week" of fat loss, I'd like you to consider this statement with a four-month or six-month timeline attached. I know we are conditioned to a "what have you done for me lately" mentality, but we are dealing with lifestyle change here, not journal entries of happy faces or frowns each day based on your scale numbers or food calculator graphs and charts.

> *Your genetically ideal weight is where you are healthy, energetic, and comfortable—whether or not it lands you on a magazine cover.*

I guarantee that making some elementary Primal changes (eliminating grains from your diet to regulate your carb intake at below a 100 grams per day average; adjusting your exercise program to refrain from Chronic Cardio and adding some brief, intense sessions to the mix) will result in a certain amount of effortless weight loss. However, there are a range of outcomes based upon individual factors (compliance rate as discussed in Troubleshooting, life stress levels, and how long and how severely you have diverged from Primal Blueprint laws before embarking on this journey). A female might effortlessly go from 185 pounds to 152 pounds in six months. At which point, she might long to drop into the 140s and find the process a bit more difficult.

One of my favorite sayings—whether it has to do with business, fitness, or balancing the varied demands and responsibilities of daily life—is, "if it were easy, everyone would be doing it." There is a reason you don't see 80 percent of American adults sporting single-digit body fat or dozens of joggers flying by in the park at a pace of six minutes per mile. If you are unsatisfied with your results after months of devoted effort, refer to the Troubleshooting tips and consider making an increased commitment to achieve superior results. Rest assured that there are no mysteries involved here, or even much genetic "good luck" that we are so conditioned to believe is important. It's all up to you and how you can direct your genes to do the right thing.

Avoiding the Three Biggest Reasons for Failure

1. Lack of awareness and/or lack of commitment to actually moderate your carb intake to "Sweet Spot" levels. If it turns out from your online pie graph results that you have been a little loosey-goosey here and there, I promise you that even a few days of Primal-style low-carb eating will cause noticeable changes in your appetite and an increase in your energy level—and lead you on the path to the promised land. Start your day tomorrow with a Primal Omelet and notice how your inclination to snack in the hours afterward is eliminated. Keep the momentum going with a Primal Salad for lunch, followed by a meat and vegetable dinner, and you'll see how these (and many other) Primal Blueprint-approved meals leverage one another to get you off the carb/insulin/stress response/sugar-craving cycle and into round-the-clock fat burning.

2. Failure to stock up on Primal Blueprint-approved foods. Dropping from several hundred grams of carbs down to 80 essentially means you can eliminate the foods that once served as major energy sources (albeit very poor, quick-burning sources) throughout your day. If you have no "logs" around (filling, nutritious, long-burning food) and your flame is petering out, your reaction might naturally be to fan the flames with wads of newspaper (cheap carbs). Make absolutely sure that you stock your home, office, car, office, and backpack with Primal Blueprint-approved snacks, such as my favorites mentioned in the Chapter 4 sidebar. (The Primal Approved—At a Glance sidebar at the end of the book summarizes healthy eating choices and also what foods to avoid.) Reach for them any time you need an energy boost or feel a sugar craving coming on.

3. Lack of awareness/commitment to Primal Blueprint-style exercise program. Many exercisers are unaware of their working heart rates and the effect they have on metabolic rate and stress levels. Because the perceived exertion of aerobic exercise (75 percent or less of maximum heart rate) is extremely moderate, most exercisers (again, misguided by Conventional Wisdom) equate significant exertion—suffering—with getting in shape. Walk through the room of a typical Spinning or Step class or along the window lineup of cardio machines and note the suffering etched on the faces of the participants. Even America's devoted exercisers—a culturally elite anomaly in the world's fattest, most sedentary nation—are quite often burning sugar and tiring themselves out from their well-meaning efforts. Remember: exercise is about the movement, not the calories burned.

Chapter Summary

1. Primal Weight Loss: You can lose one to two pounds of body fat per week (one-half to one kilogram) by targeting optimal intake levels of each daily macronutrient, fasting intermittently, doing Primal Blueprint-style workouts, and approaching the challenge with a positive, process-oriented, big picture attitude.

2. Macronutrients: Adequate protein intake (0.7 to 1 gram per pound; or 1.5 to 2.2 grams per kg, of lean body mass, depending on activity level) will preserve muscle tissue (and metabolism) during calorie-restriction efforts, avoiding the "crash and burn" effect of most diets. Maintaining the "Sweet Spot" intake of 50 to 100 grams of carbohydrates per day will moderate insulin production and allow stored body fat to be your primary energy source. Fat intake will be the main variable to ensure you are satisfied and nourished at each meal, making your weight-loss efforts effective, realistic, and even enjoyable.

3. Korgs Weight Loss: Ken and Kelly Korg can achieve their ambitious fat-reduction goals by eating delicious, nutritious Primal Blueprint-style meals. When the carb intake sweet spot is observed and protein requirements are met, ample amounts of fat will provide a high satiety factor at meals but will not result in excess fat storage thanks to low insulin levels.

4. Exercise: Exercise can complement the main variable of optimal macronutrient intake to support and accelerate weight-loss success. Increase low-level activity, make hard workouts harder (and maybe even shorter, if you've been in a chronic pattern), and understand that the commitment to changing your body requires focus and dedication.

5. Intermittent Fasting: I.F., whether deliberate or as a natural course of fluctuating mealtimes (now that stored body fat instead of ingested carbs is your preferred energy source), will create natural caloric deficits that lead to fat reduction and effortless long-term maintenance of ideal body composition. You can engage in I.F. by skipping meals, eating in a condensed window of time, eating morning and night but not in between, or engaging in planned fasts lasting for 24 hours or more.

6. Troubleshooting: If your progress slows, try being more diligent in hitting the carb intake sweet spot (using an online nutrient calculator to know exactly where you stand), moderating your life stress levels (utilizing the Primal Blueprint lifestyle laws), adopting a positive mind-set, and realizing that plateaus in your progress rate are natural and acceptable, thanks to your body's innate desire for homeostasis.

CHAPTER 9

Conclusion

Time to Party like a Grok Star!

A person will sometimes devote all his life to the development of one part of his body; the wishbone.

—Robert Frost

A s we near the end of the book, I want to call attention to the special place in my heart that Chapter 2, "Grok and Korg," occupies. I've been fascinated by the "Primal" concept for nearly two decades. (I self-published my *Training and Racing Duathlons* book using the name Primal Urge Press in 1988!) As an athlete and a coach, I've reflected on the Primal theme constantly—inspiring athletes to balance the unnatural act of endurance training with proper recovery and lifestyle support and to temper our competitive human instincts with common sense to avoid burnout.

My work in the fields of nutrition and personal training and my immersion into the health community on the Internet have enlightened me about the realities of everyday modern life for the masses. While we are making progress in some ways, I am increasingly disturbed by the seemingly inexorable drift farther and farther away from natural, healthy, evolutionary behavior in the technological world.

As my staff and I worked through the stages of Chapter 2—conceptual, research, first draft, editing, soliciting external feedback, and revisions—I finally had the chance to print a fresh copy, sit on a lounge chair in my yard, and truly "read" the material for the first time. I have to admit I was downright horrified. I questioned whether people would think the commentary was sensational or unrealistic and be turned off accordingly. I returned to my computer, reviewed all the references, conducted more research, and generally made darn sure this was an accurate and realistic picture of modern life.

Unfortunately, the draft withstood my own devil's advocate scrutiny as well as that of numerous health, medical, nutrition, psychology, and sociology experts. Family and career men in their 40s and 50s take prescriptions left and right, families frequently feel that life is too hectic and stressful to align with the broad definition of health, and teenagers often feel overpressured and disconnected from parents. Today's kids have too much body fat and too little physical fitness. We eat too much beige stuff and not enough green stuff. We avoid exercise and sit at desks all day staring at a screen in the name of increased productivity. We go home at night and stare at a bigger screen in the name of relaxation. We stay up too late and then awaken to the stressful screech of an alarm clock. We are stressed by bills, traffic, air, noise, digital pollution, the past, the future, and all kinds of anxiety we manufacture in our restless minds. Our first line of defense when our genes react as they are programmed to by these lifestyle habits is prescription drugs, which treat symptoms quickly but, over time, weaken our natural ability to achieve homeostasis.

As we bombard our genes with these lifestyle risk factors, they respond the only way they know how in an often futile attempt to maintain homeostasis and a desperate effort to keep us alive in the short term—with inflammation, early cell death, insulin resistance, atrophy, and so on. If you consider the dietary habits, activity level, and body composition of your family above-average, you can congratulate yourself while remembering that "average" is actually borderline obese (64 percent of American adults are classified as overweight, of which one-third are classified as obese).

In California, 40 percent of 10-year-old schoolchildren fail to attain a bare minimum aerobic conditioning performance standard known as the *Healthy Fitness Zone* (established by the Cooper Aerobics Institute), meaning that hundreds of thousands of "average" kids in California (what I consider a progressive, fair-weather state with a population arguably fitter than that of the United States as a whole) are technically classified "at risk" to develop serious health problems related to inactivity, because they can't complete a mile run at a slow jog. *Forty percent!* Take a big fat zero off that figure and I think you'd approximate the relevant statistic during the time of my youth.

As we reflect on how far we have drifted from Grok's simple lifestyle and ponder how we can better honor and reprogram our genes by following the Primal Blueprint, it is critical to proceed with a clean slate and a deep conviction that you are doing the right thing. This is not an easy task. Numerous elements of the Primal Blueprint flat out oppose mainstream dogma that government espouses or that big Agra and big Pharma promote with billions of advertising and marketing dollars.

One must also wonder how society has strayed so egregiously far from the healthy living that Grok enjoyed and devolved to the carb-overdosed, pill-popping, overfed, overweight, overstressed Ken Korg. How can the Conventional Wisdom that you have believed for years and decades be wrong and even dangerous? The truth is, human nature is to blame. Just like Grok, we have programmed into our genes a desire to manipulate and rule our environment for our benefit—to pursue a more advanced, more comfortable life. Our indomitable human spirit has accomplished many great things but has also created tremendous fallout from our constant quest for "progress."

Man has conquered the world. As a species, he is the fat cat. He is on top of the heap. Yet now, peak physical and intellectual performance and self-discipline are no longer requirements for survival. Man has become self-indulgent and has reverted to behaviors that provide short-term gratification. Like the miners who stripped and poisoned the land and water during the gold rush, we have done similar damage to our bodies in the name of making life easier, more convenient, and more productive.

In Eric Schlosser's *Fast Food Nation*, he reveals how the fast-food phenomenon exploded in popularity because fast food made life easier: No more cooking or lengthy waits for expensive meals! Now everyone can live the good life by dining out on delicious food! Unfortunately, the fare served up was disastrous not only to the human body but also to the human spirit—destroying a centerpiece of family fabric that was the shared home-cooked meal.

When there is interest and demand to make life easier, profit seekers often swarm in and exploit this element of the human spirit. Nowhere is this more evident than in my own field of health. While I am all in favor of capitalism and making a profit, it seems that where health is concerned, we have allowed forces to run amok to the extent that today we must question the approach, motives, and trustworthiness of many of the traditional pillars of health, human compassion, and expert knowledge.

We must admit that doctors, despite their extensive knowledge, training, and loyalty to the Hippocratic Oath, are focused on treatment rather than prevention. As with drugs, it's wonderful to have extensively trained and prepared doctors standing ready when we need them. The sad reality is that most of their business comes from dealing with symptoms—not causes—of easily preventable conditions (as evidenced by the remarkable comment from a solo family practice doc I know, who lamented that his "business was down" due to the economic recession!). The fact that doctors receive little or no training in nutrition is nothing short of abysmal.

Our government's laws, subsidies, and diet education efforts (grain-based USDA food pyramid, anyone?) are seemingly driven more by lobbyists for the beef, grain, and dairy industries than by unbiased scientific evaluation and concern for human health. In the media, the historical checks and balances provided by the impartial investigative journalist have been deemphasized and devalued by giant ratings-driven corporations. Salacious stories that elicit fear, anger, or other strong emotions are what sell, regardless of their legitimacy. Even our educational community experiences free market influences that potentially bias the objectivity and even the premise of many studies.

The Korg Komeback!

Let me reiterate my distaste for a perfectionist mentality toward diet, physical appearance, lifestyle change, and even school, career, and competitive athletics. Respecting the broad definition of health and the legacy of the simple lifestyle that our ancestors lived, we need to reject the measuring and judging forces of society and pursue fun and peace of mind in conjunction with health and fitness goals.

Admittedly, your efforts to go Primal will possibly require some serious adjustments to your comfortable modern existence. If you feel overwhelmed or take occasional exception to my strong positions, keep in mind my 80 Percent Rule as well as the suggestion to take one step at a time.

While the Korgs seem quite far down a disastrous road, they can also quite easily turn things around, step by step, with minimal pain, suffering, negativity, or disruption of the things they love to do in life. If Ken modifies his late night activities by snacking on macadamia nuts instead of cheesecake; watching less television (TiVo anyone?) in favor of reading or a quick stroll around the block with the dog; and turning the lights out at 10:30 P.M. instead of midnight, he'll fall asleep more easily and wake up refreshed the next morning, without having to rely on Ambien. This means more quality time with the kids, including *walking* young Cindy to school.

If Ken brings the macadamias, some carrot sticks, and a couple slices of beef jerky for snacks at work, and chooses lunch wisely at the supermarket deli (one-third pound of sliced tri tip stuffed inside a red bell pepper costs less than Chinese buffet), he'll maintain stable energy levels all day long, increase his productivity, and better handle workplace stress. Ken will leave the office at 6 P.M. feeling ready to enjoy and appreciate the leisure and family time options that await.

If Kelly reduces the stress of her exercise program and eats delicious, satisfying Primal Blueprint meals, she will get her blood sugar and energy levels under control and tap into her stored body fat for a steady, reliable source of energy. With a few sensible and consistently enforced limits on digital entertainment and bedtimes, Kenny can reconnect with the family, focus better in school, and consider the option to eliminate his medication.

Talk about little things making a big difference! There is no better example to illustrate this maxim than the momentum (particularly the unbridled increase in physical energy) created by healthy lifestyle changes begetting further healthy lifestyle changes.

On Your Own

Opening our eyes to the direction the bullet train carrying modern society is heading is sobering to say the least. In my opinion, the heaviest realization of all is that you are *on your own*. The imagined safety net of government, modern medicine, or the food or pharmaceutical industries looking after your health is a facade. Oh sure, you'll be cared for very, very well if something catastrophic happens (that is, if you have good medical insurance), whether it's a high-risk childbirth, serious injuries from a car accident, or one of the small fraction of cancers that are not lifestyle related. But when it comes to eating healthy, getting in shape, avoiding stupid mistakes—even building a career and a nest egg—the world can lead you astray and separate you from your cash (and other assets, such as health, sanity, etc.) in the blink of an eye.

A discernable pattern emerges when I relate the story of Grok to friends and casual acquaintances. After first expressing disbelief that Grok was leaner, stronger, and healthier than modern humans, most are captivated by the story of his uncomplicated life and the 10 surprisingly simple behavioral laws that dictated his (our) evolution. After a few moments of silence to absorb the information, people then commonly call attention to the most unpleasant aspects of Grok's life reactions ("Yeah, but didn't cavemen, like, die when they were like 30 years old—before they could even get heart disease?"), a surreptitious way of asserting their superiority over some vulnerable, primitive caveman.

It seems we are scared of what's beyond our comfort zone of comfort foods, Conventional Wisdom, typical exercise routines, and the prospect of wasting time with unstructured play. We have a tendency to get in our own way, manufacturing self-limiting beliefs and knee-jerk defense mechanisms when confronted with our frailties or the prospects of lifestyle change.

The Elitist Race

I read with amusement the occasional critiques of the Primal Blueprint eating style as being "elitist"—too expensive (eschewing inexpensive grains and switching from commercial animals and plants to the pasture-raised or organic variety) and impractical for the average person to follow. Furthermore, astute observers point out that there are not enough local, pasture-raised animal products or produce to sustain our society at its current population. My gut reaction is, "you're damn straight it's an elitist diet!" Expensive? Depends on your perspective. Eating Primal Blueprint style for the rest of your life is much cheaper than long-term prescription drug regimens or extensive doctor visits or hospital stays for cardiac bypass surgery or cancer treatments.

The evolutionary theme pops into mind here. Our increasingly sedate and sedentary modern life disguises the fact that the concept of survival of the fittest still permeates our being. Competition is everywhere in the world, with human nature programmed for "*Citius, Altius, Fortius*"—the Olympic Games motto (in Latin) meaning "faster, higher, stronger." Make no mistake, we are in a competition to achieve good health and prosperity with a massive number of entrants worldwide. Economically, you need only glance through Fareed Zakaria's *The Post American World*, to see the writing on the wall for the world's leading superpower. America is heading steadily down the pop charts while larger, hungrier, more strategically minded societies, such as China and India, will soon catch and surpass our economy. Poor investment in education and technology in favor of billions spent on military are some key reasons for our impending downfall, according to Zakaria. Imagine if all the money recently spent on bank bailouts had been channeled into diet, fitness, and health education!

> ❝*When it comes to eating right and exercising, there is no "I'll start tomorrow." Tomorrow is disease.*❞
> **—V. L. Allineare**

Over the past century of rapid technological progress, we've figured out how to manufacture and package food and mass-produce animals, producing huge profits without regard to the health, humane, or green consequences. Stepping back for a moment to grab a wide-angle view of the wide angles in the buffet line at a Vegas casino, it's evident how ridiculously out of control this situation has become. No offense, but America looks like one giant yard of fattened cattle ready for slaughter, complete with a significant percentage of "downers" (a term for sick cattle that can't stand up; they are dragged with giant hooks to slaughter).

In comparison, being "elitist" doesn't seem bad at all. Theoretically, if everyone wanted wild salmon and organic strawberries, we would indeed run out in the short term (however, demand would also stimulate increased production, thereby changing the world one person at a time through the power of our wallets). Right now, the race is on and you are welcome to participate. So suck it up and pop for the pasture-raised animal products at the farmer's market and organic leafy greens, especially if you are pregnant or have a two-year-old in his most crucial brain development stage. Come to think of it, make that especially if you are not pregnant; are age 20, 30, 40, or 50; and have an interest in enjoying a long, healthy, happy life.

> *I put a dollar in one of those change machines. Nothing changed.*
> - **George Carlin**

Around the World (or at Least to Dallas and Back) in 72 Hours

I'm often asked to reveal my lifestyle "secrets" to interested MarksDailyApple.com readers. The truth is, I'm short on secrets but big on guidelines and practical tips that will help you successfully navigate the particulars of your daily life, including the innumerable challenges to being Primal that we face in the modern world. That said, I hope my real-life experiences give you some perspective that I'm a regular guy trying to raise a family, make a living, achieve peak health and fitness levels, forage Primal foods in a modern world, and, most of all, enjoy the heck out of my life.

The exercise of keeping an accurate journal for 72 hours to produce this sidebar helped me realize that even the times when I slip from ideal are no big deal. When "stuff happens" to take you off track, it's a great opportunity to develop your "go with the flow" skills, staying positive and relaxed instead of stressed. Consider the following example from my Tuesday journal. My son Kyle called me, begging for a ride to the valley for a social opportunity while I was en route to the gym for a precious final workout before a business trip. My 30 minutes of captive teen audience time in the car was a far more precious experience than yet another workout.

When I was driving home after dropping Kyle off, I realized that the concept of hormone manipulation supersedes the need to cover all your bases on food choices and workout goals every single day. When you direct insulin, glucagon, cortisol, testosterone, growth hormone, and other agents in the correct pathways by following the Primal Blueprint, you can easily handle the unexpected because you have built a healthy, efficient foundation.

I follow the Primal Blueprint lifestyle laws naturally, thanks to family, friends, a lifelong appreciation of the outdoors, a stimulating career, and a positive attitude—one that I've worked hard to cultivate over the years. Here then are my journal entries for a three-day stretch from January 2009, featuring a business trip to Dallas bookended by typical weekdays at home in Malibu.

Tuesday—Travel Day

6:30 A.M.: Wake up and drink large cup of strong coffee with heavy whipping cream. Read paper (almost finish *LA Times* crossword puzzle—Law #10, natch!). Move to desk and answer e-mails, blog, and pack for afternoon flight to Dallas.

10:15 A.M.: Down protein shake (36 grams protein and 20 grams net carbs). Head to the gym for quick workout.

10:30 A.M.: En route to gym, son Kyle calls my cell, begging for a ride to the valley (gotta love winter break!). Return home, pick up Kyle.

11:30 A.M.: Return from valley trip with no time for workout or lunch. Depart for LAX and 3:00 P.M. flight to Dallas. Can you say, "Been there, done that?" I've flown this route 150+ times in the last 10 years. Destination: a suburban television studio (I've never once been to downtown Dallas; I hear it's nice) to tape regular appearances on my friend Doug Kaufmann's show—Know the Cause—a nationally distributed daily cable talk show on health and nutrition.

8:00 P.M.: (6:00 P.M. PST): Check into hotel, enjoy leisurely dinner at Outback Steakhouse (flank steak with asparagus and red wine—hold the potato). Time change contributes to late bedtime of 11:30 P.M.

Elapsed time stuck in metal boxes today = about six hours (counting drive to and from valley, to airport—featuring traffic jam on Pacific Coast Hwy—shuttle bus rides, and three-hour flight).

Tuesday Macronutrient Calculations

Coffee, heavy whipping cream
Protein shake (1.5 servings of
  Responsibly Slim protein powder)
Apple
Flank steak (6 ounces),
  asparagus, red wine

FitDay.com Analysis
Total Calories: 774
Protein: 88 grams, 352 calories
  (41 percent)
Carbs: 56 grams, 224 calories
  (24 percent)
Fat: 22 grams, 198 calories (22 percent)

Wednesday—Dallas Day

7:00 A.M.: Conduct short, intense Primal routine (one-minute rest between exercises): 3 × 60 pushups, 3 × 35 squats, 3 × 25 abbreviated dips between armchair and coffee table, 3 × 60-second abs planks. Elapsed time from first effort to stepping in the shower: 17 minutes.

8:00 A.M.: Breakfast of four-egg chile-chicken omelet at IHOP. Extra sour cream and Cholula hot sauce. Try as they might (and they try hard), they still can't get me to take the pancakes (or toast or English muffin) that come free with the order. Coffee with cream and packet of sugar.

9:00 A.M.: Arrive at studio for four to five hours of taping. Drink a couple bottles of water—the most water I drink all week!—to keep my vocal chords lubed.

2:30 P.M.: Late lunch with the production team. All the ribs you can eat (which isn't all that much) and iced tea at a local rib joint. I'd prefer a salad bar, but this is where the crew wants to eat and we are in Texas...who am I to say no? Skip the mashed potatoes, potato salad, corn, cornbread, applesauce, and bug juice, thus relieving my system of well over 200 grams of carbs in one fell swoop.

4:00 P.M.-5:00 P.M.: Walk the Irving Mall (low-level aerobic activity) and make phone calls the whole time. Head to airport.

6:00 P.M.: Dinner at TGI Friday's (in the terminal)—pecan crusted chicken salad and a glass of cabernet. One of my favorite travel meals. Board plane, fly home.

Wednesday Macronutrient Calculations

Coffee with cream and packet
of sugar
Four-egg chile-chicken
omelet at IHOP, extra sour
cream and Cholula hot sauce
Ribs (6 ounces) and iced tea
Pecan crusted chicken salad
and a glass of cabernet

FitDay.com Analysis
Total Calories: 2,087
Protein: 153 grams, 612 calories
(29 percent)
Carbs: 92 grams, 368 calories
(17 percent)
Fat: 123 grams, 1,107 calories
(50 percent)

Note: this was a long day of hard work, but even with the three sit-down meals, I ate fewer calories than I normally do. I often use traveling as a great opportunity to engage in Intermittent Fasting. Because the food options on the road are generally inferior or difficult to find, I hone my foraging skills and look for nothing but protein and vegetables.

Thursday—Malibu Day

7:30 A.M.: Wake up and shake off the effects of jet lag with a quick plunge in the pool (I'd estimate mid-60s temp) and a coffee with cream. Head to desk to catch up.

10:00 A.M.: Down four-egg omelet with sprinkled mozzarella cheese, sliced mushrooms, and green peppers, topped with sliced avocado and a scoop of fresh salsa. Back to desk.

11:00 A.M.: Head to gym for a "pull and sprint day."
- Four sets of cable rows starting at 20 reps at 100 pounds and adding 10 pounds per set
- 10 × 10-15 reps of wide-grip pull-ups with as little rest as possible (maybe a minute in between)
- 4 × 15 inverted rows (sort of an inverted pull-up)
- Three sets of two-arm cable curls while in squat

Jog to car, drive to beach to catch low tide. Three-minute plyometric warm-up drill followed by 10 barefoot sprint sets (each consisting of jog 10 complete strides, transition to run 12 complete strides, transition to sprint 15 strides all-out), one minute rest between. Easy jog to cool down, followed by brief "Grok squat" stretch. Gym and beach total time: 50 minutes. Head home and shower.

1:00 P.M.: Make my world-famous Primal Big Ass Salad (check video at MarksDailyApple.com) with tons of veggies and a scoop of canned salmon, drenched in olive oil-based dressing. Nothing to drink. Granny Smith apple for dessert. Back to work in the office.

4:00 P.M.: Big handful of almonds and break from desk to throw tennis ball to a very old, very slow yellow lab named Buddha. En route back to desk, a challenge is issued by Kyle. Detour from office to garage for a battle royale championship match on Wii Rock Band. Obtain perfect score of 100 on Rock Band vocals to reign supreme in Sisson family (PB Law #7, Play…and kinda sorta Law #9, Avoid Stupid Mistakes!).

7:30 P.M.: Grass-fed steak (10 ounces), three cups of steamed broccoli dripping in real butter, glass of merlot. Okay, one more. Doesn't get any better than that!

8:30 P.M.: TiVo replay of our favorite 30-minute sitcom, followed by 60-minute ESPN SportsCenter broadcast. Watch both broadcasts in only 52 minutes total.

10:00 P.M.: Five-minute outdoor walk with Buddha, retire to bed for some pleasure reading. Lights out, and out like a light, at 10:30 P.M.

Thursday Macronutrient Calculations

Coffee with cream
Four-egg omelet with
    sprinkled mozzarella cheese,
    sliced mushrooms, and green
    peppers, topped with sliced
    avocado and a scoop of fresh salsa
Primal Big Ass Salad
Granny Smith apple
Big handful of almonds
Grass-fed steak (10 ounces),
    three cups of steamed broccoli
    dripping in real butter
Two glasses of merlot

FitDay.com Analysis
Total Calories: 2,676
Protein: 168 grams, 672 calories
    (25 percent)
Carbs: 108 grams, 432 calories
    (15 percent)
Fat: 170 grams, 1,530 calories
    (57 percent)

Averages Over Three Days
(allow for rounding margin of error)

Calories: 1,842
Protein: 136 grams, 544 calories (38 percent)
Carbs: 86 grams, 344 calories (18.5 percent)
Fat: 106 grams, 954 calories (51 percent)

Rethinking Your Goals

You may have noticed by now that I emphasize a long-term approach and the enjoyment of the process of healthy lifestyle change. In discussing weight loss, I take great pains to position this eventuality as a *byproduct* of healthy eating, exercise, and lifestyle habits. We must reflect on the importance of this distinction because we are so conditioned to approaching lifestyle goals with a short-term, results-oriented approach.

We wear heart rate monitors and use GPS technology to provide objective data about whether we are reaching our goals—or failing. We use fancy training logs to record every possible bit of information about our workouts: time, distance, strength-training reps, calories burned—even "shoe mileage!" (to determine when to buy a new pair). We strain, struggle, and suffer to obtain predetermined times, paces, and distances of our workouts, thinking that our bodies and spirits will actually appreciate a robotic approach to fitness.

Consider for a moment the possibility that setting and pursuing goals is screwing us up more than it's helping. We live in a superficial world where everything we do is measured and judged, and success (and often happiness) is thus defined by what we accomplish and accumulate, rather than what kind of character we have. For athletes, the world hits us with, "how far did you run?" "what was your time?" "what place did you take in the race?" "did you beat your previous time or your opponent?" All these interrogations typically come before the more relevant questions we should ask ourselves about a workout or race: How about, "did you have fun?" Or, when my son and his volleyball team lose a competition and thereby admit it wasn't much fun, I might ask, "was it a positive experience? Did you learn and grow as a team, as an athlete and as a person through a hard-fought battle—even though it ended in defeat?"

My fervent desire to achieve my athletic goals—run in the Olympic trials, average 100-mile weeks, beat my training partners—ruined my physical health and ended my running career. When I returned to competition as a triathlete, I had a more relaxed, light-hearted attitude. I enjoyed the challenge of a new sport and pushing the limits of human endurance, just for the heck of it. Gun-shy from my injury history, I adopted a more relaxed approach. I listened to the signals from my body and backed off when energy levels declined or aches and pains crept up. I enjoyed longer, slower bike rides into the mountains, connecting with nature and enjoying a sense of adventure in exploring new routes. I built my fitness in a comfortable manner and felt refreshed, energized, and inspired about my training—a far cry from the out-and-out suffering I endured from recurring intense running sessions with a fit pack of training partners.

Lo and behold, with my casual approach I became the fourth fastest Hawaii Ironman triathlete in the world one year, avoided injuries, and had a great time. After retiring from professional racing and pursuing a "real" career, I continued competing just for kicks on the amateur level, well into my late 30s. I had no goals, structured training program or logbook. I was just having fun, inspiring my personal training clients, and mixing with the professional athletes that I coached at the time, but enjoyed by my standards excellent results—with less effort. Often I would see the "game faces" worn by others (amateurs as I now was, mind you)—tense, anxious, snapping at their loved ones, looking like they weren't having much fun or experiencing much personal growth.

It's simply no fun to predicate your happiness on whether you reach your goals. Failing to reach your goals will lead to disappointment and dwindling motivation levels. Even reaching your goals can lead to a dead end and a flawed mentality. Many "winners"—in sports or other competitive arenas, such as business—develop a distorted sense of self-worth, leaving them vulnerable to up-and-coming opponents or negligent in behaving themselves in ordinary society because of our twisted hero-worship of winners and the wealthy.

There is a phenomenon in endurance sports known as the *post-marathon blues* (or post-ironman blues for triathletes)—so common that it's been discussed in psychological journals. It seems on the occasion of the glorious achievement for which they've trained diligently for months or even years, many athletes get that "now what?" feeling that leads to a profound sense of letdown. Ideally, we would use our physical accomplishments as catalysts for continued growth (including moving on to less extreme fitness pursuits perhaps!), exploration, and challenge, not an excuse to get depressed and pig out on jelly beans in the weeks after the big event.

We must take a close look at the goal-setting process to avoid these common pitfalls and bring a relaxed, fun-first approach to our diet, fitness, body composition, career, and other lifestyle pursuits. The primary reason for switching to a Primal Blueprint eating style should be enjoyment—eat foods that taste great, stabilize your energy levels, optimize the function of all the systems in your body, provide long-lasting satisfaction, and alleviate the psychological stress of regimentation and deprivation that accompany many diets. Yes, you will look better, become stronger, have more energy, avoid illness, disease, and obesity, and enjoy other quantifiable results, but these motivators pale in comparison to the instant gratification you get at every single meal from eating the foods that your body was meant to eat.

If you have any psychological stress about your diet, reject it flat out and start eating foods and meals that make you happy, drawing upon the long list of foods and minimal logistical restrictions of the Primal Blueprint eating style. Do whatever you need to do to enjoy your life, including indulging once in a while with a clear conscience and a big smile. If you are not having fun with your current workout regimen, junk it and figure out other endeavors that turn you on. Instead of struggling and suffering to keep pace (with your peppy group exercise instructor or your training partners), adopt the Primal Blueprint suggestions to make your sustained workouts comfortable and energizing so they become fun again. Throw in some exhilarating fast activities occasionally to get you excited about pushing your physical limits and enjoying tangible breakthroughs including weight loss, more energy, and peak performance. Play once in a while. Forget the notion of consistency in this context and align your exercise program comfortably with your energy level, mood, and life responsibilities. Push yourself when you are rested and motivated and rest when you are tired.

Once you discard unnecessary goals that are mentally and emotionally stressful, you can focus your attention on process-oriented goals. Goals such as having fun, aligning workout choices with energy levels, and tackling new endeavors should define your exercise mentality. That said, great champions have an esteemed ability to blend a process-oriented approach with a strong competitive drive to achieve measurable results. It's certainly okay to aspire to specific results (e.g., losing 10 pounds or completing a 10k, marathon, or triathlon), but you must never lose sight of the concept that the rewards come from the chase, not from reaching the finish line.

You can lose 10 pounds very quickly via any number of ill-advised methods. The true joy from changing your physique comes not from a surgeon's knife, a brutal calorie-restriction diet coupled with an exhaustive workout routine, nor even accolades from the cocktail party crowd. The most lasting rewards come from the positive, fun lifestyle changes you implement to make it happen.

It is time for you to accept the grand purpose of the Primal Blueprint and reject other motivators that are confusing, petty, or contradictory to your health and well-being. To get more connected with the ideal represented by

Grok, we have to pare down, not accumulate. The power and the magic are in the simplicity—a refreshing break from the complexity of modern life, the sordid influence of ego on your endeavors and emotional state, and the pop culture messages that can easily make you feel like a loser if you aren't as tight as the beautiful person on the magazine cover.

Grok did not traffic in any of this nonsense. Granted, he was preoccupied with survival, and we surely don't need to regress to that point to enlighten our mentalities. What we can do is leverage the Primal Blueprint laws in our daily lives to become healthier, fitter, happier, and more connected with our basic nature as human beings. Make it your goal to honor your genes and your destiny to make the most of your life on earth, without attachment to any outcome.

What are you waiting for? Let's get Primal!!

Primal Approved— At a Glance

Diet

Beverages: Water (in moderation according to thirst), unsweetened tea.

Coconut Products: Butter, flakes, flour, milk, and oil offer healthful medium-chain fats; great substitute for dairy, PUFA, and wheat flour.

Coffee: Enjoy in moderation (cream and minimal sweetener okay), don't use as energy crutch.

Dairy: Raw, fermented, high-fat, and organic products are preferred (cheese, cottage cheese, cream cheese, kefir, whole milk, yogurt) in moderation.

Eggs: Local, pasture-raised, or certified organic for high omega-3 content.

Fats & Oils: Coconut, dark-roasted sesame, first press, extra-virgin, domestically grown olive, hi-oleic sunflower/safflower, marine (supplements), palm, and high omega-3 oils (borage, cod liver, krill, salmon, sunflower seed). Refrigerate and use quickly. Animal fats (chicken fat, lard, tallow), butter, and coconut oil are best for cooking.

Fish: Wild-caught from remote, pollution-free waters. Small, oily, cold water fish best (anchovies, herring, mackerel, salmon, sardines). Certain farmed fish are approved (domestic coho salmon, trout, and shellfish).

Fruit: Locally grown (or wild), organic, in-season preferred. Berries are premier choice. Go strictly organic with soft, edible skins. Moderate intake with higher glycemic/lower antioxidant values and dried fruit. Wash thoroughly.

Herbs & Spices: High-antioxidant, anti-inflammatory, immune-supporting, flavor-enhancing.

Indulgences: Dark chocolate (75 percent-plus cacao content) and red wine are best choices. Be sensible and moderate!

Macadamia Nuts: High monounsaturated, favorable O6:O3 ratio.

Meat & Fowl: Local, pasture-raised, or UDSA-certified organic critical. If you must eat conventional meat, choose the leanest possible cuts and trim excess fat to minimize toxin exposure.

Other Nuts, Seeds, and Their Derivative Butters: Cold-processed, organic if available. Refrigerate and use quickly.

Snacks: Berries, canned tuna or sardines, celery with cream cheese or macadamia nut butter, cottage cheese with nut or fruit topping, hard-boiled eggs, jerky, nuts, olives, seeds, trail mix, and other high-fat and/or high-protein, low-carb primal foods.

Supplemental Carbs: Heavy calorie burners without excess body fat looking to restock muscle glycogen can enjoy sweet potatoes and yams (instead of white or brown potatoes), quinoa, and wild rice (instead of brown or white rice).

Supplements: Multivitamin/mineral/antioxidant formula, omega-3 fish oil capsules, probiotics, protein powder, and vitamin D are great modern hacks.

Vegetables: Locally grown, organic, in-season preferred. Go strictly organic for large surface area (leafy greens) and soft, edible skins. Wash thoroughly.

Exercise

Low-Level Cardio: Two to five hours (or more) per week of walking, hiking or other low level cardio at 55-75 percent of max heart rate.

Schedule: Vary workout type, frequency, intensity, and duration, always aligned with energy levels. Be spontaneous, intuitive, and playful!

Shoes: Gradually introduce some "barefoot" time for low-risk activities to strengthen feet and simulate natural range of motion. Choose shoes with minimalist design (Vibram FiveFingers, Nike Free) to prevent cuts and other injuries. Ease into it!

Sprinting: All-out efforts lasting 8-20 seconds, every 7-10 days when fully energized. Regular, less strenuous "wind sprint" sessions for conditioning.

Strength Training: Brief, intense sessions of 30 minutes or less. Full-body, functional exercises that promote broad athletic competency.

Stretching: Minimal, full-body, functional stretches to transition from active to inactive: Grok Hang and Grok Squat.

Lifestyle/Medical Care

Medical: Rx drugs for acute conditions; aggressive lifestyle modifications before drugs! Order additional blood tests (CRP, Lp2A, A1C, fasting blood insulin) to assess disease risks.

Play: Change attitude—it's not just for kids! Enjoy daily, outdoor physical fun! Enhances work productivity and stress management.

Sleep: Minimize artificial light and digital stimulation after dark, consistent bed and wake times, calm transitions into and out of sleep. Awaken naturally without alarm. Nap when necessary.

Stupid Mistakes: Cultivate hypervigilance and risk management skills, avoid multitasking and overly stressful or regimented lifestyle practices. Focus on peak performance!

Sunlight: Fear not the mighty orb! Expose large skin surface areas as long and often as possible without burning.

Use Your Brain: Engage in fun, creative intellectual pursuits to stay sharp and enthusiastic for all of life's challenges.

Primal Avoid—
At a Glance

Diet

Baking Ingredients: Corn meal, starch, and syrup; other starches and syrups; flours; powders (gluten, maltodextrin, milk); sweeteners (dextrose, fructose, lactose, malitol, xylitol); yeast.

Beverages: Bottled, fresh-squeezed, or refrigerated juices (Odwalla, OJ, Ocean Spray, etc.); "energy drinks" (Red Bull, Rock Star, Monster, etc.); almond, rice, soy, and other flavored "milks"; powdered drink mixes (chai, coffee, or hot chocolate flavored); soft drinks and diet soft drinks; sports performance drinks (Gatorade, Vitamin Water); sweetened cocktails (daiquiri, eggnog, margarita); sweetened teas (Snapple, Arizona).

Coffee: Avoid excessive use or as energy crutch in place of adequate sleep and healthy lifestyle habits.

Condiments/Cooking Items: Honey mustard; jams and jellies; ketchup; mayonnaise and lite mayonnaise spreads; low-fat salad dressing; and anything containing high fructose corn syrup; other products made with sugary sweeteners and/or PUFA oils.

Dairy: Limit or avoid conventional and GMO milk products due to hormone, pesticide, antibiotic, allergenic, and immune-suppressing agents. Avoid ice cream, non-fat/low-fat milk, processed (American) cheese and cheese spreads, and sweetened low-fat/non-fat/frozen yogurt.

Eggs: Limit mass-produced eggs (fed with grains, hormones, pesticides, and antibiotics). Find local, pastured eggs at farmer's market!

Fast Food: Avoid chemically treated, deep fried, insulin-stimulating, devoid of nutritional value fare: French fries, onion rings, deep fried foods, burgers, hot dogs, chimichangas, chalupas, chorizos, and the rest of the industrialized fare we are inundated with daily.

Fish: Avoid most fish from farms (especially imports), polluted waters, objectionable catch methods, or from top of food chain (shark, sword, etc.— concentrated contaminants).

Fruit: Limit or avoid GMO, remote grown, or conventionally grown with soft, edible skins. Stick with local, in-season, high-antioxidant fruit (berries, stone fruits), especially if you are trying to reduce body fat.

Grains: Avoid cereal, corn, pasta, rice, and wheat; bread and flour products (baguettes, crackers, croissants, Danishes, donuts, graham crackers, muffins, pizza, pretzels, rolls, saltine crackers, swirls, tortillas, Triscuits, Wheat Thins; breakfast foods (Cream of Wheat, dried cereal, French toast, granola, grits, oatmeal, pancakes, waffles); chips (corn, potato, tortilla); cooking grains (amaranth, barley, bulgur, couscous, millet, rye); pretzels; puffed snacks (Cheetos, Goldfish, Pirates Booty, popcorn, rice cakes), and all other baked or processed high-carb foods. Even avoid whole grains due to higher levels of objectionable phytates, lectins, and gluten.

Indulgences: Avoid high-carbohydrate (sugar or flour-based), heavily processed treats: cookies, cake, pie, brownies, candy, candy bars, ice cream, donuts, popsicles, and other frozen desserts.

Legumes: Alfalfa, beans, peanuts, peanut butter, peas, lentils, soybeans, and tofu. Less objectionable than grains, but still contain anti-nutrients. Consider them supplemental carbs—unnecessary and possibly counterproductive to health and weight management.

Meat & Fowl: Limit or avoid commercially grown, grain-fed ranch animals (with concentrated hormones, pesticides, and antibiotics). Limit or avoid pre-packaged processed products (breakfast sausage, dinner roasts, lunch meats); smoked, cured, or nitrate or nitrite-treated meats (bologna, ham, hot dogs, jerky, pepperoni, salami).

Oils: Avoid trans and partially hydrogenated, all PUFA (canola, etc.) buttery spreads and sprays; margarine, vegetable shortening, and deep fried foods.

Processed Foods: Energy bars; fruit bars and rolls; granola bars; protein bars; frozen breakfast, dinner, and dessert products; and packaged, grain/sugar-laden snack products. If it's in a box, package, or wrapper, think twice!

Sweets: Brownies; candy; candy bars; cake; chocolate syrup; cookies; donuts; ice cream; milk chocolate; milk chocolate chips; pie; sugar/sweeteners (agave, artificial sweeteners, brown sugar, cane sugar, evaporated cane juice, HFCS, honey, molasses, powdered sugar, raw sugar, table sugar); sugar/chocolate coated nuts and trails mixes; popsicles and other frozen desserts; syrups; and other packaged/processed sweets and treats. The less you consume, the less you'll want!

Supplements: Avoid cheap, bulk-produced supplements with additives, fillers, binders, lubricants, extruding agents, and other synthetic chemicals.

Vegetables: Limit or avoid GMO, remote grown, or conventionally grown with large surface areas or edible skins (leafy greens, peppers).

Exercise

Chronic Cardio: Avoid a consistent schedule of sustained cardio workouts at medium-to-difficult intensity (above 75 percent of max heart rate).

Schedule: Avoid consistent application of stress with insufficient rest (compromises health, energy, and motivation levels). Consistency is *not* key when it comes to fitness!

Stretching: Avoid static, isolated muscle group stretches of "cold" muscles in favor of simple, brief, dynamic stretches.

(continued)

Primal Avoid— At a Glance

(continued)

Medical/Lifestyle

Medical: Limit or avoid prescription medication for lifestyle-related health problems. Reframe "fix it" mentality into a "prevention" mentality.

Sleep: Don't burn the candle at both ends. Avoid excessive evening digital stimulation, morning alarms after insufficient sleep, or fighting off a much-needed nap with caffeine.

Stupid Mistakes: Avoid multitasking, zoning out, or trusting that the world will keep you safe. Don't blame others for your stupid mistakes.

Bonus Material

Primal Blueprint Common Stumbling Blocks and Quick Tips

We've analyzed hundreds of threads and thousands of posts on the MarksDailyApple.com forum and have come up with this list of most common challenges. Next to each concept is a quick tip that might help your effort and prompt you to refer to the book over time for additional guidance.

Breakfast ideas: Omelet or other egg dish, smoothie, and more flexibility to eat whatever you want or skip breakfast when your fat-burning genes are fine-tuned.

Budget issues: Look at the big picture and prioritize expenses. Your budget impact might actually be reduced by getting rid of processed carbs and sweetened beverages and hitting your local farmer's market.

Dealing with non-Primals (spouses, kids, etc.): Set an example through action, not talking. Refrain from arguing the particulars with resistant folks and let your results and your energetic disposition speak for themselves.

Dining out: Be assertive and request menu flexibility to piece together suitable meals, centered around animal protein. You can stay Primal-aligned at most any restaurant by making some careful choices and requests.

Eliminating Chronic Cardio: Balancing stress and rest is the key to fitness progress! Adopt an intuitive approach to exercise in favor of compulsively logging miles or reps in the name of "consistency."

Finding good snacks: Review list of my favorites on page 134. Discover your own favorites from the extremely broad list of Primal-aligned options.

Getting enough fat: Inadequate fat intake is likely influenced by decades of cultural programming to minimize intake of all fats, despite the health benefits of many. Eat as much fat as you desire to enjoy meals and achieve satiety.

Getting enough sleep: Implement the sleeping tips detailed in Chapter 7, and in the Primal Blueprint hacks that follow, with particular attention to a calm, quiet, dark final two hours before bedtime.

Giving up diet soda: Artificial sweeteners confuse the brain's appetite center, triggering sugar cravings and even insulin surges. Try flavoring carbonated water with a generous squeeze of lemon and a bit of salt to get your carbonation fix.

Giving up grains: Face it—grains are bland-tasting. It's the stuff you put on grains that makes them taste good! Reframe your perspective about what you really need and reject rigid SAD traditions. Eggs for dinner? Steak for breakfast? Knock yourself out!

How to engage in Intermittent Fasting: The best bet for novices is to eat dinner, then delay breakfast the following morning until hunger sensations are compelling. See how long you can comfortably last without food, then enjoy a delicious Primal-approved meal. Check your progress each month, as your ability to regulate energy without ingested calories provides a good indication of how well your genes have been programmed to be a fat-burning beast.

Lack of quick/easy food: Advance planning is important, since the modern world will not provide very well for your Primal needs on the go. Create a stash of easily transportable Primal snacks (jerky, apples, macadamia nuts) so you can always have ready-to-go options available.

Learning to cook: Start with simple recipes, build your confidence, and get ever more creative over time. Check out *Primal Blueprint Quick and Easy Meals* for a simple, fun, non-intimidating way to get into a Primal groove in the kitchen. Keep your kitchen well-stocked to make things easy.

Listening to body: Cultivate an intuitive approach to eating, exercise, sleep and other Primal behaviors. This means you must reject external influences (superficial cultural messages, peer pressure, judgmental family and friends), and answer to yourself first and foremost.

Listening to hunger signals: Eat when you're hungry, finish when you're satisfied. Give yourself permission to eat whatever you want, whenever you want, as much as you want (within Primal guidelines of course) to achieve dietary satisfaction and promote health. Slow down your eating pace to really tune in!

Managing expectations: Focus on the intrinsic value of living Primally, and don't attach your happiness or self-esteem to the results. Take what your body gives you each day (energy, motivation, health, etc.) and never force results on an unnatural time schedule. Trust that the immediate sensations you experience from promoting optimal gene expression (more energy, regulated appetite, hormone, and immune function) will translate into long-term results with body composition and other peak performance goals.

Managing stress: Minimize insulin production, eliminate chronic exercise, and align sleep habits with circadian rhythm. Build momentum with these three big ones, and let further lifestyle refinements fall into place.

Overthinking things: Some passionate Primal folks actually go overboard and become inflexible and anxious about their adherence to Primal guidelines. This type of mentality, however well-intentioned, can compromise mental and even physical health. Accept that there is a range of potential outcomes—from magazine cover model to ordinary but extremely healthy. Don't get bogged down with details when you are honoring the most important big picture principles of Primal living.

Packing lunch/preparing meals: Cook large portions ahead of time, then refrigerate or freeze to have quick access to great meals on the go. Chop and store veggies to facilitate quick salad preparation. Portion out barbeque or crock pot meat dishes for quick reheating.

Playing more: Schedule a grand outing and involve others. Get involved with kids—the world's foremost experts on play. If you're really out of practice, start small with a five-minute break from work or a quick stop at the park on the way home.

Reading food labels: Should you really be reading labels?! Emphasize plant and animal foods and minimize consumption of wrapped, packaged, canned, and frozen foods. That said, make avoiding refined carbs and chemically-altered fats a priority when you read labels.

Resisting temptations: Why resist? Reject the struggle-and-suffer mentality and enjoy life! An occasional well-chosen treat is absolutely Primal-approved. Honor the 80 Percent Rule and don't stress about perfection or obsess about resisting temptations. Go with the flow and calmly return to your center if you happen to get thrown off track.

Scheduling meals: What for?! You will enjoy more flexibility with your schedule, shopping, and planning as you become more fat-adapted. The need to fuel with unfavorable options just because your body needs some calories will quickly diminish as you become expert at burning stored body fat.

Sourcing Primal ingredients: Backyard garden or rented urban plot, farmer's markets, Co-ops, specialty grocers, or Internet if you live in a Primal-challenged area.

Supplements: The best categories to supplement a healthy diet in stressful modern life are: multivitamin/antioxidant, omega-3 fish oil, probiotic, high-protein meal replacement, and vitamin D for the sunlight challenged.

Sweet tooth: High cacao-content dark chocolate (75 percent or above) is a Primal-approved treat that will satisfy your sweet tooth and provide an antioxidant boost.

Variety in diet: The Primal guidelines afford tremendous variety in food choices. However, there is no rule that says you must eat a broad variety of foods. Personally, I'm a creature of habit and enjoy repeating my favorite Primal-approved meals frequently. If you're inclined to experiment and shake things up, go ahead and enjoy yourself!

Working out consistently: Consistency is overrated! Focus on balancing stress and rest intuitively. Take what your body gives you each day instead of blindly following a regimented workout pattern. Don't ever feel guilty for skipping a workout!

Working out motivation: People who can't get or stay motivated to exercise generally view it as painful and overly stressful. Do workouts that are fun and make you happy. Head out the door for a hike, haul off a few PEM exercises on a whim, or sleep in 'till brunch if your body wants you to. Don't worry about burning a certain number of calories or following a certain pace; build momentum naturally with workouts that are fun and enjoyable.

Primal Blueprint Hacks

Law #1: Eat Plants and Animals: Transforming your dietary habits is not easy, even for the most disciplined among us. The pull of comfort foods, cultural forces misaligned with health and balance, and our innate resistance to change must be skillfully negotiated. The Five Favorite Meals strategy can help keep you focused and satisfied as you leave your old dietary habits in the dust. Find Primal breakfast, lunch, and dinner meals, and convenient snacks that you really love and use these as a foundation for going Primal. There are probably a dozen distinct omelet variations you can create from the starting point of cracking eggs into a mixing bowl.

While my eating habits vary wildly from day to day (see pages 278-281 for a 72-hour journal), I'd say my entire diet revolves around a mid-day Big Ass Salad that I make on many days of the week. Some days I'll hit it around noon, having skipped breakfast or had a quick morning shake. Other days I'll enjoy it in the late afternoon, providing such satisfaction and nourishment that dinner essentially becomes optional.

If you're fond of macadamia nuts, prepare some baggies for your desk, briefcase, car, or home, and make them your go-to afternoon snack. Building productive and easy to implement habits such as centerpiece meals or Primal snack stashes should mitigate the chances of backsliding into quick-energy sweetened beverages or power bars when hunger strikes.

Summary

1. Make Primal eating simple and convenient by establishing some go-to breakfast, lunch, and dinner meals, and favorite snacks. Cycle through your five favorites as you build momentum going Primal. Always keep Primal-approved snacks around!

Law #2: Avoid Poisonous Things: Out of sight, out of mind. What better hack to implement here than to simply avoid exposing yourself to health-compromising foods? This is particularly true when it comes to the struggle to wean children away from cultural traditions into a somewhat Primal eating pattern. Establish firm guidelines for what is allowed in your home and don't deviate from it. If the T-ball team wins the championship and all are compelled to celebrate with hot fudge sundaes, your kid should go ahead and enjoy life to the fullest. This is different from stocking caramel sauce, chocolate syrup, and vanilla ice cream in your home for daily doses.

If you find yourself in the midst of tempting foods and are compelled to indulge, do so with a clear conscience and a total focus on the enjoyment that your treat provides. Often, when you reject the silly mind games of guilt and rebellion, you'll discover that those few moments of gustatory pleasure experienced when the treat hits your taste buds are simply not worth the long-term negative consequences of digestive distress or acting in a manner incongruent with your big picture life goals.

Summary

1. Keep offensive foods out of your home and stay away from junk food establishments.
2. If you must indulge, do so with a clear conscience and total focus on the pleasure and satisfaction it provides. With taboos eliminated, you may realize that it's not really worth it, and that Primal-approved substitutes can provide similar satisfaction.

Law #3: Move Frequently at a Slow Pace: Own this idea about aerobic exercise: it's not about the calories; *it's about the movement*. If you are a cardio enthusiast, slowing down your workouts will promote fitness more than a chronic pattern of workouts that compromises hormone, immune, and metabolic function. Apply your impressive levels of discipline and motivation not only to getting out the door and putting in the hours, but to backing off when you know you really should. You won't get fat if you include more rest days and recovery sessions in your schedule, I promise! Remember, 80 percent of your body composition success is influenced by diet, and 100 percent of your fitness progress is influenced by common sense.

If you aren't the type to be found in a Spinning class or crossing the finish line in your town's 10k road run, focus on taking incremental measures to accumulate more total movement in everyday life. Contrary to what certain fitness pundits might spout, those 30-second hops up three flights of stairs, five-minute walks around your corporate campus, and 15-minute strolls through the neighborhood with the dog definitely add up. You really can become aerobically fit without having a gym membership or a fancy spandex outfit. Just get out and move!

So many people get stuck here because we've been conditioned to believe that there is no intermediate category between couch potato and aerobics queen. Tomorrow, hack into your daily lifestyle routine and discover five ways that you can replace mechanized or sedentary habits with physical movement.

Once in a while, go for an extended outing such as a hike that is paced comfortably enough such that you'll actually enjoy it and look forward to doing it again. If you're nature-averse, make your hike of the urban variety. You can even arrange a one-way journey to a fun destination such as a farmer's market and get a ride back home.

Summary:
1. Slow down cardio workouts to avoid falling into a chronic pattern.
2. Take incremental steps to increase overall daily movement—work breaks, errands, evening strolls, etc. Even a five-minute walk or ascending a few flights of stairs builds habits that support a more active lifestyle.
3. Get out for extended outings once in a while and enjoy nature or urban adventures.

Law #4: Lift Heavy Things: Again, let's make things simple so there are no excuses or hurdles to making law #4 a fun, comfortable, and consistent part of your lifestyle. The fitness/gym/bodybuilding scene is so laden with hype, complexity, intimidation, and "broscience" (you know, science dispensed by bodybuilding bros) that even looking at a dumbbell or strapping into a spaceship-style strength-training contraption at the gym can be completely unappealing to all but the most fervent enthusiasts.

Hear this in counter-argument to the broscience that says you need "muscle confusion," workout days cross-referenced against specific body parts, or multimillion dollar, 30,000 square foot venues and top dollar personal trainers to develop an impressive physique: *you can get extremely fit in just two intense workouts a week, lasting no more than 30 minutes.* No equipment is necessary (except perhaps a pull-up bar) and you use nothing more than your own bodyweight for resistance.

The Primal Essential Movements (PEMs) are four simple, safe, full-body functional exercises that can be done anywhere—backyard, park, or even a cramped motel room. These four exercises—pushups, pull-ups, squats, and planks—work the entire body in a functional manner to develop broad athletic competency. The PEMs are scalable to all levels of fitness through a series of progression exercises that are easier than the baseline essential movement. For example, chair-assisted pull-ups or knee pushups will allow a novice to simulate the resistance and muscle recruitment of the PEM while doing an appropriate number of repetitions to build full-body strength.

Strive to complete one full-length PEM session and one abbreviated PEM session each week, on days when energy, motivation, and immune function are strong. A full-length session involves two or more sets of maximum repetitions of each of the four Primal Essential Movements. An abbreviated PEM workout involves a single set of maximum repetitions in each exercise. Start with two to five minutes of easy cardiovascular exercise before you commence your PEM exercises. After each exercise, take a 30-60-second break to get your breathing rate back to near normal. A full-length PEM should take less than 30 minutes to complete, while an abbreviated PEM should take less than 15 minutes.

Summary:

1. Keep it simple with the PEM: pushups, pull-ups, squat, and plank. Use the progression exercises appropriate for your fitness level to achieve an appropriate number of reps.
2. Strive to conduct one full-length PEM (two to three sets of max reps for each PEM) and one abbreviated PEM (one set, max reps for each PEM) per week.

Law #5: Sprint Once in a While: If you are a fitness novice or otherwise intimidated about sprinting, try a few preparatory sessions where you simulate a sprint workout at 75 percent of maximum intensity. Known as "strides" or "wind sprints" in running parlance, you complete a series of efforts of the same duration and rest interval as recommended for a sprint workout, but at significantly less than maximum effort. Whether you are on an exercise bike or actually running, these sessions will prepare your muscles and nervous system for eventual workouts at maximum effort.

Almost everyone can eventually enjoy the optimal gene expression benefits of all-out sprinting when you conduct prep sessions at incremental intensities from 75 percent on up to eventually 100 percent, and utilize low- or no-impact exercises if running carries a high injury risk for you.

Summary:

1. Sprint once every 7-10 days when 100 percent rested and motivated.
2. To prepare for the strenuous nature of sprinting, conduct lower intensity "strides" or "wind sprints" and choose low- or no-impact options.
3. Refer to the forthcoming Sprint Workouts Suggestions for details.

Law #6: Get Adequate Sleep: As soon as it gets dark, minimize artificial light in your home by using bare minimum lamps and overhead lighting, switching out a few key lights to yellow bulbs or donning yellow or orange lens sunglasses. The tinted bulbs and lenses allow plenty of light in, but do not disrupt the production of the sleep hormone melatonin in the manner that white light bulbs and digital screens do.

Melatonin production has been triggered by darkness for two million years, so when you blast your eyeballs with digital stimulation from Netflix or YouTube, cortisol levels can spike and carbohydrate cravings can occur, leading to sleep deprivation and excess body fat storage. Mellow things out after dark by choosing relaxing endeavors such as reading, strolling, talking, and board games instead of digital entertainment. Create an ideal sleeping environment: simple, quiet, as dark as possible, clutter-free, cool (65°F seems to be the preferred sleeping temp), and used exclusively for sleeping.

When you implement calm, relaxing evenings, you set yourself up for success on the other end: waking up naturally, without an alarm, feeling refreshed and energized. Even if you're convinced that you're not a morning person, exposing yourself to direct sunlight as soon as possible after awakening will help elevate serotonin and suppress melatonin, kicking your body into high energy mode for a busy day.

Summary

1. Minimize light: Minimal indoor lighting and yellow bulbs or lenses after dark.
2. Install f.lux: Visit stereopsis.com and download a free program called f.lux for your computer. F.lux alters the "color temperature" of your computer screen to align with ambient light—easier on the eyes after dark.
3. Minimize digital stimulation: Especially in the final two hours, choose reading, conversation, board games, or neighborhood strolls instead of going from screen to bed.
4. Bedroom: Get rid of all clutter and maintain a simple, stress-free environment. Get blackout curtains and keep the temperature around 65°F.
5. Blindfold: A handy resource for napping and eliminating potential light distractions during your evening sleep period.
6. Napping: Whenever you fall behind on sleep, a 20-30 minute nap can help rejuvenate energy and brain function extremely well.

7. Morning: Awaken naturally, close to sunrise, and expose to direct sunlight ASAP.

Law #7: Play: Let's hack this in two ways: taking a few mini-play breaks throughout the day lasting 5-15 minutes and scheduling grand play outings once in a while that involve exciting new adventures with family and friends. There are few rules or restrictions to mini play breaks, except to let go of inhibitions and cultural pressure that discourage anything out of the ordinary. Don't be afraid to get strange looks from co-workers when you start playing waste-basket hoops or attempt to juggle some tennis balls in the office courtyard. Don't let the hectic pace of modern life stand in your way here—start modestly if you must with a five-minute endeavor. Once you become comfortable departing from your daily routine, you may experience bursts of creativity. When in doubt, hang around kids and you'll be playing in no time.

For your grand outing, take a few moments to jot down a wish list of adventures you and your loved ones might like to try. Rank them in order of priority, being realistic with your time and budget. Then, take a couple of initial steps today toward making it happen—schedule your rock climbing lessons, grab a hiking map from the state park Web site and plot out a route, or rent or purchase necessary gear. Plan the big day and stay accountable by involving others and getting a firm handle on logistics so the adventure is not too daunting when the time comes.

Law #8: Get Adequate Sunlight: For maximum vitamin D production, expose large surface areas of your skin (arms, legs, torso) to direct sun for about *half the amount of time you think it takes to get slightly burned*. This is a highly individual estimate based on time of year and day, skin pigment, latitude, reflectiveness of the ground surface, and other variables. Nevertheless, guesstimating the halfway mark is a pretty low-risk endeavor, so make a strong effort to expose as much skin as possible to direct sunlight during the months of the year when the sun's rays are sufficient to manufacture vitamin D (year-round in the tropics; around eight months in the Continental USA). Take vitamin D supplements during the winter months, particularly if you have climate, pigment, or lifestyle challenges to obtaining adequate sunlight during the summertime. Even a sincere effort to obtain sufficient vitamin D from diet will fall well short. Get some sun!

To mitigate skin cancer concerns or reduce the cosmetic appearance of aging, cover frequently exposed, sensitive skin areas (face, neck, hands) with clothing or sunscreen—they contribute minimally to vitamin D production anyway.

Summary
1. Expose large skin surface areas to direct sunlight during strong sunlight months for half of "burning time."
2. Cover face, neck, and hands to prevent long-term overexposure.
3. Supplement with vitamin D during winter months if necessary.

Law #9: Avoid Stupid Mistakes: Reject the concept of multitasking as a big fat lie. The human brain is literally incapable of multitasking. Instead, we divert our attention quickly back and forth between stimuli, making us more stressed, less focused, and more likely to make mistakes. We need little reminder that texting and driving is foolish, but when you cut other corners while juggling your hectic daily schedule, bad things can happen. Is talking on a hands-free cell phone while driving cool? Many don't think twice about this, but your brain is significantly less focused on the road, and thus you are less safe, when you're blabbing on the phone.

Cultivate hypervigilance and risk management skills by taking nothing for granted—not even a quick ride through town to the supermarket. Your own and other's lives are in your hands each time you get behind the wheel; do you *really* need to have a conversation at the same time? Focusing on a single task at a time throughout your day—even if some or many of them are mundane—will give you the discipline and resolve to stay focused when the stakes escalate, such as every time you turn the key and hit the road.

Summary
1. Multitasking is literally impossible for the human brain. Concentrate on a single task at a time to increase productivity and reduce stress.
2. Cultivate hypervigilance and risk management skills by taking nothing for granted. Respecting the importance of even mundane tasks will hone your focusing skills and minimize mental stress from attempts to multitask.

Law #10: Use Your Brain: Engage in creative intellectual pursuits that counter the grind of daily responsibilities. Give yourself permission to have fun once in a while, or more often than that, knowing that creative brain use will enhance your performance in your core areas of responsibility and economic contribution.

Get the most out of your brain by strictly filtering and editing the excessive amount of stimulation you are exposed to in daily life and taking frequent breaks away from tasks of intent focus to refresh brain function.

Summary

1. Find creative intellectual pursuits to balance the daily grind: music, language, crosswords, Sudoku, model airplanes, fantasy sports leagues, or whatever else interests you.
2. Find ways to stimulate and challenge your brain throughout the day: adding up numbers in your head or remembering names of acquaintances.
3. Treat your brain kindly: take frequent breaks to refresh focus and avoid burnout.

Primal Essential Movements

To experienced gym goers, this routine of the most basic movements might seem a little bland. However, if all you ever do is pushups, pull-ups, squats, and planks you can still become as rock solid as the guys and gals in the Bowflex commercials. Retired football legend, Heisman Trophy winner, and Olympic bobsledder Herschel Walker (who was once traded by the Dallas Cowboys to the Minnesota Vikings for—counting eventual draft picks—a total of *19* other players!), reportedly never touched weights, instead relying on pushups (with his wife riding on his back—captured by a memorable *Sports Illustrated* photo) and 2,000 sit ups per day to develop his massive—and extremely functional—physique.

Begin your strength-training sessions with a two- to five-minute warm-up of low-intensity cardiovascular exercise (walking, jogging, stationary cycling, or other cardio machine at 55-75 percent of maximum heart rate). You should break a light sweat, indicating elevated body temperature and breathing rate. Conclude each workout with a two- to five-minute cool down to allow sufficient time to return your breathing rate to normal. Be certain that you have medical clearance before attempting any strenuous workout, including those described in the Primal Blueprint. If you don't have a proper overhead bar for pull-ups, improvise using railings, stairwells, door frames, park playgrounds, tree branches—anything that can support your weight.

Next to each exercise are levels of "mastery" for males and females. The mastery levels represent one set of maximum effort. Your first PEM workout should be an assessment session to determine, by trial and error, your maximum effort level for each essential movement. If you can't complete the mastery number of reps for a particular Essential Movement, drop down to the appropriate progression exercise to enable a sufficient number of repetitions to be completed at your workout. As you improve to achieve mastery level with your progression exercise, bump up to the next progression exercise or the baseline movement. Advanced strength trainers can integrate numerous adaptations to increase the degree of difficult beyond the baseline Essential Movements, including donning a weighted vest for the entire PEM session.

Males – Primal Essential Movement mastery
- 50 Pushups
- 12 Pull-ups (overhand grip)
- 50 Squats (thighs parallel to ground)
- Plank: 2 minutes holding the Forearm/Feet Plank position

Females – Essential Movement mastery
- 20 Pushups
- 5 Pull-ups (overhand grip)
- 50 Squats (thighs parallel to ground)
- Plank: 2 minutes holding Forearm/Feet Plank position

Pushups (lats, pecs, triceps). Mastery = Male 50, Female 20: Assume pushup plank position (arms extended below you, hands forward, body straight). Lower to ground—chest touching first! Keep body dead straight, core and glutes tight, head and neck neutral to torso. Elbows bend backwards at 45-degree angle as you lower.

Easiest Progression – Knee Pushup (M50, F30): Do pushups starting from a plank position on your knees.

Next Progression – Bench Pushup (M50, F25): Do pushups with hands resting on a bench or other object elevated from ground.

Pull-ups (back, lats, pecs, biceps). Mastery = Male 12, Female 5: Grasp bar (or tree branch) at shoulder width with overhanded grip. Elbows tight, chin tucked, shoulder blades retracted to protect spine. Lead with chest up, keeping lower body quiet. Raise your chin over the bar and gradually lower all the way until your arms are straight (or just before straight if you have joint issues).

> **Easiest Progression – Chair-Assisted Pull-up** (M20, F15): Start with your leg loosely positioned on a support chair underneath the bar. Engage your upper body muscles and raise yourself up to the bar. Use just enough leg force to assist getting your chin over the bar. You probably only need to use one leg, but can use two if necessary. Yes, *everyone* can do pull-ups!

> **Next Progression – Chin-Up** (M7, F4): Many find the chin-up to be slightly easier than a pull-up, particularly if you have wrist, elbow, or shoulder issues. Simply invert your grip on the bar so your palms face you and raise yourself until your chin is over the bar.

Squats (lower body). Mastery = Male 50, Female 50: Feet shoulder-width or slightly wider apart. Toes forward or naturally pointed outward slightly. Lower yourself by extending your butt out and bringing thighs to just below parallel to the ground. Try to maintain a straight spine (it will travel from a 90-degree to a 45-degree angle), but resist the urge to lean forward. Use your quads to absorb the load both sitting and standing. Go down in a smooth and steady movement until your thighs are about parallel to the floor. Return to a standing position without locking your knees, making sure your knees track in line with your feet.

> **Easiest Progression – Assisted Squat** (M50, F50): Hold pole or other support object while lowering into and raising up from squat position. Use support object as little as possible.

Planks (core and lower back, as well as shoulders, triceps, hip flexors). Mastery = Male 2 minutes, Female 2 minutes: Hold pushup plank position while resting your elbows on the ground. Maintain position until failure. An optional movement to stimulate the oblique abs is to lean on one extended arm and rotate body into sideways plank position, preserving a straight line from your head to toe. Hold until failure, and then repeat on other side.

Easiest Progression – Forearm/Knee Plank (M 2 minutes, F 2 minutes): Assume plank position with forearms and knees resting on ground. Tense core and glutes during exercise.

Next Progression – Hand/Feet Plank (M 2 minutes, F 2 minutes): Assume plank position a la pushup starting point, with extended hands and feet on ground.

PEM Isolation: For a unique challenge, set an ambitious numerical goal for a single PEM and make that your entire workout one day. Perform reps until failure, then rest as needed and tackle additional reps, counting your accumulated total to reach your goal. For example, some mornings I'll aspire to do 200 decline pushups. These might accumulate in sets as follows: 60, 30, 50, 25, 25, and 15. I might do half the sets in 10 minutes, then get sidetracked for 20 minutes before I finish off the last several sets.

PEM Sprint Workout: This is a fun session that's over with quickly and integrates strength training and sprinting. It's a great challenge to all of your muscle groups and your cardiovascular system.

- One set maximum effort pushups, then immediately sprint 80 meters. Rest 30-60 seconds until breathing returns to normal.
- One set maximum effort plank, then bunny hop 40 meters. Rest 30-60 seconds.
- One set maximum effort pull-ups, then sprint 80 meters. Rest 30-60 seconds.
- One set maximum effort squats, then bunny hop 40 meters (wow!).

Sprint Workout Suggestions

Begin each workout with a five-minute warm-up of low-intensity walking or jogging (55-75 percent of maximum heart rate) followed by light stretching. Conclude each workout with a five minute cool down identical to the warm-up. Be certain that you have medical clearance before attempting any strenuous workout, including those described in the Primal Blueprint.

Novice Sprint Workout - Strides and 75% Sprints. Six times warm-up strides of 8-15 seconds each (you'll need around 50-100 meters of space), with a 20-second rest period between strides. Focus on maintaining good running form and don't worry about your speed. These are just warm-ups for your main sprint efforts. After your warm-up strides, do six sprints, lasting 8-15 seconds each, at 75 percent effort. Take a one-minute rest period between sprints or otherwise enough to be fully recovered and achieve normal respiration before beginning your next sprint.

After two to three sessions over a few weeks time, increase your sprint efforts to full speed. Use a moving start (jog up to starting line and then begin sprinting) instead of a static start, to minimize injury risk. The range of 8-15 seconds is personal preference. Naturally, shorter sprints will be at faster speeds. I like to include both shorter and longer duration sprint sessions into my schedule. Pay attention to the difference between leg fatigue and pain. If you experience any acute pain or tightness, particularly in your hamstrings, wrap up the workout immediately with an easy cool down and ice the offended area.

Sprint Workout #1 - Strides and 100% Sprints. Strides and sprint workout as described for novice workout, except build to 100 percent effort on the sprints.

Sprint Workout #2 - Hill Repeats. Six to eight times hill sprints lasting 8-20 seconds at 75-100 percent effort. Recover by walking or trotting down the hill. Return to normal breathing before beginning next effort.

Sprint Workout #3 - Accelerations. Six to eight times 30-second sprints with the first 10 seconds at medium effort, second 10 seconds at hard effort and third 10 seconds at full sprint. One to two minutes recovery between efforts. You can use a running track and do 150-meter repeats—accelerating every 50 meters (start at turn apex, accelerate at straightaway, accelerate again at middle of straightaway, finish at traditional finish line) or any other course you can mark with 1/3 distance intervals.

Sprint Workout #4 - Technique Drills.

- **Strides:** Four times eight-second strides at 75 percent effort. Ten-second rest between efforts. One-minute rest before next exercise.
- **Skipping:** Two to four times 50 meters. Drive knee as high as you can (try to hit your chest), taking off and landing on opposite leg. Then launch off, and land, with opposite leg, driving other knee high into chest—like an exaggerated skip. Strive for maximum height instead of length. Fifteen-second rest between efforts. One-minute rest before next exercise.
- **Bounding:** Two to four times 50 meters. Take as long a stride as possible, focusing on keeping your balance rather than speed. Thirty-second rest between efforts. One-minute rest before next exercise.
- **Bunny Hopping:** Two to four times 50 meters. Take off on both legs and jump up and forward. Focus on achieving a good balance between height and length. Swing arms to assist effort and ensure a balanced landing. One-minute rest between efforts (you'll need it, trust me). Two-minute rest before next exercise.
- **Full Sprint:** Two to four times 50-meter full sprint. One-minute rest between efforts.

Sprint Workout #5 - Stair Drills.

Conduct this workout on stadium or building stairs. Your flight of stairs should take 8-20 seconds to ascend. Take 30 seconds rest between each exercise, or more or less as needed to feel refreshed and get your breathing under control.

- Four times warm-up stair climbs at 75 percent effort. When you reach the top, return immediately down the stairs at a comfortable pace, then ascend again.
- Two times single stairs. Ascend one stair at a time with rapid leg turn over. Descend comfortably and repeat effort.
- Two times bounding stairs. Ascend by skipping as many steps as you can. Focus on keeping your balance rather than speed. Drive arms for balance and leverage. Descend comfortably and repeat effort.
- Two times hopping stairs. Take off and land on both legs, taking either one or two stairs at a time. Use handrail if you are concerned

about slipping and proceed with caution. Descend comfortably and immediately repeat effort.

- Two times one-legged stairs (caution: very advanced exercise). Ascend stairs by hopping on one leg, one stair at a time. Using a handrail for support is highly recommended.
- Four times full speed stairs. Skip desired number of stairs with each stride to get to the top as fast as possible. Descend comfortably and recover completely between efforts.

Sprint Workout #6 - "Grokball" This workout, inspired by MarksDailyApple.com regular Grant Peterson, is a refreshing example of the simplicity of fitness in a culture that habitually tries to make things more complex than they need to be. In the amount of time it takes to get through the basic set-up instructions of your heart rate monitor owner's manual, you can capture the essence of Grok with this primal effort.

Take a five- to ten-pound medicine ball (depending on your own body-weight and strength level) to an ample sized athletic field. After a five-minute light jog, grab the ball and throw it down the field. Sprint after it, pick it up and throw it again, completing repeat trips up and down the field. Discover numerous variations on the throw—overhead like a soccer throw-in, under-hand like an old school free-throw, sideways one-armed like a discus thrower, sideways two-armed like a hammer thrower, roll like a bowling ball (one- or two-handed), or face backwards and throw over your head two-handed (watch out for little kids at soccer practice with the latter).

Be extremely careful to keep your spine and neck in a neutral position every time you throw. Your legs and core muscle groups will provide the most leverage and receive the most training effect from the throws. Your spine and neck should always be in a straight line (angle to the ground might vary from perpendicular to 45 degrees depending on your throwing style)—don't curve your back or neck fore-aft or side to side. Make sure that the force of your effort is absorbed by your legs and core muscles.

Begin with gentle throws that will give you a form check. As you fatigue after a few lengths of the field, you will have to be especially diligent about maintaining proper body position for your throws. When you notice that your ability to maintain correct form becomes compromised due to fatigue, it is time to stop the workout; the same goes if you experience any acute pain in your muscles or joints. Finish your session with five minutes of easy jogging.

Cycling Sprint Workout #1 - Interval Ladder. Take a five-minute warm-up on bike at 55-75 percent of maximum heart rate. Sprint 15 seconds, rest 15 seconds. Then a 30-second sprint with a 30-second rest. Then 45-second sprint, 45-second rest. Then 60-second sprint, 60-second rest. After the 60-second effort, sprint 45, rest 45, and so on to complete the ladder workout. Five minutes easy pedaling cool down.

Cycling Sprint Workout #2 - "One for Two." Six to eight times one-minute all-out with two-minute recovery between efforts. The extended recovery time in this workout helps improve power—the number of watts you can produce at maximum intensity. The interval workouts (#1 and #3) are more focused on developing oxygen-carrying capacity, since recovery intervals are shorter in relation to work efforts.

Cycling Sprint Workout #3 - Tabata Intervals. Tabata is a workout system where you achieve four minutes of intense effort in sprinting, weight lifting, or any other maximum effort exercise, using the consistent work/rest ratio of 20-seconds sprint, 10-seconds rest, 20-seconds sprint, 10-seconds rest—repeated for 4 minutes. That alone is a sufficient workout, but some people like to pedal slowly for a few minutes and then repeat the six-minute Tabata session.

A Few Words About Diets and Dieting

While it's encouraging to notice the increasing mainstream acceptance of the Primal/paleo/ancestral health eating style, we are still swimming upstream against the massive forces that have entrenched a grain-based diet into Western culture. If you are struggling in your mind about who is "right," I believe any confusion can be alleviated when you consider a larger context and the different paradigm the Standard American Diet operates in. When you consume a grossly excessive amount of carbohydrates in comparison with our ancestors, the Conventional Wisdom blather actually holds true: eating fat will make you fat (and clog the pipes of your inflamed organism); eating regularly scheduled, macronutrient-balanced meals is necessary to stabilize energy; and burning tons of calories through chronic exercise is necessary to try and stave off fat accumulation over the years.

It's only when you reject the flawed starting-point assumptions that you can see the Primal Blueprint in the proper perspective. You don't require carbohydrates to survive—any scientist will confirm this. If you are eating Primally, your fat-burning genes are up-regulated; you don't need regular meals to get through the day. If insulin and glucose are not running rampant in your bloodstream, causing inflammation and comprehensive cellular damage, then eating fat—lots of fat (of the right kinds)—will support health and provide an excellent source of long-lasting energy.

If you are still conflicted, the best thing to do is to try ditching grains and sugars for 21 days and see how your body reacts. Or, if you have been struggling with weight management, check out the Success Stories link at MarksDailyApple.com to get a sense of the transformation people are experiencing when they go Primal—often on the heels of years of frustration of trying to play the game by Conventional Wisdom.

Beyond this glaring distinction between Primal eating and a grain-based, high-carb diet there are certain other points to clarify. Vegetarians will have objections to my emphasis on meat, but these objections are almost entirely countered (saving the philosophical ones, which involve a personal belief system and not a dietary quality debate) by emphasizing local, pasture-raised animal products and consuming high-antioxidant vegetables and fruits along with your meat.

If you've seen research suggesting that meats and high-fat diets are unhealthy, this conclusion is likely heavily influenced by eating overcooked or heavily processed meat laden with nitrites and other toxins; consuming high-fat foods in conjunction with moderate- to high-carb diets (so insulin drives the fat into storage and promotes systemic inflammation that allows ingested cholesterol and saturated fat to cause trouble in your arteries); consuming trans and hydrogenated fats (troublemakers who get the whole class blamed for their bad behavior); and obtaining insufficient high-antioxidant foods such as fresh organic produce.

Some dieticians argue that the avoidance of whole grains and legumes compromises nutrient intake, since these foods have long occupied a prominent position in the diet recommended by Conventional Wisdom. We know already that grains and legumes stress the insulin response system and are far inferior sources of vitamins and minerals—particularly on a per calorie "bang for your buck" basis—than to those found in plants and animals. Furthermore, a grain-based diet results in excessive fiber consumption and health risks associated with the aforementioned anti-nutrients (lectins, glutens, and phytates)—on a noticeable allergic level and a more insidious sub-clinical level.

Those in the low-fat camp might shudder at all the fat Primal enthusiasts enjoy from animal meats, eggs, fish, avocados, macadamia nuts, coconut products, butter, and olive oil. However, we know that heart disease is related more to the insulin and inflammatory elements of your diet than it is to fat intake. The continued popularity of the sentiment that too much fat is bad for you simply blows my mind. It's time to separate once and for all good fats from bad. Fortunately, the health dangers of trans and partially hydrogenated fats in most vegetable oils are now well accepted, as are the health benefits of consuming omega-3 fats, and more attention is being paid to the health risks of eating excessive PUFA oils.

We're getting there, but we need to also recognize that saturated fat is not evil either—unless you wolf down too many carbs in conjunction with them or rely exclusively on feedlot animals (hormones, pesticides, antibiotics, poor O6:O3 ratios), cook them wrong, or fail to consume high-antioxidant plant foods.

Dr. Ron Rosedale, author of the *Rosedale Diet* and acclaimed for reversing type 2 diabetes, obesity, and heart disease through diet, says, "a high complex carbohydrate, low saturated fat diet is an absolute oxymoron. A high complex carbohydrate diet is nothing but a high glucose diet, or a high sugar diet. Your body is just going to store it as saturated fat (since we have very limited glycogen stores in muscle and liver), and the body makes it into saturated fat quite readily."

The Biggest Losers

"Who will be the biggest loser this week?"—goes the tag line of the popular boot camp weight loss competition television program. The answer is definitely the public. You simply can't lose 10 or 20 pounds of body fat in 10 or 20 days—period. It's a parlor trick. Most of the weight lost is from reduced water retention (four grams of water bond with every gram of stored glycogen in the body). Some of the weight lost is precious muscle, leaving only a small fraction of the impressive total as actual body fat. What's more, at the "finish line" of extreme, unsustainable crash diet/workout efforts, big losers are left depleted, exhausted, and prone to a rebound effect of overeating and underexercising. This is the human organism's survival instinct kicking in and trying to restore, replenish, and recover from the stress of an extreme experience like a crash diet.

You may have heard the oft-reported government survey figure that 97 percent of dieters gain the weight back within five years. More amusing is a recent study from Dr. Traci Mann, a UCLA psychology professor, who tracked the long-term success rate of participants in 31 popular diets. The study reported that 41 percent of participants gained back more weight than they lost within one year. While Mann admitted the number seemed "depressing," she also revealed that "we have strong reasons to feel that this number *under-represents* the true number of participants who gained back more weight than they lost." Among them were people dropping out of contact due to embarrassment and people crash-dieting right before the study period ended to save face!

What a complete mess we are in. We need to take a step back and adjust our collective mentality to approach the subject of healthy eating with a fresh perspective. There is no reason why any of us should suffer from excessive body fat, emotional stress, or disappointment on the subject of eating. I am advocating a variable, intuitive eating style that includes a tremendous variety of delicious foods and minimal (from one point of view anyway!) restrictions. Furthermore, I am not irresponsibly pitching the Primal Blueprint eating style as the end-all secret to good health and longevity. The other Primal Blueprint laws go hand in hand with optimal eating habits to produce best results. Ignoring them is recipe for failure. For example, an extreme endurance athlete immersed in a stressful training program (burning carbs for hours on end every day) will probably crash and burn if he suddenly switches to eating Primal Blueprint style. For such an athlete, we must first address the issue of sensible training methods before turning our attention to dietary habits.

Primal Blueprint Internet Resources

I've taken advantage of the infinite capacity of the Internet to augment this book with continually updated supporting material. The direct links are as follows:

Primal Blueprint Text References:

marksdailyapple.com/the-book/references/primal-blueprint-text-references/

Primal Blueprint Suggested Reading:

marksdailyapple.com/the-book/references/suggested-reading/

Primal Blueprint Shopping and Information Resources:

marksdailyapple.com/the-book/references/primal-blueprint-resources/

Primal Blueprint Q&A: *Everything You Always Wanted to Ask...but Were Afraid to Know*

marksdailyapple.com/the-book/references/questions-and-answers/

    All About Grok
        Dispute About Recent Human Evolution
        Details About Genes Directing Cellular Function
        Reconciling Evolutionary Rationale with Religious Beliefs
        Grok and Korg Nicknames
    Diet
        Differing Scientific Conclusions
        Insulin-Balanced Meals
        Fiber
        Diet Sodas
    Exercise
        Compliance for Low Body Fat Athletes
        Cortisol
        Natural vs. Synthetic Human Growth Hormone and Testosterone
    Lifestyle
        Getting Kids' Buy-In
        Prescription Drugs

Primal Blueprint Comparisons to Popular Diets

INDEX

to avoid, 288
to enjoy in moderation,
141-144, 286
danger, avoiding, 31
Danger Zone, 99
dark chocolate, 134, 151-152
Darwin, Charles, 32, 36
"Darwin Awards," 228-229
death
causes of, 9-12
from old age, 11
depression, health and, 90
Devany, Art, 232
diabetes
nuts, seeds, and, 147
type 2, 83
Diamond, Jared, 2, 36, 165
diary. *See* food diary
diet
of early humans, 42-43
insulin and, 72-75
LDLs, HDLs, and, 84
low-fat, 7
for Metabolic Syndrome,
89
metabolism and, 8
nutrition and, 53
plants and animals in, 117
Primal Blueprint and, 22-
23, 69
Primal Blueprint com-
pared to popular,
315
of primal families, 40
vegetables as center of,
131
Western, 107
dietary fiber. *See* fiber
digital media, 55, 60-63
dinner
in Kelly Korg eating plan,
250
in Ken Korg eating plan,
246
disease. *See also* heart
disease; specific
conditions
modern illness and, 46
reduced risk factors for, 68
disease pyramid, 166-167
DNA, genetic triggers

and, 19
Dobzhansky, Theodosius, 15
dried fruit, 134, 138
drinking, before sleep, 219
drinks. *See* beverages; specific drinks
drugs. *See* medications;
specific types
Dumbest Generation, The
(Bauerlein), 231

E

eating
binge eating, 47
condensing daily period
for, 260
food types and, 22-23
frequency of, 106-108
health and, 51-52
Intermittent Fasting and,
237, 259-262
in Primal Blueprint, 65-
113
before sleep, 219
volume and, 72
eating well, Primal Blueprint
on, 105-109
*Eating Well for Optimum
Health* (Weil), 105
Eaton, Boyd, 17
EGF. *See* epidural growth
factor (EGF)
eggs, 128-129, 134, 286
avoiding, 288
Conventional Wisdom vs.
Primal Blueprint
on, 3
80 Percent Rule, 109-110, xi
elitism, in Primal Blueprint,
274, 275-277
endocrine system, 77
energy
aerobic exercise and, 190
macronutrients and, 93
stable levels of, 274
strength-training workouts
and, 198
swings during day, 108
workouts and, 200
energy levels, 47, 48
environmental contaminants,

in fish, 126
epidural growth factor
(EGF), 143
epigenetics, 20
equipment, athletic shoes as,
209-210
evolution, 15-19, 36
family life of modern hu-
mans and, 43-57
family life of primal
humans and, 39,
40-44
halting of, 19
nutritional sources and,
164-166
sleep and, 215
exercise, 179-234, 287. *See
also* workouts
by adolescents, 55
to avoid, 289
cardio, 4, 61, 187-196
classes in, 44, 48
committing to, 266
compliance with pre-
scribed programs,
62
increasing, 9
insulin sensitivity and, 75
maximum effort sprints
and, 28
Metabolic Syndrome and,
89
Primal Fitness program
and, 179-212, 237
ramping up activity, 254
slow-movement, 26-27
sprinting and, 204-208
strength training and,
27-28
walking as, 40-41
wash-board abs and, 256
weekly schedule for, 257-
258
exercise plan, for weight loss,
252-258

F

family life
comparison between pri-
mal and modern-
day, 39-58

PRIMAL ESSENTIAL MOVEMENTS
Workout Log

PEM Workout Date: _____ Success score (1-10): _____

Location: _____ Duration: _____

Reps completed:

Pushups set 1: _____ Set 2: _____

Squats set 1: _____ Set 2: _____

Pull-ups set 1: _____ Set 2: _____

Plank (time) set 1: _____ Set 2: _____

Progression exercises used (describe any):

Pushups: _____ Pull-ups: _____

Squats: _____ Plank:_____

Comments: _____

_____

· ·

PEM Workout Date: _____ Success score (1-10): _____

Location: _____ Duration: _____

Reps completed:

Pushups set 1: _____ Set 2: _____

Squats set 1: _____ Set 2: _____

Pull-ups set 1: _____ Set 2: _____

Plank (time) set 1: _____ Set 2: _____

Progression exercises used (describe any):

Pushups: _____ Pull-ups: _____

Squats: _____ Plank:_____

Comments: _____

_____

PRIMAL ESSENTIAL MOVEMENTS
Workout Log

PEM Workout Date: _____ Success score (1-10): _____

Location: _____ Duration: _____

Reps completed:

Pushups set 1: _____   Set 2: _____

Squats set 1: _____   Set 2: _____

Pull-ups set 1: _____   Set 2: _____

Plank (time) set 1: _____   Set 2: _____

Progression exercises used (describe any):

Pushups: _____ Pull-ups: _____

Squats: _____ Plank:_____

Comments: _____

_____

· ·

PEM Workout Date: _____ Success score (1-10): _____

Location: _____ Duration: _____

Reps completed:

Pushups set 1: _____   Set 2: _____

Squats set 1: _____   Set 2: _____

Pull-ups set 1: _____   Set 2: _____

Plank (time) set 1: _____   Set 2: _____

Progression exercises used (describe any):

Pushups: _____ Pull-ups: _____

Squats: _____ Plank:_____

Comments: _____

_____

PRIMAL ESSENTIAL MOVEMENTS
Workout Log

PEM Workout Date: _____ Success score (1-10): _____

Location: _____ Duration:_____

Reps completed:

Pushups set 1: _____   Set 2: _____

Squats set 1: _____   Set 2: _____

Pull-ups set 1: _____   Set 2: _____

Plank (time) set 1: _____   Set 2: _____

Progression exercises used (describe any):

Pushups: _____   Pull-ups: _____

Squats: _____   Plank:_____

Comments: _____

_____

• •

PEM Workout Date: _____ Success score (1-10): _____

Location: _____ Duration:_____

Reps completed:

Pushups set 1: _____   Set 2: _____

Squats set 1: _____   Set 2: _____

Pull-ups set 1: _____   Set 2: _____

Plank (time) set 1: _____   Set 2: _____

Progression exercises used (describe any):

Pushups: _____   Pull-ups: _____

Squats: _____   Plank:_____

Comments: _____

_____

PRIMAL ESSENTIAL MOVEMENTS
Workout Log

PEM Workout Date: _____ Success score (1-10): _____

Location: _____ Duration: _____

Reps completed:

Pushups set 1: _____   Set 2: _____

Squats set 1: _____   Set 2: _____

Pull-ups set 1: _____   Set 2: _____

Plank (time) set 1: _____   Set 2: _____

Progression exercises used (describe any):

Pushups: _____   Pull-ups: _____

Squats: _____   Plank: _____

Comments: _____

_____

· ·

PEM Workout Date: _____ Success score (1-10): _____

Location: _____ Duration: _____

Reps completed:

Pushups set 1: _____   Set 2: _____

Squats set 1: _____   Set 2: _____

Pull-ups set 1: _____   Set 2: _____

Plank (time) set 1: _____   Set 2: _____

Progression exercises used (describe any):

Pushups: _____   Pull-ups: _____

Squats: _____   Plank: _____

Comments: _____

PRIMAL BLUEPRINT
Sprint Workout Log

Sprint Workout Date: _____ Success score (1-10): _____

Location: _____

Activity: _____

Total Duration: _____ Reps: _____

Duration or distance_____ Rest Interval: _____

• •

Sprint Workout Date: _____ Success score (1-10): _____

Location: _____

Activity: _____

Total Duration: _____ Reps: _____

Duration or distance_____ Rest Interval: _____

• •

Sprint Workout Date: _____ Success score (1-10): _____

Location: _____

Activity: _____

Total Duration: _____ Reps: _____

Duration or distance_____ Rest Interval: _____

• •

Sprint Workout Date: _____ Success score (1-10): _____

Location: _____

Activity: _____

Total Duration: _____ Reps: _____

Duration or distance_____ Rest Interval: _____

PRIMAL BLUEPRINT
Sprint Workout Log

Sprint Workout Date: _____ Success score (1-10): _____

Location: _____

Activity: _____

Total Duration: _____ Reps: _____

Duration or distance_____ Rest Interval: _____

. . . .

Sprint Workout Date: _____ Success score (1-10): _____

Location: _____

Activity: _____

Total Duration: _____ Reps: _____

Duration or distance_____ Rest Interval: _____

. . . .

Sprint Workout Date: _____ Success score (1-10): _____

Location: _____

Activity: _____

Total Duration: _____ Reps: _____

Duration or distance_____ Rest Interval: _____

. . . .

Sprint Workout Date: _____ Success score (1-10): _____

Location: _____

Activity: _____

Total Duration: _____ Reps: _____

Duration or distance_____ Rest Interval: _____

PRIMAL NOTES

PRIMAL NOTES

PRIMAL NOTES

PRIMAL NOTES

PRIMAL NOTES

PRIMAL NOTES

PRIMAL NOTES